Mental Health in Africa and the Americas Today

A Book of Conference Proceedings

Edited by

Samuel O. Okpaku, M.D., Ph.D.

Chrisolith Books
2907 Belmont Blvd.
Nashville, TN 37212

ISBN: 0-916085-01-5

First printing, 1991.

Typesetting and Book Design: Dina E. John
Cover Design: Nancy Apple
Editorial Assistant: Patricia Buie

PRINTED IN THE UNITED STATES OF AMERICA

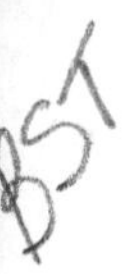

For Anire, Aubrey and Temisan

Contents

About the Book

THE BOOK

This volume represents the proceedings of the first joint meeting of the African Psychiatric Association, the American Psychiatric Association and the Black Psychiatrists of America. This historic conference was most appropriately held in Nairobi, Kenya in 1986.

Some contributors to the volume include Professors T. S. Asuni, S. Acuda, Ayo Binitie, F. Earls, C. Nadelson, C. Pierce and J. Talbott. It is a fascinating and highly instructive manual for western trained mental health professionals and policy makers as it provides a vivid description of mental health in African, American and Caribbean Societies.

For example, the chapter by pioneering African psychiatrist Professor T. S. Asuni of the internationally renowned Aro Village Psychiatric Hospital in Nigeria provides some important insights into the innovative strategies he uses in the treatment of the African mentally ill. He and his colleagues share their experiences in the optimal use of available local resources coupled with strategies that use patients' families, relatives and the general community as therapeutic allies. This report enables the reader to gain a more complete understanding of the often quoted successful outcome of the treatment of schizophrenic patients in these societies as compared to the results obtained in industrialized societies.

Some commentators rather superficially describe African psychiatry as "the psychiatry of the psychoses". In fact, such commentaries are simplistic in nature and show gross misunderstanding of the local conditions. Furthermore, it seems inappropriate to assume that the evolution of psychiatry in Africa will, of necessity, have to parallel the evolution of psychiatry in the western world. The indigenous African psychiatrists, even those with western training, are firmly grounded in their cultural heritage and its continuity.

It is useful therefore to compare the African approach with the current admission criteria and managed care which appear to be the major preoccupations in American psychiatry. The African model of brief psychotherapy is equally fascinating as is the use of psychiatric nurses and mental health para-professionals as important team members. This volume therefore is a must for mental health professionals, practitioners and policy makers who are engaged in contemporary, multicultural and transcultural settings.

The chapters by the African contributors provide further basis for comparisons and contrasts with psychiatry in the American and Canadian contexts. (For example, in 1986 Nigeria, with a population of 100 million inhabitants was estimated to have 50 qualified psychiatrists. In the United States of America the corresponding figures were respectively, 200 million and 50,000.)

In addition, the volume draws attention to the low priority given to mental health as a component of public health services. It also emphasizes the importance of the role of mental health services delivery as an integral part of primary health care.

This book will undoubtedly be a useful handbook for the experienced as well as the psychiatrist in training.

THE CONFERENCE AND THE PARTICIPANTS

For many of the Afro-American participants the occasion was a homecoming and a pilgrimage. For the Anglo-American participants it was equally moving. These moments are illustrated by the following comments:

Afro-American: "For me this was the most psychologically, socially, and racially - the best experience that I have experienced in my life...."

Anglo-American: "I particularly enjoyed meeting so many Black colleagues, since my usual routine, professional and social, allows or provides few opportunities to meet Black colleagues."

For most participants, the total experience was truly a transcultural event.

Acknowledgements

The publication of this book has involved the assistance and support of a number of individuals. A partial list includes the following individuals:

Professor S. W. Acuda, (Past Secretary, African Psychiatric Association, University of Kenya, Nairobi, Kenya)

Professor Ayo Binitie, (Past President, African Psychiatric Association, University of Benin, Nigeria)

Fran Baker, M.D., MPH, (Associate Professor of Psychiatry, University of Texas San Antonio, Texas, U.S.A.)

Felton Earls, M.D. (Professor of Psychiatry, School of Public Health, Harvard University, Cambridge, Massachusetts, U.S.A.)

William Lawson, M.D., Ph.D., (Medical Director, Department of Mental Health, Tennessee, and Assistant Professor of Psychiatry, Vanderbilt University School of Medicine, Nashville, Tennessee)

George Mahay, M.B., B.S., F.R.C. Psych., (Senior Lecturer, Dept. of Psychiatry, University of Barbados, Barbados)

Ms. Ellen Mercer, (Coordinator, International Office, American Psychiatric Association, Washington, D.C., U.S.A.)

Jeanne Spurlock, M.D., (Deputy Medical Director, American Psychiatric Association, Washington, D.C., U.S.A.)

Olugbenga Jacob Adesida, (Editorial Staff, Third Press, New York, U.S.A.)

Ms. Patricia Buie (Buie Art Associates, Tokyo, Japan and Nashville, Tennessee, U.S.A.)

Joseph Okpaku, Ph.D. (Publisher, Third Press, New York, U.S.A.)

Thomas Okpaku, M.A., (Consultant, Chrisolith Books)

Ms. Jane Weaver, (Editorial Consultant, Fairfax, Virginia, U.S.A.)

Further acknowledgement is hereby given to Richard A. Fields, M.D., (Past President, Black Psychiatrists of America), Professor Ezra E. H. Griffith (Past President, Black Psychiatrists of America), Professor Robert O. Pasnau (Past President, American Psychiatric Association), Melvin Sabshin, M.D. (Medical Director, American Psychiatric Association), Professor Harold Vitosky (Chair, International Committee, American Psychiatric Association), for their encouragement and assistance.

Sincere gratitude is extended to the American Psychiatric Association, the African Psychiatrists Association and the Black Psychiatrists of America Association for permission to publish this book of proceedings.

My gratitude is also extended to Ms. Sherry Bransford, Ms. Sharon Bratcher, Ms. Karen Cunningham, Ms. Julia Reid, and Ms. Amy Sibulkin for their assistance in the preparation of the manuscript.

My thanks also go to those anonymous individuals who have in various ways helped in bringing to completion the publication of this book.

Samuel O. Okpaku, M.D., Ph.D.

Preface

This volume represents a significant portion of the papers presented at the first joint conference sponsored by the African Psychiatric Association, the American Psychiatric Association and the Black Psychiatrists of America. The conference was held in Nairobi, Kenya, in September, 1986. In light of the rapid pace of scientific development, one is tempted to imagine that the contents of the presentations may no longer be relevant. The reader will find clearly that this is not so. The contents of this volume provide a kaleidoscopic view of mental health in Africa, the United States and Canada and the Caribbean.

Furthermore, as the only participant at the conference, with membership in the three organizing societies, I felt strongly that this unique occasion, with the largest single gathering of psychiatrists anywhere in Africa should be recorded in a book of proceedings. The collection of the papers and the subsequent editorial work took considerably longer than was anticipated. Hence, the delay in publication. The reader will nevertheless find the volume justifiable and useful from a variety of perspectives.

This collection of papers presented mostly by individuals who are experts, high government officials or influential members of the participating organizations, gives an overview of the critical issues of concern to psychiatrists and mental health professionals on both sides of the Atlantic. In the United States and Canada, priority areas include treatment and services to the chronic mentally ill, the excessive hospitalization of children and adolescents, dual diagnosis, including alcohol and drug abuse, suicide and fragmentation of funding and services. On the African side, there are issues of lack of trained professionals, lack of drugs and psychiatric correlates of social change. In terms of the presentations, several observations could be clearly made. Firstly, the relevance of the cultural context to psychiatric practice cannot be over-emphasized. An example is the result of the World Health Organization study on schizophrenia, indicating a better outcome for such patients in the developing world. Another point is that the various countries were at different stages of industrialization and there was a huge gap between the most affluent countries and the poorest in terms of economic and manpower resources. Nevertheless, there was a pervasive reference to a common lack of resources irrespective of economic power or industrialization. Simply to illustrate this point, we may wish to compare Nigeria and the United States. The population of Nigeria is estimated at about 100 million, and that of the United States as about twice that much. The number of psychiatrists in the United States is estimated at about 50,000 and the corresponding number for Nigeria is probably, at best, in the hundreds. These two nations differ tremendously in gross national product and annual budgets.

In spite of these disparities, there was an underlying reference to the magnitude of the needs for services and the corresponding low priority given to mental health funding irrespective of the countries involved. Perhaps more fascinating than the issue of resources, are the creative attempts being made to provide relief to the human suffering inflicted by mental illness in its ubiquity.

In terms of research, several observations are relevant. It is true that many of the participants from the African side lamented the lack of research resources. My observation from their presentations, in fact, implied a need for a more optimistic view. The clinical challenges and the research potentials in these two cultures remain great. The clinical materials presented at the conference provided an excellent spectrum of opportunities for research, some of which can only be carried out within the particular cultural context. There remain, therefore, ample opportunities for nosological and basic psychiatric research with populations whose illnesses are relatively free of contamination with substance abuse. Bearing in mind the overarching role of culture in the definition of health and the appropriateness of services, there are further opportunities for useful research endeavors. Therefore, the apparent "lack of research opportunities" requires a closer examination.

It should be reassuring to the African psychiatrist that not all American psychiatrists are in academic institutions and that there are no ideal institutions for research. I believe that a more critical issue for some of the African psychiatrists therefore, is the feeling of relative isolation and the relative lack of a critically supportive environment that nurtures competitive research. Some of this frustration may be relieved by developing local interdisciplinary teams.

Another observation has to do with international and cross-cultural collaboration. We are currently witnessing major political and economic changes that continue to point to a greater emphasis on cultural psychiatry and cross-cultural work. Mass voluntary migration , refugee problems, social change, and rural-urban shifts are relevant issues for cross-cultural approaches.

However, the potential contribution of African psychiatry to mainline psychiatry should not be perceived as only relevant in the domain of socio-cultural psychiatry. There are numerous opportunities for biological and basic research. There are various centers either investigating or capable of contributing to current frontline researches on the genetics and biochemistry of the major psychiatric syndromes. The opportunities for international collaboration with these African centers are made more attractive because of unduly burdensome bureaucracy or social advocacy in the United States. Examples are the liability issues, debates about animal research and informed consent for research involving humans.

Other areas of potential collaboration include the role of primary care in mental health services and alternative service delivery systems. In the United States the relevance of primary care to mental health service delivery is becoming more apparent with an ever increasing cost of health care and the pressure for more cost effective services will grow. African patterns of service delivery, which interdigitate primary care and psychiatric services, serve as useful models.

In view of the above, therefore, for the students of international and cross cultural mental health, this volume will serve as a useful reference point. For individuals interested in collaborative endeavors, the names and addresses of the participants may serve as possible sources of contact. At a time when various American Medical Specialties including the American Psychiatric Association and The Educational Council for Foreign Medical Graduates have initiated an International Medical Scholars Program to facilitate the training of selective candidates, it is envisaged that such a volume will be useful in identifying potential recruitment or training sites.

Lastly, for the participants and their families, who experienced a truly transcultural phenomenon, the volume will, I hope, always remain a memorable souvenir.

Samuel O. Okpaku, M.D., Ph.D

Vanderbilt University
Nashville, TN 37212

Introduction

The volume is divided into five sections. Each chapter focuses on a dominant theme.

Section I: Historical and Sociocultural Perspectives

This set of papers addresses various aspects of the development of modern psychiatry in Africa and historical commentaries on mental health in the United States with respect to Afro-Americans. The general observations are instructive particularly in light of earlier observations by Rousseau and even more recently by Bean who stated: "In a world where far more than half the inhabitants live under the menace of hunger, serious disease and early deaths, where small pox, malaria, plague, cholera and undernutrition affect many hundreds of millions, the situation of psychiatry is not unlike that of public health in the pre-Pasteur period of our part of the world." Within the same context, the comments of J. H. Orley and Aubrey Lewis are relevant.

J. H. Orley stated that: "There does seem a tendency for some writers, especially psychiatrists, to talk of 'Africa' and the 'African' when, in fact, they are referring only to their own experiences and to their research amongst the patients with whom they have worked. Thus, they give the impression of making valuable generalizations about Africa when they are doing nothing of the such."

Aubrey Lewis stated that: "There is a risk of putting too much stress on the cultural aspect of strange forms of mental disorder."

The above observations need to be heeded not only within the African context but elsewhere as well.

A further point of note is the area of 'racism' and 'pluralism' in contemporary United States. The negative consequences in terms of distorted images and negative stereotyping, inaccessibility to services, and reduction in human potential remain major challenges to enlightened mental health professionals and agencies.

Section II: Adult and General Psychiatry

This section addresses aspects of adult and general psychiatry. Topics covered range from the role of biological psychiatry in Africa, the possible role of EEG in the diagnosis and treatment of psychoneurotic disorders in Nairobi as well as the relationship of psyche and soma as viewed by American psychiatrists. Once again the role of cultural factors cannot be ignored in the full appreciation of these papers.

Section III: Child Psychiatry

This section presents four papers on child psychiatry. Aspects of mental health service delivery to children and adolescents in Africa, United States and Great Britain are discussed.

Section IV: Alcohol and Substance Abuse

This section consists of a set of papers which address issues of substance abuse ranging from alcoholism in Afro-Americans to the differential abuse of artane and khat in certain parts of Africa. These papers again highlight the sociocultural context of substance abuse behavior. The human suffering and the economic cost of substance abuse are underscored by the current experiences in the United States. The need for governments and practitioners in less wealthy nations to explore and adopt preventive measures to limit and deter substance abuse cannot be over-emphasized. Unfortunately some of the African countries are on the distribution routes of illicit drugs.

Section V: Training, Education and Service Delivery

The papers in this section, like the preceding ones, reveal certain assumptions that are likely to be held about developed vs developing countries. The need for comprehensive training in dealing with the multiple problems of physical and mental illnesses as well as the ravages of poverty and racism are very instructive.

SECTION I:

Historical and Sociocultural Factors

Chapter 1

The Mentally Ill in Modern and Traditional African Societies

by

Ayo Binitie, MD, (London), DPM, MRCPsych, FNMC, FWAPC,
Professor of Mental Health,
Head, Department of Mental Health,
University of Benin,
Benin City, Nigeria

ABSTRACT

African villages are served by traditional healers, who are thought to ward off evil spirits and keep the forces of nature in balance. Witches also play a central role in traditional African life; they are believed to punish social transgression. Since the introduction of Western European culture, some Africans have adopted Western practices, received extensive schooling, and become an elite westernized minority. More common, however, has been the transitional life style: combining African traditional beliefs with Western religion and practices. Important forms of psychiatric care introduced into Africa have involved a village or neighborhood milieu that accommodates relatives. Traditional healers may also have an important role in psychotherapeutic situations or in treating aggression. An African may turn to both a traditional healer and a hospital when ill, illustrating both the flux in African society and the need for culturally sensitive treatment.

AN AFRICAN VILLAGE

The object of my quest was a remote African village unspoiled by modernity. I saw the village up on the hill set against the lush green of the forest around it. Here and there a coconut palm swayed Africa's invitation to the Europeans.

As we approached the village, I noticed there is a bridge across the rivulet. The bridge, I later learned, was built by communal effort. I wondered why they took the trouble. They could have stayed on this side of the river. It may be that in the remote past, when slave raiding was important, the river was a natural barrier ensuring defence and security. The houses neatly grouped together in two long rows with a main street down the center may have been constructed with this object in mind. The inhabitants can remember as far back as 150 years.

Between 30 and 40 houses are arranged on the hillside, about 50 yards from the river. The approach to the bridge is a slightly curved road. The main street intersects the road to the bridge, and the longer end contains about 25 houses. The shorter end extends about 30 yards and contains about 10 houses. The houses all have mud walls and thatch roofs made from coconut and oil-palm fronds, which are readily available in the village. The houses are constructed in more or less similar fashion.

Outside each house is a veranda 3-4 feet wide and about 2-3 feet off the ground. In the evenings family members sit and exchange views and tell stories in the moonlight. The entrance to the house is to one side or the other of the long veranda and leads to the main reception area. Another door leads from the reception area to the back yard. Usually, two or three rooms are entered from the reception area.

The population of the village is about 200. The inhabitants are either old or very young. There are about 50 men aged 40 to 60 years or above. The women number about 60. They are younger, and some are still of child-bearing age. The children are numerous, all under seven years, and go about with their mothers, assisting with household chores. Quite a few men have more than one wife, but the majority have only one. The men report that their grown-up children have left for various towns and cities in search of employment or education. They aim to better the lot of their fathers and village. They hope to return to the village in the distant future. At the time of my visit, there was still no evidence of their achievements in the cities or in the village. Maybe they have not succeeded or maybe they have turned their backs on the village. Perhaps they, too, like the government, have forgotten the village and the villagers.

The villagers are traditionally farmers, but not much farming can be seen now. There is much land but little cultivation. The crops planted are cassava, plantains, and a little cocoyam. Rubber trees are abundant, testimony to the rubber boom. However, there is no one to tap them. There is poverty in the environment and wretchedness in the faces. Productive capacity has declined markedly. The barns are empty; so are the houses. Living is precarious. Parasite infestations are common. The children have large heads and potbellies, evidence of malnutrition.

SOCIAL ORGANIZATION AND TRADITIONAL HEALERS

The village head, or Odionwere, owes allegiance to the traditional group ruler some miles away. An Odionwere is a son of the area and is the oldest living individual in the defined area. According to this gerontocracy, the next oldest becomes the deputy. The social system is organized in terms of age groups. The class of elders is normally followed by the warrior class, which comprises young men in their prime and is known as the class of youths. This frequent ceremony for passage from childhood to adult life is impressive.

In the village are two part-time traditional healers. They are part-time because they also farm. They see themselves as witches and wizards destined to ward off evil forces and to keep the forces of nature in balance and harmony. You hear them say, you young educated people are knowledgeable in books, but you do not really understand or know the world. We pray for you. We pray that the world does not know you or become interested in your affairs. There is much more to the world than meets the eye. There are mighty spiritual forces.

Asked how they know of the existence of such forces, which cannot be seen, they say, we know of the existence of such forces because of various events and happenings, which you mortals cannot explain or know about. Before any events occur here in the visible world, it has first happened in the spiritual world; the fates of people are decided and all activities concluded first, before they begin to happen here. All the spirits, both good and evil, are created by God Almighty himself. Everyone comes into the world with a destiny that must, to a larger or smaller degree, be fulfilled. Traditional healers hold communion with the spirits and ferret out the destinies of men, make appropriate sacrifices, and ameliorate or change the fortunes of men.

This is the lot of traditional doctors. Communicating with the spirits in this way is a hazardous occupation. The priests have to have special spiritual preparations for this role if they are not to come to harm.

There are various kinds of spirits. Some are the souls of men who once lived on earth but have not found a resting place. These spirits haunt the sites of their former activities. They may appear in their usual forms or enter and trouble people known to them. They cause fevers, nightmares, and misfortunes to those visited. There are usually reasons for the pestilence of such spirits. A traditional healer handling such cases has to fortify himself so that he himself does not become infected with these afflictions. Traditional healers also give food to recently departed ancestors to appease them so that they will cast a favorable eye on the present generation and protect and guide them.

Traditional healers balance the forces of nature in this way. They constantly seek to chase out evil forces and capture the good. A man is good if spirits surround him and the ancestors look with favor on his activities. Such a favored person must constantly make sacrifices to please his ancestors and to protect his destiny or head. Otherwise, evil forces will become jealous and compete and take over his soul and head.

WITCHES AND WIZARDS

Witches and wizards play a central role in African cosmology and day-to-day life. A survey of a sample of medical students showed that they all believed that witches are present in the community, and they cited many examples of confessional statements reported in the popular press.

Central to the idea of witches is the belief that they can do harm from a distance without being in physical contact with their victims. Witches exist to do harm. They terrorize the victims through their capacity to cause illness, misfortune, childlessness, poverty, and death.

Witches are female. Male witches are called wizards. Witchcraft is believed to be acquired by consuming "witches' substance" in food or drink. People are not born witches—they acquire their characteristics— but witchcraft is more common in some families than others. This is so because the "substance" is more readily available in families with witches. The witches meet mainly at night, on top of tall trees. At these meetings they decide on the victims. The witches meet and suck the blood of the victims, not in the real body but in the spirit. Witches return home at the end of their nightly journeys and resume their earthly selves. The legend is that witches select as their victims members of their own families, share in the feasts of others, and offer victims from their families at the appropriate time.

Witches are provoked by the victims' acts of commission and omission: sudden acquisition of wealth, rudeness to elders, boasting, offending elders, sudden success, selfishness, greed, failure to invite strangers to share in food, failure to greet, acquisition of property without appropriate placation of ancestral spirits, and usurpation of the rights of the first born. The general belief is that some infraction or impropriety, however slight, is usually the provocation for witchcraft. Even exceptional beauty may be considered an offense. However, on rare occasions there is no cause at all except that it is the turn of the particular witch to offer a victim and she can find no one at fault and has to victimize an innocent person. The offending witch frequently confesses before or after such a grave miscarriage of the witches' code.

Witches in a traditional society are judicial agents serving to warn and punish offenders. Witches are viewed as agents of socialization, helping to equilibrate society by preventing social greed and unscrupulous behavior. Traditional African societies believe firmly in the agencies of these spiritual forces and rely on the priests and healers to tame the forces around them. Goodness and evil are not inherent. A person becomes good or bad when the witches and wizards interfere with his head, his ancestral spirits, and his local gods and goddesses. The forces for good and evil are in the environment. It is the task of the individual to use the existing social institutions to trap the good and keep out the bad.

WESTERN CULTURE IN THE AFRICAN SETTING

The Western European culture was introduced into Africa as the occupying powers established imperial control and mastery over the African continent. Naturally, the new rulers brought with them their own institutions and social system. Many of the African subjects introjected this new way of life and set out to acquire the ways and mores of the new culture. This chain of events produced the educated westernized Africans.

The characteristics of the westernized Africans include a prolonged period of schooling (over 15 years in most cases), Christian religion, and work in the wage sector of the economy. They occupy the higher administrative positions in the government, medicine, law, universities, and occasionally, business. The majority have spent prolonged periods in Europe. They admire the Western ways of life and institutions and desire to replicate them in Africa.

In Europe, an important arsenal of westernization is the Protestant ethic. The doctrine proclaimed by Max Weber emphasizes honesty, hard work, frugality, and the belief that accumulated surpluses be used to produce more wealth. The educated Western African elite nominally share these beliefs.

Westernized Africans wish for and have housing, clothing, and a consumption pattern that approach those of the European. They are essentially city or town dwellers. The members of this group differ from their European counterparts, however, in that they have no overriding material or philosophical interest in westernization. Their common denominator is the capacity to afford and maintain a Western way of life for themselves and their children. The overriding group interests or philosophy make the group a predatory class, pursuing its pleasure and wants.

THE TRANSITIONAL GROUP

Probably the transitional group is not a group at all but rather, people who have left the traditional social systems of their ancestors and are now pursuing the Western way of life but for one reason or the other have not yet achieved it. They are limited by their education and social opportunities. Many in this group embrace the religion of the metropolitan powers but usually understand African traditional religion and vigorously share its system of belief.

The most important attribute of the transitional group is the desire to be like the educated Western elite. Catering to this group are the revivalist churches, which practice divination and the casting out of witches, wizards, and evil forces but do not use the divination system of traditional systems. Instead of the diviners' board, they use the Bible. The song and dance follow traditional patterns, but the hymns are taken from Christian hymnals. Practitioners have visions or dreams, hear voices, and speak in tongues. These experiences enable the practitioners to be warned of impending dangers and catastrophes. The religious system, which has been reported by Peel (1968), has proved highly popular, meeting the spiritual needs of a society that is in a state of flux.

EMPIRICAL STUDIES

There have been many empirical reports from Africa about psychiatric care: Shelley and Watson (1936), Gordon (1936), Laubscher (1937), Collomb (1956 & 1965), Lambo (1956, 1960, 1961 a, and 1961b), Field (1960), Bohannan (1960), Prince (1960), Forster (1962), Leighton, et al. (1963), Margetts (1965), Swift (1969), Asuni (1969), Boroffka (1969 & 1970), and Binitie (1971a, 1971b, & 1981).

These reports concerned themselves with whether Western diagnostic categories usefully apply to African patients. They discussed the types of disorders seen and whether these conform to the patterns seen in Europe. The reports also dealt with the types of institutions that treat the patients. Some reports have also concerned themselves with care of patients in the traditional African setting. Some reports also dealt with innovative therapeutic systems. So important is the topic of delivery in mental health care that in 1969 the Association of Psychiatrists in Africa organized a special workshop, "The Delivery of Mental Health Care." It was clear that the conference was concerned with furthering Western-type institutions in Africa. The participants recognized that the models of the West would have to be used but would have to be modified to suit local conditions. The conference participants concluded that the basic unit of care was the mental hospital but warned that these hospitals should not be too large. The disadvantages of large hospitals are bureaucracy and impersonal treatment, and every effort should be made to avoid them.

Boroffka (1970) reviewed psychiatry in Nigeria and traced its history from traditional times to the advent of colonialism and to the current forms of social psychiatry and therapeutic communities. He quoted the then Oba of Benin: "Lunacy has been regarded in Benin as a desperate disease that needed desperate treatment. In the olden times, lunatics were not allowed to roam about but were chained at home to avoid being a nuisance and a menace to the public, and while in chains they were given the best possible treatment. There were no asylums or any recognized public institutions where lunatics were treated. The house of the relative and his treatment at the expense of his relative afforded the only asylum."

Boroffka pointed out that all institutionalized mental patients were imprisoned in the early years of colonialism. Later, asylums were established and provided custodial care. Much later came psychiatric hospitals and psychiatric outpatient services, where patients voluntarily seek treatment.

In another article Boroffka (1969) wrote: "Transcultural psychiatry started as early as 1904, with Kraepelin's observations from Java, and continued up to the works in recent years by him, Carothers, Margetts, Witthower, and many others, including the study by Leighton, Lambo, et al., "Psychiatric Disorders among the Yoruba." It has established beyond doubt that the same mental disorders known in Western countries do exist elsewhere and that, as far as figures are known, incidence and prevalence do not seem to vary substantially all over the world."

Alternative forms of care have been reported by Lambo, Binitie, and Swift. Lambo (1961b) first reported on the village system at Aro. Reports of variants of the village system have come from Binitie

(1971b), who described a therapeutic neighborhood in Benin, and from Swift (1969), who described the building of a new village for psychiatric rehabilitation.

ARO VILLAGE EXPERIMENT IN NIGERIA

The development of Aro Village proceeded in phases. In the first phase, it was used as quarters for patients about to be admitted to the hospital one mile away and for the relatives accompanying them. After the patients were admitted, the relatives continued to stay there and visit the hospital. For some patients bed space was not immediately available. Such patients could return to the hinterland and wait until beds were available, or they could stay at Aro Village. Over time it became apparent that patients who entered the hospital in this way did well. Furthermore, because of the rural setting and the familiarity of the environment, they felt comfortable in the village. Fortunately, no untoward incidents resulted from this arrangement; Lambo initially feared that an explosive situation might develop.

During the next phase, it became official policy to house relatively unsophisticated patients and their relatives in Aro Village. The nurse and staff of the hospital went down to the village to administer treatment. Patients took part in the activities of the village, and some of them earned their living in the usual occupation of the area, petty trading.

The third phase of the development of Aro Village began when the village was handed over to the University of Ibadan after the transfer of Professor Lambo. The village became severed from the main hospital and had to set up its own therapeutic unit. A vigorous rehabilitation program has since been added. Resident psychiatric nurses are in charge of day-to-day operations and psychiatrists from the university, 50 miles away, visit twice a week to supervise the center.

The need for a treatment center for relatively unsophisticated patients still existed, however. Therefore, the current superintendent, Professor Asuni, developed another village adjacent to the Neuropsychiatric Center at Aro. The impact of this new treatment arrangement has been widespread and has led to the spread of this system of care throughout Africa. This treatment system allows treatment in a rural community without the excessive expense of infrastructural facilities.

In Tanzania, Dr. Swift set up a new village 25 miles from Dodma. Swift's village was established specifically to care for psychiatric patients. It differs from the Aro experiments in that it involved no villagers besides the patients and their guardians.

THERAPEUTIC NEIGHBORHOODS IN USELU-BENIN

The experiments in alternative systems of care in Aro were conducted in the relative calm of a rural setting and the absence of population pressures, which create competition for living space. Doubts have been expressed as to whether this experiment could prove successful in an urban setting. The establishment of a new psychiatric facility in Uselu- Benin provided an opportunity for experiments in an urban setting. Landlords around the hospital at Uselu were induced with higher-than-usual rents to accommodate patients and their relatives. The hospital guaranteed the rents, and the landlords agreed to cooperate. Patients were accordingly admitted along with their relatives, who were to care for them. Hospital staff were posted to this situation to look after patients admitted there.

The findings in the neighborhood showed that, given adequate patient care, the neighbors were tolerant of the patients' odd behaviors. It was also found that the patients could be treated without additional restraint in this setting.

Our experience showed that mothers formed the largest number of relatives who accompany patients to live in the neighborhood. The choice of the mother is strategic in that the fathers are freed to earn a living for the family. The mothers can look after and perform chores for the patients that fathers might find difficult.

TRADITIONAL THERAPEUTIC SYSTEM

Reports about psychiatry in Africa mention the role of traditional healers in the care of not only psychiatric disorders but physical ailments as well. Field (1960), in her study of rural Ghana, showed the central role played by the traditional healers in rural life, for both the prevention and treatment of disease. Traditional healers operate from shrines and are consulted there by their clients. Sacrifice is prescribed to ward off evil, and potions and draughts are given to cure sickness and encourage health. Reports from all parts of Africa suggest that the role of traditional healers is similar. Western-trained personnel have suggested that traditional healers are very good with psychotherapeutic methods because of their thorough understanding of the culture within which they operate. Concerning their power to tame the witches and control the forces of evil in the communities, explanations have also been offered. The role of witches in a traditional society and the kinds of persons usually attacked by witches were described earlier in this paper. Alland (1965), in a study conducted in the Ivory Coast, found that witches kill their victims out of envy or jealousy. Male informants (wizards) invariably listed property as the primary cause of envy, while females listed fecundity.

"It is my conclusion that aggressive feelings generated by strains in the social system but suppressed during socialization find their outlet in beliefs associated with witchcraft," Alland stated.

In my example, the terms in which aggressive sentiment is expressed appear to be borrowed from an available cultural vocabulary conditioned by socialization and directed by social structure.

These views were previously expressed by Gluckman (1944) in a review of Evan Pritchard's book *Witchcraft, Oracles, and Magic Among the Azanda:* "The fundamental point is that the African is born into a society which believes in witchcraft and, therefore, the very texture of his thinking from childhood on is woven with magical and mystical ideas....The witch wants to hurt people he hates, has quarrelled with, one of whom he is envious . . . charges of witchcraft thus reflect personal relations and quarrels."

Nadel (1952) came to similar conclusions."The witchcraft here examined are casually as well as conspicuously related to specific anxieties and stresses arising in social life."

There have been reports on the use of drugs by traditional healers. Prince (1960) reported on the use of rauwolfia alkaloids in the treatment of psychiatric disorders. Margetts (1965), also reporting from Nigeria, found native healers who used drugs and restraint for the treatment of psychiatric disorders. There is now much intense research in the field. Sofowora (1979) has summarized some of the ongoing research and research findings in this area. African traditional healers continue to use, on an empirical basis, herbs and medications that have been handed down to them through generations of ancestors.

DISCUSSION

This paper has touched on a number of ongoing social changes within the communities in Africa. The participants interact within the social milieu unaware of the various social forces that shape their lives, their interaction patterns, and the social networks and psychology that weave the fabric of life in Africa.

The educated elite strive to be European, to adopt a European attitude to life, establish European institutions, and lead a genteel, sophisticated Western life. Within the culture, however, powerful social forces emphasize his Africanness. He himself may be Europeanized, but his mother, father, sisters, aunts, and other relations constantly return him to his roots. He is the leader of his tribe, his family, and his clansmen, who believe in the omni-presence of evil forces within the community. They regularly, force him to make concessions to his African ancestry. They make sacrifices for him to ward off the machinations of evil forces and witches. They pressure him into taking another wife to accord with ancient beliefs; successful men, he is told, have more than one wife. He has to make concessions and assist less fortunate members of his clan. His attempt to westernize is constantly frustrated. If he is ill with any ailment, he chooses Western institutions, such as the hospital, but his relations, who feel that they know better, consult the oracles on his behalf and, if possible, forcibly remove him to a traditional treatment center.

The African traditional culture bathes him, soothes him, and eventually, envelops and engulfs him. He struggles on, ultimately becoming a hedonist, living only for the remnants of the Western way of life with none of the supporting social institutions.

The true traditional African feels secure in his culture but finds no material satisfaction. His institutions provide spiritual satisfaction and an understanding of the environment within the framework of the world as seen through traditional eyes. If he seeks the material comforts of the Western ways, he loses his Africanness and is enmeshed in a new world where no solace is offered and no security is possible. The young, strong, and vigorous desert this system in search of the new Western way. In times of trouble, most revert to the traditional ways or join the new group of religious revivalist sects.

The transitional group, caught between the old and the new, have tried to synthesize a new way that incorporates the ways of old with the new. They have borrowed freely from the Christian and Islamic religions but utilize the traditional African vehicles of divination, ritual songs, and dance and the expulsion of evil spirits. The priests in this sector have visions. Instead of using the traditional divination tray, they use the Bible or Koran for the casting out of the devil, witches, wizards, and evil forces. The sudden popularity of such institutions in recent times attests to the need these priests fill in the community.

Inevitably, there are tensions and conflicts between these three systems. Within the health sector, the conflict between Western doctors, the carriers of the Western therapeutic ideal, and the traditional healers is sometimes fierce. In general, given the power and prestige of the Western doctors, it would appear that they are winning. In terms of sheer numbers of people treated, however, the traditional healers have the advantage. Traditional healers are secure in the knowledge that many of the transitional types revert to the ancient ways in times of crisis.

The entire social system, and hence the institutions within the system, are in flux. The majority of citizens no longer know quite where they belong. In the course of a single episode of illness, it is not unusual for an African to run through the entire spectrum of available therapeutic systems. This may be done either simultaneously—where the oracle is consulted, prayers are said, and the patient is taken to the hospital—or in rotation—as the patient and his relatives are exposed to first one system and then the other.

REFERENCES

Asuni, T.: Methods of delivering mental health care. Presented at "The Delivery of Mental Health Care,"Kampala, Uganda, April 14-17, 1969.

Binitie, A.: Experiments in the development and planning of psychiatry in the Bendel States of Nigeria. Psychopathologie Africaine 1971a.

Binitie, A.: A study of depression in Benin City Nigeria. MD thesis, London University, 1971b.

Binitie, A.: Psychiatric disorders in a rural practice in the Bendel State of Nigeria. Acta Psychiatrica Scandinavica 64:273-280, 1981.

Bohannan, P. (ed.): African Homicide and Suicide. Princeton, N.J., U.S.A., Princeton University Press, 1960, 1981.

Boroffka, A.: Different ways of starting mental health care. Presented at "The Delivery of Mental Health Care," Kampala, Uganda, April 14-17, 1969.

Boroffka, A.: Psychiatry in Nigeria today and tomorrow. Nigeria Medical Journal 7(4):36-39, 1970.

Carothers, J. C.: The African Mind in Health and Disease: A Study in Ethnopsychiatry. World Health Organization Monograph Series No. 17, Geneva, Switzerland, WHO, 1953.

Collomb, H.: Introduction a la psychiatric-tropicale. Medicine Tropicale 16:141-151, 1956.

Collomb, H.: Psychiatrie en Afrique (experience Senegalese). Psychopathologie Africaine, vol. 84, 1965.

Field, M. J.: Search for Security: An Ethnic- Psychiatric Study of Rural Ghana. New York, U.S.A., W. W. Norton, 1970.

Forde, D.: African Worlds. Oxford, England, Oxford University Press, 1963.

Forster, E. F. B.: The theory and practice of psychiatry in Ghana. American Journal of Psychotherapy 16:7-51, 1962.

Fortes, M., and Dietertan, G.: African System Thought. Oxford, England, Oxford University Press, 1965.

Gluckman, M.: The cogie of African science and witchcraft, an appreciation of Evan Pritchard's "Witchcraft, Oracles, and Magic Among the Azande." Rhodes Hivingstene Journal, 1:61-71, 1944.

Gorden, M. L.: Inquiry into the correlation of civilization and mental disorders in the Kenya Native. East African Medical Journal 12:325-327, 1936.

Lambo, T. A.: Neuropsychiatric Observations in the Western Region of Nigeria. 1956.

Lambo, T. A.: Further neuropsychiatric observations in Nigeria, with comments on the need for epidemiological study in Africa. British Medical Journal 5214:1696-1704, 1960.

Lambo, T.A.: A form of social psychiatry in Africa. World Mental Health 13:190 1961a.

Lambo, T. A.: A plan for the treatment of the mentally ill in Nigeria: the village system at Aro. Edited by Linn, L. 1961b.

Laubscher, B. J. F.: Sex, custom and psychopathology. Routledge, Keegan and Paul, London, England, 1937.

Margetts, E. L.: Traditional Yoruba healers in Nigeria. Man 102:572-573, 1965.

Nadel, S. F.: Witchcraft in four African societies, an essay in comparison. American Anthropologist 54:18- 29, 1952.

Peel, J. D. Y.: Adadura: A Religious Movement Among the Yoruba. Oxford University Press, Oxford, England, 1968.

Prince, R.: The use of rauwolfia for the treatment of psychoses by Nigerian nature doctors. American Journal of Psychiatry 117:147-149, 1960.

Prince, R.: Indigenous Yoruba Psychiatry, in Magic, Faith, and Healing: Studies in Primitive Psychiatry Today. Edited by Kiev, A. New York, U.S.A., Free Press, 1964.

Shelley, H. M., Watson, W. H.: An investigation concerning mental disorder in the Nyasaland native with special reference to primary ecological and other contributory factors. Journal of Mental Science 84:701-730, 1936.

Sofowora, A.: African medical plants, in Proceedings of a Conference, Edited by Sofowora, A., Ile-Ife, Nigeria, University of Ife Press, 1979.

Swift, C. R.: Village settlements for convalescent psychiatric patients. Presented at "The Delivery of Mental Health Care," Kampala, Uganda, April 14-17, 1969.

Chapter 2

Development of Psychiatry in Africa

by

Tolani Asuni, Professor,
Department of Psychiatry,
College of Medicine,
University of Lagos,
Lagos, Nigeria

ABSTRACT

African countries inherited the philosophy and practice of psychiatry of the colonial powers, and that influence has remained largely because of the extreme shortage of trained indigenous personnel. The first Pan-African Psychiatric Conference was held in 1961, and the African Psychiatric Association was formed in 1972. Other professional organizations available to African psychiatrists include the World Health Organization, the World Psychiatric Association, and the World Federation of Mental Health. Because psychiatrists in Africa are so scarce, few national psychiatric associations exist. Most psychiatrists are based in hospitals, and they primarily treat psychosis. Generally, they head teams of mental health professionals, and the trend is toward decentralization of psychiatric services from overcrowded hospitals to small, scattered facilities staffed by other members of the psychiatric team. Another trend is the formalization of traditional psychiatric practice or its incorporation into Western practice; many of the traditional approaches have psychotherapeutic value. The formal Western type of psychiatry practiced in Africa uses physical treatments primarily and only superficial psychotherapy. Relatives are usually involved in treatment and help convince patients they have been ill. Efforts to train psychiatrists in their own countries or regions are intensifying, and more exposure to psychiatry is being given in medical schools. Research is difficult because of the lack of funds, poor data collection and follow-up, and shortage of personnel and facilities.

HISTORICAL INTRODUCTION

I recognize the problem of generalizing for the whole of Africa. All the same, I am familiar enough with the situation to venture broad generalizations, which are valid even though there may be some exceptions.

COLONIALISM

Africa is a big continent. Culturally, the area north of the Sahara is Arabic and the area south of the Sahara is African. In this context the Republic of South Africa is left out. Liberia is the only country that has never been under any colonial domination, but it has had very close contact with the United States, a world power. Ethiopia was under Italian domination for a while. The result of the colonial domination is that these countries have inherited the philosophy and practice of psychiatry bequeathed by the colonial powers. These powers include Great Britain, France, Belgium, Spain, and Portugal. Germany's influence waned after the First World War, when its colonies were taken over and mandated to other powers, whose influence superseded that of the Germans. Only in the last three decades have most of these countries become independent. But the pervasive influence of the colonial powers still remains to varying degrees, depending on the situation in each country.

PSYCHIATRIC PERSONNEL

One of the major reasons for the continuing colonial influence is the extreme shortage of trained indigenous personnel in all fields, especially psychiatry. In addition, most of those who have received training have done so in the colonizing countries. Only recently have personnel begun going to other countries for their training. With no or very few trained indigenous personnel, it is easier to continue with the inherited tradition. There are, however, some exceptions to this tendency.

These exceptions include the late Tigani El Mahi of the Sudan, T.A. Lambo, and myself; we initiated new programs under different circumstances. These innovations were based on the cultural perspectives in our own countries. I will come back to these innovations later.

During the Colonial era, all psychiatrists in Africa were foreigners from colonizing countries. Their writings on psychiatry in Africa reflected not only the tradition in their own countries but also their own interpretation and perspective of the African situation. One outcome of this bias was the erroneous report that depression was rare in Africa. This conclusion, of course, also reflected the general impression of the happy savage, as stated by Rousseau, the French philosopher, and the impression that the African's brain was less developed than that of the European *(Carothers, 1953).*

The first African psychiatrist was Tigani El Mahi of the Sudan. He trained in Great Britain and returned to his country in the late 1940's or early 1950's. The second was B. Forster of Gambia, who, however, worked in Ghana after training in Great Britain. The third was T.A. Lambo of Nigeria, who returned home about 1954 after receiving his training in Great Britain. Then came a crop of Africans, including me, mostly from Nigeria. There are still very few psychiatrists in Africa, even though the number is increasing. Some countries still do not have a single indigenous psychiatrist.

PSYCHIATRIC CONFERENCES

On the initiative of T.A. Lambo and with my assistance, the first Pan-African Psychiatric Conference was held in the Aro Village

Hospital, Abeokuta, Nigeria, in 1961. At this conference, the indigenous African psychiatrists were outnumbered by distinguished participants from the United States, Canada, Great Britain, Germany, Norway, and The Netherlands. The indigenous African psychiatrists included one each from Ghana, Mauritius, and Lesotho; two from Sudan; and four from Nigeria. They were about all the African psychiatrists at the time. Of course, many Western psychiatrists working in Africa also participated in the conference. They came from Senegal, Kenya, and other countries. The conference had a positive impact on psychiatry in Africa and certainly gave international visibility to African psychiatry.

The next congress was held in Dakar, Senegal, in 1968 on the initiative of the late Dr. Henry Collomb. French participants outnumbered all others. It was at this conference that the idea of formalizing the organization of African psychiatric conferences came up.

AFRICAN PSYCHIATRIC ASSOCIATION

Instead of depending on the initiative of individuals, it was considered desirable to form the African Psychiatric Association to take responsibility for organizing conferences on a regular basis. The association was formed in 1972. As no country had any national psychiatric association, individual membership was the only option. The association held annual workshops in different African countries in East Africa, in West Africa, and in Anglophone and Francophone countries. It held conferences once every 4-6 years. These meetings were meant to give psychiatrists working either single-handedly or in relative professional isolation, the opportunity to meet with their colleagues to share their experiences and ideas and to provide stimulation, encouragement, and support to each other. It was also meant to call the attention of authorities, of the host country in particular, so that they could give support and encouragement to the few psychiatrists in their territories.

In addition to the regular individual membership of the African Psychiatric Association, provisions were made for associate and other forms of memberships. The changes would open membership to psychiatric nurses and non-African psychiatrists who had worked in

Africa or who had a special interest in African psychiatry.

PSYCHIATRIC JOURNALS

Psychiatrists in Africa published their professional and academic papers outside Africa, in European and North American journals. Very few were published in medical journals in East and West Africa.

There have been two psychiatric journals in Africa. The older of the two is Psychologie Africaine, which is published by the Dakar group. As expected, most of the articles in this journal are in French and address mainly the French African situation.

The African Psychiatric Association started the African Journal of Psychiatry to give a broader perspective. Articles are published in the original English and French languages. Summaries are given in both languages.

Psychopathologie Africaine is encountering some difficulty in continuing publication. The African Journal of Psychiatry is also having problems in getting the publication out regularly. For this and other reasons, African psychiatrists continue to submit their articles to journals published outside the continent.

While on the subject of publications, it is relevant to draw attention to some differences between the French and English articles and papers on psychiatric matters. English publications appear to be more scientific and pragmatic, whereas the French appear to be more philosophical and discursive. It also appears that a larger proportion of the articles by Francophone authors relate to psychoanalytic concepts than those by Anglophone authors. This is evidently a reflection of the difference between British and French psychiatry and of the respective influences on authors who trained in Great Britain and France.

INTERGOVERNMENTAL ORGANIZATIONS:

WORLD HEALTH ORGANIZATION

The African Regional Headquarters of the World Health Organization (WHO) is located in Brazzaville, Republic of the

Congo. It does not serve the whole of the African continent, as some countries in North Africa belong to the European region and some countries in Northeast Africa belong to the Mediterranean region.

In addition, Brazzaville is the only regional headquarters that does not have a mental health expert on its staff on a regular basis to look after mental health matters in the region. This may be due to apparently low priority member states give to mental health in the context of the region's more devastating health problems.

It is encouraging, however, that the planners of the 1973 annual regional meeting of the member states were persuaded to have a technical discussion on "The Place of Mental Health in the Development of Public Health Services in Africa." The meeting was held in Lagos, Nigeria, and the delegation from the member states was taken to see the Aro Neuropsychiatric Hospital in Aro, Abeokuta, Nigeria. In addition, the regional office has sponsored African psychiatrists' participation in professional meetings.

The initiative in mental health matters in the region appears to have been taken by the central headquarters of WHO in Geneva, Switzerland. An example of this initiative is the Action Group Program, which involves mostly countries in eastern and southern Africa.

THE ORGANIZATION OF AFRICAN UNITY

This organization does not appear to have any major program for health matters, let alone mental health. It did, however, organize a meeting for mental health experts in Africa some years ago.

NONGOVERNMENTAL ORGANIZATIONS:

WORLD PSYCHIATRIC ASSOCIATION

Although the World Psychiatric Association (WPA) is mainly an association of national psychiatric associations, there is a provision for individual memberships. Since there are few national psychiatric associations in Africa, most Africans join on an individual basis. As WPA has an official relationship with WHO, the association is usually invited to participate in the regional WHO meetings in an observer capacity. WPA nominates an African if there is one on the committee (and there is usually one) to represent it in the regional meetings. Through this participation psychiatric issues can be raised in the meeting. In fact, it was through this participation that WHO was persuaded to sponsor discussion of a psychiatric topic in 1973.

The World Federation of Mental Health (WFMH) consists of national mental health associations and individual members. It is not an exclusively psychiatric association, as membership includes all related mental health professions.

Since psychiatrists in Africa are the most vocal in support of mental health, they play a recognized role in WFMH. Two successive vice-presidents for Africa were psychiatrists. To facilitate its work in Africa, the organization is considering the division of the region into subregions.

NATIONAL PSYCHIATRIC ASSOCIATIONS

In view of the fact that there are very few psychiatrists, if any, in most African countries, it is understandable that the feasibility of national psychiatric associations is poor. The psychiatric association in Nigeria, however, has a membership of slightly over 50. This is, perhaps, the largest number in any one country except Egypt and other North African countries. The Kenya Psychiatric Association was launched in 1986 with a membership of 26 psychiatrists.

AFRICAN PSYCHIATRY IN THE 1980s:

PSYCHIATRIC SERVICES

Psychiatric service is an integral part of the health service in African countries, but psychiatry is not usually represented in the ministries of health. It is treated like any other specialty. The most senior psychiatrist in the service is usually consulted on psychiatric matters. He/she is based in a psychiatric hospital.

The fact that psychiatry is hospital-based does not mean that the activities of psychiatrists are limited to the psychiatric hospital. They extend their work to the community, as in the case of psychiatrists in the Aro Neuropsychiatric Hospital in Nigeria, and they do liaison psychiatry by going into general hospitals close to their bases. In fact, some areas, such as Lagos State of Nigeria, where there is no state psychiatric hospital, the psychiatrists are based in the general hospitals.

One general statement that can be validly made is that psychiatry in Africa is the psychiatry of psychosis. This does not mean that we do not have other forms of psychiatric ailments. But psychosis is the most disturbing, not only to the individual but also to the community. Psychosis does not lend itself readily to containment, as do other psychiatric disturbances. Furthermore, there are traditional and cultural ways of dealing with minor psychiatric disturbances that cannot be contained. Therefore, psychiatric services are mainly based on the psychiatry of psychosis, although awareness that psychiatry has a wider function is beginning now to bring patients with neurosis and adolescence problems to the psychiatrists.

In view of the great demands on the few psychiatrists in Africa, it is not realistic to expect psychiatrists to devote all their time to any particular aspect of psychiatry. Most psychiatrists can, therefore, be called generalists who may, however, focus on particular subspecialties that interest them or to which they are exposed by the nature of their assignments. It should, therefore, not be surprising to find an African equally experienced and knowledgeable in child and adolescent psychiatry, forensic psychiatry, and liaison psychiatry at the same time.

The psychiatrist theoretically works in a team with nurses, psychiatric social workers, psychologists, and occupational therapists. In reality, not all members of the team are represented in the service, mainly because of the shortage of trained personnel. In view of this shortage, it becomes necessary for the available members of a team to be flexible in their roles. Nurses may have to do some social work, particularly when relatives visit sick family members in the hospital. They may have to supervise the work the patient has brought back from the occupational therapy department. This particular example has the advantage of allowing the nurses to know their patients better, as it adds another dimension to their interaction.

The leadership of the team is vested in the psychiatrist, who has the responsibility of coordinating the team. To do this effectively, he/she should be familiar with the scope of each profession in the team without assuming to be an expert in these other areas.

The trend in the provision of service in countries where there are enough psychiatrists for the basic operation is to relieve the congestion in the usually overcrowded psychiatric hospitals, to decentralize the service, and to have psychiatric facilities scattered all over the country. Indeed, WHO has recommended that other members of the psychiatric team, especially nurses, staff small psychiatric stations and treat psychiatric cases to the best of their ability under the supervision of the few psychiatrists available. By doing so, there will be wide psychiatric coverage of the population, even down to the grass-roots level.

WHO's recommendation is based on the fact that there are more nurses and assistant medical officers than psychiatrists and their training is shorter than that of psychiatrists. To facilitate the implementation of this recommendation, nurses can be allowed to prescribe basic drugs (Swift and Asuni, 1975).

PSYCHIATRIC PRACTICE

Social, economic, and cultural factors must be addressed in psychiatric practice everywhere if the practice is to be relevant, appropriate, credible, and effective. The personality of the psychiatrist and the type of training he/she has had are also influential. This is an area where generalization for the whole of Africa may be hazardous.

In Africa, there are two broad types of psychiatric practice. One is the informal traditional psychiatric practice; the other is the formal Western type. There is a move to formalize the traditional psychiatric practice in a number of African countries, while in a few, such as Mozambique, the traditional psychiatric practice is banned. The move to formalize the traditional practice is based on the premise that traditional methods are more aligned with the culture of the people and that they are more accessible and more acceptable to the people. These are strong arguments. The formalization goes further. Incorporating and/or assimilating traditional practitioners in the formal health delivery system is being considered seriously.

Some psychiatrists are wary about this trend. The major reason is that not enough studies have been done about traditional practice to justify the move. In-depth studies of the practice are needed to identify its strengths and weaknesses which can be used to guide the collaboration and cooperation with formal Western psychiatric practice. Even if traditional practice is considered an alternative that gives the people an option other than the formal practice, which is relatively scarce, it is still necessary to know the areas of competence of traditional healers.

The traditional practice varies from country to country. Among the Yorubas of Nigeria, attempts have been made to classify the practice. One class includes the use of herbs, primarily after divination for diagnosis. It is believed that some of the herbs may prove to be very effective in the treatment of not only psychiatric disorders but also other medical ailments. On the basis of this belief, at least two centers have been created to look into the pharmacology of the medicinal herbs used by traditional healers. The centers are in Dakar, Senegal, and in Ife, Nigeria.

Over 20 years ago it was established that one of the potent herbs used in the treatment of psychosis was Rauwolfia serpentina (Prince, 1960). The psychotherapeutic principles involved in its use depend on the cosmic view held by the people. In some cases it is closely linked with the religious belief of the people, while in others it is associated with the people's philosophy regarding their relationship to the spirit world. In some cases, membership in a cult is important and the patient is conditioned to live with his/her symptoms. The objective of psychotherapeutic intervention in this case is acceptance of the patient by the group members.

The range of problems handled by traditional practice is sometimes very wide and varies from social to personal. To this extent, it is similar to psychotherapy in the West. One major difference is that traditional practice does not focus on the individual exclusively, as Western psychotherapy tends to do; neither does it tend to deal with the unconscious in the same way as Western psychotherapy, if at all (Dawson, 1964; Field, 1960; Messing, 1959; Turner, 1964; Jahoda, 1972; Zemplenia, 1966; Whisson, 1964; Prince, 1964; Orley, 1970).

It is easy to understand how traditional therapists can be effective in cases of neurosis. Therein may lie their strength, especially when it comes to psychotherapy.

Another type of informal practice is that carried out by religious bodies (Asuni, 1967a, 1967b, & 1973), mostly the syncretic religious bodies, which claim not only the healing of the soul but also the healing of mental illness. There is no doubt that they are able to give support, comfort, and solace to the troubled mind, but their claim to do more still needs to be verified. There are different levels of psychotherapeutic religious intervention. The simplest is prayer to potentiate other forms of intervention, such as formal westernized practice. This form of intervention may be universal. The second level is participation in group activity, such as dancing and keeping vigil, which may have some cathartic effect. The third level is the laying on of hands and the use of holy water and oil. These may have placebo effects. Whatever it does, the practice is worth looking into closely because it is used by a large number of people. I have found (Asuni, 1973) that the practice is patronized by people with a range of problems from purely social to mainly psychiatric.

One interesting observation is that some patients use one or both of these informal practices along with the formal westernized practice. Indeed, psychiatrists in Africa should be aware of this and accept it as long as it does not conflict with their objective and mode of practice, especially in terms of medication.

The practice of the formal Western type of psychiatry is the one that has always been recognized by the governments. It was inherited from the colonial days, as rudimentary as it was then; the asylums were later renamed psychiatric hospitals. The practice developed along the line of Western psychiatry, with a mainly eclectic approach and less emphasis on classical or neoclassical psychotherapy.

Physical forms of treatment—chemotherapy and electroconvulsive therapy—are used extensively. The psychotherapy used is superficial, and no attempt at interpretation is made. It does not usually delve into the unconscious. Attempts at deep-insight psychotherapy have usually proved futile. In any case, it is so time-consuming that patients get impatient, terminate treatment, and go elsewhere. Further, it can reach only a very few of those who need it (Kiev, 1972). An experiment with inpatient group psychotherapy as an adjunct to physical therapy (Asuni, 1967) was found useful. It did not follow any particular school of psychotherapy.

Patients who have been exposed to Western culture may respond positively to the types of psychotherapy techniques practiced in the West.

Even though African psychiatry has not made an issue of family psychiatry, it is extensively used. It is almost inconceivable to treat patients, especially psychotic patients, in isolation from their families. In fact, in most cases the participation of the family, and sometimes friends, is demanded before treatment is started or during the treatment process. Since very few, if any, supportive services are available outside the hospital, the participation of relatives is essential for rehabilitation. In any case, it is usually relatives or friends who accompany the patients to the hospital.

Even in some developed countries where supportive social services are available to varying degrees, the role of relatives in the management of functional illness is now being appreciated (Kuipers and Bebbington, 1985). Relatives are useful in early identification of and consequently intervention in psychotic illness. They are available to give necessary information. Their participation in the treatment program enhances the patient's coping mechanisms and facilitates his/her rehabilitation.

Since the type of deep-insight psychotherapy practiced in Europe and North America is not usually practiced in Africa, the treatment objective is the patient's realization that he/she has been ill and his/her recognition of the pathological experiences, such as delusions and hallucinations, as symptoms of the illness. In other words, it is not enough for the psychotic patient to lose the psychotic symptoms and behave normally. Efforts are made to help him/her trace the development of these symptoms. This has a preventive effect. Later, incipient relapse can be quickly nipped in the bud.

If psychopharmacological, milieu, and other forms of treatment have not succeeded in making the patient realize that he/she has been ill, we conduct what we call a confrontation interview, during which the relatives are invited to relate the abnormal behavior and statements of the patient. This sometimes has a dramatic effect. The patient, on hearing this report, becomes penitent and begs the relatives for forgiveness for his/her abusive, insolent, and aggressive behavior. Another effect of the confrontation interview is that it reassures the relatives that the patient is well enough to be discharged from the hospital and puts them in an understanding and accepting frame of mind.

It is only fair to admit that in some cases the patient does not regain insight through this process. The reaction of unresponsive patients is unshakable denial. In such cases, we have to be satisfied with improvement in behavior.

Another example of innovation is the treatment of patients, especially traditional patients not as westernized, in villages near the hospital. These patients are boarded with their relatives in nearby villages while they attend the hospital for consultation and a hospital-based treatment program. During their stay in the village, they participate in communal village activities and assist their relatives in providing food and water and in other domestic chores, depending on their mental state. This ensures the participation of relatives in the treatment program and enhances surveillance after the patients return home.

In one or two places, such as the Aro Neuropsychiatric Hospital in Abeokuta, Nigeria, which became known internationally partly because of the innovative Aro Village, the town has expanded to engulf the villages around. Consequently, the character of the villages has been lost.

Attempts are under way to treat as many patients as possible, no matter how disturbed, on an ambulatory basis. However, some relatives, having come to the end of their tether after expending a lot of effort, time, energy, and money on consulting one traditional healer after another, try to dump their sick relatives in the hospital. Psychiatrists generally try to avoid the dumping and persuade the relatives that the hospital is for active treatment and not asylum.

Very few psychiatrists are in private practice or have connections with hospitals in which they can hospitalize patients who need it. There are no private psychiatric hospitals. There are, however, psychiatric departments in large university teaching hospitals, some of which provide a degree of privacy because of their small size.

TRAINING OF PSYCHIATRISTS

To be a psychiatrist, one needs to have recognized psychiatric training and certification. The training of African psychiatrists has been done mostly in Western countries. Recently psychiatrists have received training in Eastern countries. Efforts are now being intensified to train psychiatrists locally, in their own African countries and in neighboring countries if the training facilities in their own areas are not adequate. It is appreciated, however, that it is necessary to send residents abroad, usually to Western countries, to broaden their outlook and to expose them to areas in which local training is weak.

In addition to the future benefits of training residents in the environment in which they are going to work, service is also a consideration. Doctors do render service while they are in training. Training abroad means that their countries are deprived of their service, which the countries cannot readily afford.

Those trained abroad, without previous exposure to psychiatry in their own countries, usually try to practice in the mode of their training. They accept the cultural and other differences that have been emphasized in their training. It takes them some time to readjust to their local situations, which are different from the places where they were trained.

PSYCHIATRIC ORIENTATION FOR MEDICAL STUDENTS

Most medical schools in Africa have departments of psychiatry or sections of psychiatry within the departments of medicine. Depending on the training program, the time given to psychiatry varies from 4 to 12 weeks. The trend is to allow more time for psychiatry, especially where the time allocated for psychiatry is currently relatively short.

This exposure to psychiatry is often preceded by lectures in medical psychology. A wide spectrum of clinical psychiatry is taught, but case demonstrations depend on the clinical facilities available in the teaching hospitals. Where there is a local psychiatric hospital, the medical students are often taken there for teaching purposes, and the staff of this hospital is involved in teaching medical students.

RESEARCH IN PSYCHIATRY

This academic activity is not confined to the medical schools. Psychiatrists with academic flair, who are in the health service also carry out research, sometimes using the clinical material in their hospitals. This material covers a wider range of psychiatric diagnoses than is available in psychiatry departments of teaching hospitals. It is also available in greater quantities. In fact, the earlier publications on psychiatry in Africa came from psychiatrists in the health services before the establishment of medical schools with psychiatry departments.

Research requiring advanced technology is not common in Africa for obvious reasons. Epidemiological research on a large scale is also expensive, and the study done by Leighton, et al. (1963) in Nigeria has not been repeated elsewhere in Africa.

It is surprising that, in spite of the many problems facing research workers in Africa, psychiatrists are able to carry out research and publish their work in reputable journals. The problems confronting researchers include inadequate and unreliable demographic data, poor case notes, difficulty in following up cases, shortage of personnel, poor secretarial services, poor library facilities, and difficulty in subscribing to journals because of strict foreign-exchange control.

It is even more surprising that the few psychiatrists available are called on to administer programs, provide service, and teach at the same time. Needless to say, some do more than others, but on the whole they all have more varied responsibilities than their counterparts in the developed countries of the world.

REFERENCES

Asuni, T.: Nigerian experiment in group psychotherapy. American Journal of Psychotherapy 12:95-104, 1967a.

Asuni, T.: Religious conversion and psychoses. International Mental Health Research Newsletter 9(4):608, 1967b.

Asuni, T.: Sociomedical problems of religious converts. Psychopathologie Africaine 9:223-236, 1973.

Carothers, J. C.: The African Mind in Health and Disease: Study in Ethnopsychiatry. World Health Organization Monograph Series No. 17. Geneva, Switzerland, WHO, 1953.

Dawson, J.: Urbanization and mental health in a West African community, Magic Faith, and Healing: Studies in Primitive Psychiatry Today. Edited by Kiev. Free Press, New York, USA., 1964.

Field, M. J.: Search for Security: An Ethno-Psychiatric Study of Rural Ghana. New York, USA, W.W. Norton, 1970.

German, G. A.: Aspects of Clinical Psychiatry in Sub- Saharan Africa. British Journal of Psychiatry 121:461- 479, 1972.

Jahoda, G.: Traditional healers and other institutions concerned with mental illness in Ghana. International Journal of Social Psychiatry, 7, 1972.

Kiev, A.: Transcultural Psychiatry. Free Press, New York, USA, 1972.

Kuipers, L., Bebbington, P.: Relatives as a resource in the management of functional illness. British Journal of Psychiatry 147:465-470, 1985.

Leighton, A., Lambo, T.A., Hughes, C. C., et al.: Psychiatric Disorder Among the Yoruba. Ithaca, N. Y., U. S. A., Cornell University Press, 1963.

Messing, S. D.: Group therapy and social status in Zar cult of Ethiopia, in Culture and Mental Health. Edited by Opter, M. K.; Macmillan, New York, U.S.A., 1959.

Orley, J. H.: Culture and Mental Illness: A Study From Uganda. Nairobi, Kenya, East African Publishing House, 1970.

Prince, R.: Indigenous Yoruba psychiatry, in Magic, Faith, and Healing: Studies in Primitive Psychiatry Today. Edited by Kiev, A. New York, U.S.A., Free Press, 1964.

Swift, C. R., Asuni, T.: Mental Health and Disease in Africa. Churchill Livingstone. London, England, 1975.

Turner, V. W.: A Ndembu doctor in practice, in Magic, Faith, and Healing: Studies in Primitive Psychiatry Today. Edited by Kiev, A. New York, U.S.A. Free Press, 1964.

Whisson, M. G.: Some aspects of functional disorders among the Kenya Luo. Ibid.

Zemplenia, A.: La dimension therapeutique du culte des Rab. N'dep, Tuuru et Samp. Rites de possession Chez les lebou et woloff. Psychopathologie Africaine 2(3):295- 441, 1966.

Chapter 3

Social Consequences of Psychosis for Psychotic Patients In Western Province, Kenya, After Treatment

by

G.P.M. Assen, MD,
Department of Psychiatry,
Faculty of Medicine
University of Nairobi,
Nairobi, Kenya

ABSTRACT

This study tested the hypothesis that treatment of African psychotic patients by traditional healers is followed by better social reintegration than treatment by modern medicine. Nineteen patients in the Luhya tribe of Kenya were treated by traditional healers, four were treated by prayer healers, and 23 matched patients were treated in a hospital psychiatric ward. The author describes the diagnostic and treatment characteristics of the patients and the improvements in their scores on the Present State Examination and Disability

Assessment Schedule. The neuroleptics used in the hospital shortened the patients' hospital episodes, but illness beliefs were not addressed, decreasing the likelihood of compliance after discharge. The author describes the social consequences of psychoses for the Luhya, which depend on the quality of treatment, the patient's behavior, and community norms and values. Outcome of hospital treatment might improve if hospital staff adapt their explanations of treatment to these beliefs.

INTRODUCTION AND HYPOTHESIS

Previous studies have established that the epidemiology of psychiatric diseases in Africa is comparable with that in Western countries (Giel and Van Luijk, 1969; German, 1972). Research in Kenya confirms this finding (Ndetei, 1980; Acuda, 1982). Only limited services can be offered, however, owing to a serious shortage of medical means and manpower in mental health care in Kenya (Otsyula, 1973; Ndetei, 1980).

During my preparation of this research project, the World Health Organization (WHO) pleaded strongly for the integration of traditional healers in modern medicine, especially in primary health care (WHO, 1978a and 1983).

There has been little systematic research on the effect of treatment by traditional healers (Kleinman, 1977). The successful case studies mentioned in the literature (Kiev, 1964; Kleinman, 1980) mostly concern patients with neurotic problems, and little grande psychiatrie is mentioned. Exceptions are the reports by Harding (1973), who mentioned the use of herbs with rauwolfia by traditional healers, and Field (1960). This scarcity of material was a reason to start this study on the efficacy of treatment by traditional healers of psychotic patients.

Patients seen at a traditional healer's compound were compared with patients admitted at a psychiatric ward of a general hospital. The following questions were posed:

- What happens with patients treated by a traditional healer and with patients treated at a psychiatric ward?
- Is there a difference in social reintegration after treatment?

- What is the attitude of the community concerning the different types of treatment?
- Is it advisable to encourage the treatment of psychotic patients by traditional healers?

Traditional healers share the world view of their patients and are, therefore, close to the emotions and experiences of relatives. Healers share their beliefs about the role that supernatural powers play in the origin of diseases, including madness (Mbiti, 1969; Wagner, 1970). The traditional healers are acquainted with symptoms by which madness presents itself and with the possible social consequences (Rappaport and Drent, 1979).

This study was designed to test the hypothesis that treatment by traditional healers provides a better chance for social reintegration of psychotic patients than treatment by modern medicine. The practical importance is to determine whether it is possible to integrate traditional healers into the official mental health care system.

METHODS:

DEFINITIONS

I have used the following definition of a traditional healer:

The traditional healer is recognized by his or her own community as competent to provide a variety of health services by using plant, animal, and mineral substances, as well as other methods based on social, cultural, and religious background. He or she also utilizes the prevailing knowledge, attitudes, and beliefs in the community about physical, mental, and social well-being, and the causes of disease and disability. (Good and Kimani, 1980)

During this study, the important role of prayer healers in treating (psychotic) patients became clear. Therefore, they were included in this research. The hypothesis applied to them was the same as that for the traditional healers.

A prayer healer treats people by means of praying only; no herbs or medicines are used. He may use rituals.

The following definition of a psychotic patient was used:

A patient with a mental disorder in which impairment of mental function has developed to a degree that interferes grossly with insight, ability to meet some ordinary demands of life, or to maintain adequate contact with reality....It is not an exact or well-defined term. (WHO, 1978b)

Resocialization was defined as a process of being taken up in and by the community, in which both the community, by its acceptance, and the patient, by his own actions and behavior, play reciprocal parts.

It was assumed that treatment by a traditional healer, a prayer healer, or the psychiatric ward is able to influence both the patient and the community.

SELECTION OF PATIENTS AND TRADITIONAL HEALERS

Patients treated by traditional or prayer healers who were psychotic patients and 15 years old or older who belonged to the Luhya tribe. Each patient was required to be admitted to traditional or prayer healer's compound.

In the area covered by the research in Western Province, Kenya, there was one hospital with a psychiatric ward, the Provincial Hospital in Kakamega. A patient treated at this ward was included in the study if he or she was comparable with one of the patients seen at a traditional or prayer healer's compound. The following qualifying characteristics applied: sex, age, marital status, education/profession, diagnosis made by the investigator, and number of psychotic episodes (a distinction was made between patients who were having their first psychotic episode and patients who had had two or more psychotic episodes).

No retrospective cases were included because disease histories and symptoms thus obtained are not always reliable.

The traditional and prayer healers belonged to the Luhya tribe. Each one selected had a reputation for treating psychotic patients or had a very busy practice, which provided ample opportunity for encountering psychotic patients. Furthermore, only traditional and prayer healers who treated psychotic patients (in most cases) on their own compounds were selected. This was to ensure the observation of the patient and his treatment. Moreover, residing in the healer's compound resembled admission to the psychiatric ward of the

Provincial Hospital. Patients were in both cases taken out of their sometimes pathological home situations.

QUESTIONNAIRES

The following questionnaires were used:

- Present States Examination (PSE). This instrument was designed by WHO to assess a patient's symptoms during the 4 weeks before the semistructured interview (Wing, 1975).
- Disability Assessment Schedule (DAS). This questionnaire, also developed by WHO, assesses the patient's behavior and social functioning in his particular social and cultural background (WHO, 1980).
- Open-ended questionnaire. This was designed especially for this study to obtain information that could not be obtained with the PSE or DAS, such as previous and present disease history, choice and expectation of treatment, cultural concepts of psychoses, life history, and family and social circumstances. This questionnaire was used with the patient and his/her relatives, neighbors, and village elders to assess the clinical diagnosis and the social integration at the start of the study and after 6 months of follow-up.

PATIENT'S PARTICULARS

Nineteen patients (eleven male, eight female) were treated by traditional healers, and four (three males, one female) were treated by prayer healers. These 23 patients were matched with patients treated at the psychiatric ward in Kakamega. Tables I and II offer some interesting comparisons.

Table I

DISTRIBUTION OF MATCHED PAIRS ACCORDING TO AGE, SEX, AND MARITAL STATUS

	TRADITIONAL HEALER[1]						PRAYER HEALER[2]						HOSPITAL A[3]						HOSPITAL B[4]					
	M[5]		S[6]		D[7]		M		S		D		M		S		D		M		S		D	
Age	m[8]	f[9]	m	f	m	f	m	f	m	f	m	f	m	f	m	f	m	f	m	f	m	f	m	f
15–25	–	–	5	3	–	–	1	1	–	1	–	–	–	1	4	2	–	–	–	1	2	–	–	–
26–35	1	1	1	–	–	1	–	–	–	–	–	–	1	1	1	–	3	–	1	–	–	–	–	–
36–45	–	2	–	–	2	–	1	–	–	–	–	–	1	2	–	–	–	1	–	–	–	–	–	–
46–60	2	1	–	–	–	–	–	–	–	–	–	–	1	1	–	–	–	–	–	–	–	–	–	–
Total	3	4	6	3	2	1	1	1	1	–	1	–	3	5	2	3	1	1	1	1	2	–	–	–

[1] Patients treated at a traditional healer's compound.
[2] Patients treated at a prayer healer's compound.
[3] Patients treated at the psychiatric ward, matched with the patients treated at a traditional healer's compound.
[4] Patients treated at the psychiatric ward, matched with the patients treated at a prayer healer's compound.
[5] Married.
[6] Single.
[7] Divorced. All divorces mentioned above were a result of this psychotic episode.
[8] Male.
[9] Female

Table II
Profession During Last Year Before the Present Psychotic Episode

	TRADITIONAL HEALER[1]		PRAYER HEALER[2]		HOSPITAL A[3]		HOSPITAL B[4]	
PROFESSION	M	F	M	F	M	F	M	F
STUDENT, Primary School	1	2	1	–	1	3	1	–
STUDENT, Secondary School	1	1	–	–	–	–	–	–
HELPING AT HOME[7]	5[8]	–	1	–	7	–	1	–
FARMER	2	–	–	–	–	–	–	–
HOUSEWIFE	–	5	–	1	–	5	–	1
EMPLOYED	2	–	1	–	3	–	1	–

1 Patients treated at a traditional healer's compound.
2 Patients treated at a prayer healer's compound.
3 Patients treated at the psychiatric ward, matched with the patients treated at a traditional healer's compound.
4 Patients treated at the psychiatric ward, matched with the patients treated at a prayer healer's compound.
5 Male.
6 Female.
7 Helping at home. The patient has no responsibility for work yet.
8 One patient in this group has been in prisn most of the time of the last year before this treatment.

OBSERVATIONS AND RESULTS:

CONCEPTS AMONG THE LUHYA ABOUT PSYCHOSES

Psychotic patients are clearly recognized by the Luhya as mentally disturbed or mad. They call this disease lilalu. According to the Luhya, all patients who were suffering from lilalu were psychotic. The Luhya consider psychosis a disease of the head; the brain is thought to be disturbed (Assen, 1983).

The cause is usually believed to be an evil spirit, esishieno or omusambwa, or witchcraft. Sometimes the Luhya say it is due to cerebral malaria. The traditional healer performs his treatment according to the believed cause of the disease (obtained by divination). In general, they believe an evil spirit causes madness, lilalu, but the reasons for the evil spirits' actions vary.

DESCRIPTION OF TREATMENT

Treatment by Traditional Healers. The traditional healer tries to neutralize the power of the evil spirit or witchcraft over the patient and tries to cool down the disease in the patient's body. His treatment may consist of rituals, herbal treatment, and protective medicines (hirizi, a kind of amulet or protective herb). Most traditional healers tie the patient if he is aggressive.

Treatment by Prayer Healers. To the prayer healers of the Church of God, one of the many independent churches of Kenya and included in this study, the cause of lilalu may be evil spirits, witchcraft, or just a disease. In general, the independent churches say, "A disease is believed to be a punishment of God for sin or a testing of faith. A third possibility identifies sickness entirely with the work of the adversary. The way is opened for the Devil's activity by human sin" (Kenya Churches Handbook, 1983).

The prayer healer may divine from the Bible.

The treatment consists of praying for the patient and shouting to the evil spirits, or shetani, to go away. When the patient is cured, the prayer healer goes to the patient's compound to burn all the traditional things, such as gourds for the spirits and siphons for drinking beer (hirizi).

Also, prayer healers perform rituals as part of their treatment. However, they are usually less extensive and are mostly closing ceremonies (rites of passage).

Treatment at the Psychiatric Ward in Kakamega Hospital. In the Provincial Hospital of Kakamega in Western Province, there is a small psychiatric ward. It has 22 beds for 11 men and 11 women. In 1983, 59 patients were admitted to the ward. It serves a population of about 5 million people, who live in three provinces.

Only psychotic patients were admitted to the psychiatric ward at Kakamega. Because of the lack of means for conducting other therapies, such as occupational, drugs were the main therapeutic factor. Neuroleptics, especially chlorpromazine, were important in shortening psychotic episodes, keeping the patients quiet in the small and crowded ward, and preventing aggressive outbursts.

Table III

DIAGNOSTIC CATEGORIES OF PSYCHOTIC PATIENTS TREATED BY TRADITIONAL OR PRAYER HEALERS OR IN A PSYCHIATRIC WARD IN KENYA

Diagnostic Group	Traditional & Prayer healers	Hospital
Substance-induced psychosis	3	3
Nonaffective functional psychosis	16	15
Bipolar	4	5

PSYCHIATRIC DIAGNOSIS

The clinical diagnoses were made according to DSM-III (American Psychiatric Association, 1980), and the patients were then classified as having substance-induced psychoses, nonaffective functional psychoses, or bipolar disorder. According to ICD-9, the nonaffective functional psychoses consist of schizophrenia and all its subtypes, the paranoid psychoses, and other nonorganic or reactive psychoses. Table III compares the diagnostic classifications of the patients treated in the two settings.

PRELIMINARY PSE QUESTIONNAIRE RESULTS

Some questions could not be answered in such a way that a score could be made by seriously ill patients who had florid hallucinations and delusions, strongly deviant behavior, or profound disturbances in thought. Sections of the PSE lacking data were not processed. Only scores obtained by observation were processed. These are the sections concerning behavior, affect, and speech, and a total score for these three sections was calculated. I will mention the following conclusions about these items:

1. In both groups of patients, between the beginning of the treatment (T1) and the followup at 6 months (T2), symptoms improved in most patients.
2. The patients treated in the hospital showed fewer observable symptoms on these sections of the PSE at T1 than the patients treated by traditional or prayer healers. A possible explanation could be the fact that a traditional healer gives less structure to the patient than the hospital staff, which may generate more deviant behavior. Also, hospital staff may be able to give the patient feedback about deviant behavior more easily than can a traditional healer. Another explanation of the low scores of the patients treated in the hospital might be an initial effect of chlorpromazine.
3. The changes in scores between T1 and T2 of the patients treated in the hospital were smaller than the changes in the scores of the patients treated by traditional or prayer healers. Because the initial values in the two groups were different, however, changes in scores cannot be compared. This difference in score might change the initial difference in scores rather than reflect a difference in treatment efficacy.

DAS RESULTS

The results mentioned here concern the items of self-care, under activity, social withdrawal, participation in household activities, affective and sexual relationships (or heterosexual relationship when the patient is single), social contact outside the household, work performance and efforts to get a job, and interest in and information about the outside world and overall adjustment.

There were improvements in both groups and for all items measured by the DAS:

1. In both groups, the number of patients who had improved was bigger than the number of patients who had deteriorated. This was true for all items.
2. The number of patients with improved overall adjustment scores was the same in both groups.
3. The number of patients who were treated in the hospital and showed improvement was higher in the areas of affective and sexual relationship (or heterosexual relationship), social contact outside the household, and work performance or trying to get a job.

At T1, fewer patients treated by traditional or prayer healers had positive scores on the DAS—i.e., showed less social dysfunctioning—and this concerns all above-mentioned items of the DAS. However, these patients scored higher on the observational items of the PSE (indicating more symptoms) than the patients treated in the hospital.

SOCIAL REINTEGRATION

We can distinguish the following determinants of social reintegration:

- Quality of treatment.
- Community norms and values that may give rise to stigmatization or acceptance of lilalu patients.

- The patient's behavior, which may evoke more permissive or more rejective behavior from the community.

These elements are interdependent, and the last two in particular are inseparable.

The Treatment. In treating a patient, we can distinguish between treating disease and treating illness. Disease, according to Kleinman (1980), refers to a malfunction of biological and/or psychological processes. The term illness has a wider meaning and includes the psychological experience and meaning of the perceived disease. A disease can be cured. Illness requires additional care.

Cure. Traditional healers use herbs to cool down the disease in the body of the patient. The herbs of the traditional healers included in this study did not have a clear sedative effect.

Prayer healers use only prayers to chase away the evil spirits in order to cure the patient.

In the hospital, treatment with neuroleptics had a clear effect on delusions and hallucinations. The patients complained sometimes of being sedated too much and, because of that, were not able to function properly. Other complaints were a dry mouth or hypersalivation.

Care. We can distinguish the following care aspects in treatment:

- Providing daily care, such as food and sanitary care.
- Performing rituals to neutralize underlying causes of disease and to mark transition to the healthy state.
- Evoking trust.

In the daily care of psychotic patients at the traditional healers' compounds it was striking that, if the patients failed to care for themselves, the relatives of the patients were supposed to be responsible. If they did not perform this task, nobody would.

Josephina, a 17-year-old girl diagnosed as having schizoaffective disorder, failed to perform self-care tasks. Her mother took care of her at the traditional healer's. She brought water to wash the girl, dressed her, and brought her food. One day, Josephina's mother went home to check on the other children. When she returned a few days later, she found the girl sitting unwashed, in her own feces and urine.

Patients treated by prayer healers were cared for. Some prayer healers did not like frequent visits by relatives to check on the patients. Because, they explained, "It might be due to their blood [that the patient is sick], and if they talk with the patient, he may get a lot of thoughts when they leave and the disease may increase again."

In the hospital, the daily care of the patients is carried out by nurses and by other patients. Food is supplied by the hospital. The traditional healer may perform rituals during the illness, as well as in a closing ceremony (rite of passage). Usually, the prayer healer only performs the latter ones. Healing rituals move through three separate stages. The sickness is labeled with an appropriate and culturally sanctioned category. The label is then ritually manipulated (culturally transformed). Finally, a new label (e.g., sending away an evil spirit, cured, well) is applied and sanctioned as a meaningful symbolic form that may be independent of behavioral or social change (Kleinman, 1980).

Emmanuel, a 40-year-old man with schizophrenia, disorganized type, was back from prison. His family wanted a ceremony to send away the evil spirits, which were, according to the divination of the traditional healer, still present in Emmanuel. Late in the evening a traditional healer came to perform a ritual. All members of the extended family were present. After Emmanuel sat on a sheep, herbs were given to everyone, and all the family members jumped three times over the sheep. Then, the sheep was killed. The skull of the sheep was stuffed with herbs and was placed over the door to prevent the evil spirits, the emisabwa, from entering anyone of the family again. As extra prevention, the whole compound was sprinkled with a mixture of the sheep's blood and the herbs of the healer.

Traditional healers share with the patient and his relatives their beliefs about the role supernatural forces play in causing diseases, including lilalu. The treatment of a traditional healer is adapted to this way of thinking. This may increase the patient's trust in the treatment (Kleinman, 1977; van der Hart, 1978; Rappaport and Drent, 1979), which is important to making a treatment successful (Nawas et al., 1980). The treatment in the hospital has no link with the concept and experience of disease by the family or the patient.

Often Luhya informants said that lilalu is an "African disease that can only be cured in an African way. It is caused by evil spirits that you cannot see in the blood, so the hospital is unable to cure that disease." Orley (1970) encountered a comparable concept of African diseases among the Baganda in Uganda.

If a patient is ill and treated in the hospital, he expects to be healthy when discharged. He will accept taking medication for about a month afterward, but if he needs to use it for a long time, as is necessary for chronic psychotic patients, then the Luhya conclude that the hospital is not able to cure the disease.

It is important to keep in mind that, according to the beliefs of Luhya, someone is not cured when he uses medication. If someone has suffered from lilalu, it is important to the Luhya to be able to declare the patient cured. If not, relatives and community members will remain fearful that the person is doing something shameful, which they contribute to lilalu, even if under normal circumstances they would consider the same behavior acceptable. Without an official declaration of cure they may also fear that his spirit after death will be particularly harmful.

Interaction of the Community and the Patient. The social consequences of an episode of madness are determined by the behavior of the patient during and after treatment and, by the disease history. The kind of treatment the patient receives has no direct influence on the social consequences of his disease.

An aggressive patient will be approached in a manner different from the way a withdrawn, depressive patient is approached. People will fear a patient if he is aggressive and will not sit in his compound. This also partly isolates the relatives who stay at the same compound. Such a patient cannot participate in community life. At home, he may be tied up occasionally or continuously, depending on his actions. In one case, a verbally aggressive male patient was tied up at home as a preventive measure because he was making threats. Afterward, he said that being tied up made him extremely aggressive.

If a patient is not aggressive, people will not fear him and he will be tolerated. People may give him food, money, or cigarettes. If relatives receive an invitation, for example, to a wedding, the invitation is not meant for the patient. But if he goes, he will not be chased away.

Mothers warn their children not to go near a lilalu patient. Because, as a woman said, "You never know what such a patient may do." Such a warning applies for several months after a patient is cured. If a patient behaves abnormally, it can provoke laughter in others. The behavior is especially shameful if it has a sexual aspect. Because, according to the Luhya, the patient himself does not know what he does, his behavior is more a shame to the family than to the patient. As soon as the patient behaves normally again, the shame for the family is over. However, people may talk about it for a long time.

The aspect of disease history that concerns the community is whether the illness is a first episode or a recurrence. In the case of a recurrence, the community will be cautious about the effect of treatment, which may be only temporary.

A cured patient will not be quickly laughed at because of his previous disease, as the Luhya are afraid that anger will make the disease return. On the other hand, because of his previous disease, a cured patient who wants to speak with the subchief of the baraza, a public meeting place, may be laughed at secretly and not taken seriously by those who disagree with him on a point, irrespective of the sense or value of his words. The same might happen to the patient's relatives, as the husband of a 60-year-old patient suffering from a bipolar disease told me: "When I say something on the baraza and others do not agree with me, they can say that my head is like my wife's. We are not less liked by other people on outside, but inwardly they do not like us because of this disease. "

If a patient has been psychotic when still single, it will be difficult to find a partner, especially in his own area, because people fear a return of the disease. If the disease has been cured for a long time and if it was only one psychotic episode, that person may still find a partner. If lilalu starts during marriage, it may cause a divorce. This happened to four patients in each group in this study.

This study does not show clearly what lilalu means for people with jobs. In the group of patients treated by traditional or prayer healers, there were three employed patients at the start of this psychiatric episode. All three were still ill at the 6-month follow-up. One of them was fired because he did not attend work for a long time. It was not yet clear what would happen to the others.

Three of the four patients treated in the hospital who had jobs at the start of this psychotic episode returned to their original work. One of them, a teacher who held the position of assistant headmaster, asked for a transfer to another school. Although he denied that it had to do with his cured lilalu, he strongly gave that impression. The fourth was a cook who found a job elsewhere.

Two persons treated by traditional healers and three treated in the hospital had lost their jobs during previous psychotic episodes.

Stigma is a mark of shame or disgrace imposed on someone by the community on the basis of the community's norms and values. The word dates back to classical Greece. The Greeks used the term stigma for the brand imprinted on a person to distinguish him socially from others and to differentiate him negatively. Setting a stigmatized individual apart is frequently justified as a rational and practical necessity. More likely, the motives that induce the community to expel the stigmatized individual from normal patterns of intercourse are often indefinable sensations of discomfort, frustration, or fear in the presence of a person who is not the same—i.e., reactions of aversion (Bijleveld, 1978). The Luhya may react this way to aggressive psychotic patients.

Family members try to keep the patient at the compound as much as possible, sometimes by tying him up. This is to guarantee the safety of the patient. In this way, the patient cannot get lost or cause an accident. On the other hand, it also protects the relatives against shameful behavior by the patient in front of the community. The more the patient displays shameful behavior, the longer the community will remember it. A patient who worked in Nairobi and went to his home area for treatment during a psychotic episode told me, "Here in Nairobi, it is quite different from home. People do not know me here and they won't talk about me; but at home everybody knows that I have been suffering from this disease, and almost all people came to check on me. Many more people visited our compound than at other times. Now they are still talking about it and, even after many years, they will still know it . . . . In the old times, it would also have been a problem for my children to get married because I have been suffering from this disease. But, in these days, that won't be a problem anymore."

Explanations of the shamefulness of the diseases make it clear that the Luhya notion of what is shameful has to do with deviation from normality. To modern medicine, this condition is a physical or psychiatric disease, but what counts with the Luhya is the visible abnormality. Any illness that gives the skin a different color or changes the appearance of a limb from a normal appearance may give rise to shame. Any illness that induces behavior that is not normal—

e.g., collapsing in the presence of people or walking naked—is shameful. Suffering from lilalu is shameful to the Luhya.

Following is a brief summary of the reasons why people fear lilalu and why it is considered shameful:

- Lilalu can make a patient roam the countryside and run to unknown places, where he may die.
- Without knowledge of his death, relatives cannot give him a proper burial.
- A patient may injure many people, even attack his mother sexually.
- A mad person may beat an innocent person then relatives of the innocent become angry and may beat the madman to death.
- A man may walk naked, even when his in-laws are present or in the markets.
- A mad person may speak words no one understands.
- Madness separates a patient from his family.
- A madman cannot work or produce food. If people do not give him food to eat, he will die.

Bijleveld (1976 & 1978) studied the stigmatization of leprosy patients among the Luhya. He gave people a list with seven diseases and asked them to list these in order of seriousness. Madness was fourth, after leprosy, tuberculosis/asthma, and epilepsy. They considered venereal disease, emisambwa (possession by potentially harmful spirits), and elephantiasis less serious.

Bijleveld also asked people what treatment they considered most effective for the seven diseases. Of those interviewed, 33% considered madness incurable. Of the other 67%, 42% thought modern treatment most effective and 58% thought traditional treatment was effective. Madness was the disease feared most; 32% of those interviewed feared madness most, and 27% feared epilepsy most. The unpredictability and violence of a madman's actions and the scant hope that his condition can be remedied are the reasons insanity tops the list (Bijlveld, 1976).

The respondents were also asked which disease was the most shameful; madness occupied the fourth place with 15%, after venereal disease, leprosy, and epilepsy.

CONCLUSIONS

The traditional and prayer healers usually consider an evil spirit the cause of psychosis. The herbs used by traditional healers for treatment have no effect on the course of psychosis. They may have some effect on symptoms. Both traditional and prayer healers share their patients' beliefs about diseases. This evokes the patient's trust in the ability of the healer.

In the hospital, neuroleptics are effective in shortening psychoses. The effect of neuroleptics is reduced because the hospital does not address the patient's, relatives', and community's ideas about psychoses. The medical staff of a modern hospital is not used to talking about the cultural aspects of diseases to the patient and his relatives. Nor is the staff of the hospital used to explain the treatment of psychosis or to offer health education to the patient and his relatives in terms of cultural concepts. For these reasons, the patient will not appear for follow-up until he is officially cured. Because of this lack of understanding, the patient does not recognize the importance of taking medicine after the delusions and hallucinations have disappeared.

For the hospital staff, it is important to adapt the explanation of the treatment of the patient's beliefs—e.g., the Luhya know a preventive measure against evil spirits, the so-called hirizi. One kind of hirizi the Luhya use only during treatment by a traditional healer; the other kind they should, according to the advice of the traditional healer, wear their whole lives. In explaining the use of tablets, health care staff could make use of this example by telling the patient that medicines are to cool down the disease but are also a protection, just like the hirizi. As Kleinman (1980) stated, "Failure to heal illness is not articulated in the health professional's system of evaluating the efficacy of healing, but is articulated in patient noncompliance and dissatisfaction, subsequent use of alternative health care facilities, poor and inadequate care and medical-legal suits....What is needed in modern health care system, in developing and developed societies, is systematic recognition and treatment of psychosocial and cultural features of illness. That calls for fundamental reconceptualization of clinical care and restructuring of clinical practice. If appropriately trained, the modern health professional (not necessarily a physician) can effectively and systematically treat both disease and illness;

whereas, in many instances, indigenous healers can neither systematically nor effectively diagnose and treat disease."

REFERENCES

Acuda, S. W.: Presentation of psychiatric illness in East Africa. Postgraduate Doctor (Africa) 4(1):20-23, 1982.

American Psychiatric Association: Diagnostic and Statistical Manual of Mental Disorders, 3rd ed. (DSM-III). Washington, D.C., U.S.A., APA, 1980.

Assen, G. P. M.: Traditional treatment of psychoses; experience among the Luhya in West Kenya. Presented at the Postgraduate Congress in Psychiatry, Moshi, Tanzania, 1983.

Bikleveld, I.: Leprosy and Other Diseases in the Three Wangas: Community Thought Patterns About Health Care and Their Consequences for Emergent Patients. Amsterdam, The Netherlands, Royal Tropical Institute, Department of Social Research.

Bijleveld, I.: Leprosy in the Three Wangas, Kenya: Stigma and Stigma Management. Amsterdam, The Netherlands, 1978, Royal Tropical Institute.

Eniosho, O. A., Bell, N. W.: Mental Health in Africa. Ibadan, Nigeria, Ibadan University Press, 1982.

Field, M. J.: Search for Security: An Ethno-Psychiatric Study of Rural Ghana (1960). New York, U.S.A., W. W. Norton, 1970.

Fuller, E.: What Western psychotherapists can learn from witchdoctors. American Journal of Orthopsychiatry 42:69-76, 1972.

German, G. A.: Aspects of clinical psychiatry in sub-Saharan Africa. British Journal of Psychiatry 121:641-479, 1972. J Psychiatric Symptoms, 2nd ed. Cambridge, England, Cambridge University Press, 1975.

World Health Organization: The Promotion and Development of Traditional Medicine. WHO technical report series no. 622. Geneva, Switzerland, WHO, 1978a.

World Health Organization: Glossary and Guide in International Classification of Diseases, 9th revision (ICD-9). Geneva, Switzerland, WHO 1978b.

World Health Organization: Disability Assessment Schedule, revised version. Geneva, Switzerland, WHO, 1980.

World Health Organization: Traditional Medicine and Health Care Coverage. Geneva, Switzerland, WHO, 1983.

Chapter 4

Acute Psychosis and Rapid Social Change in Swaziland

by

E. A. Guinness, MD, MBBch (Cantab), MRCPsych,
Swaziland Mental Health Services
Swaziland 1982-1987

ABSTRACT

The nature and precipitants of acute reactive psychosis in Swaziland are explored. Of 101 patients studied, 75% had underlying anxiety or depression; their psychoses were culturally prescribed reactions to acute-on-chronic stress. In many cases, a hysterical dissociative state seemed to be the mechanism. However, acute reactive psychosis is related to schizophrenia in that it can recur or become more prolonged if the stresses persist. Occasionally it heralds the onset of chronic schizophrenia.

A population group at risk for acute reactive psychosis—anxious secondary school students—was further explored in a field study. Students are affected by several aspects of the transition from traditional life-styles to Western industrialization: the change from peasant status to a cash economy (represented by the financial investment in the student), the breakdown in extended family support systems, and dissonance between traditional beliefs and Western cultural influences.

The author draws parallels between the hysterical psychosis described by Freud and Charcot in the nineteenth century and acute transient psychosis in Africa. This phenomenon may be seen as part of the evolution of psychiatric symptoms during a period of rapid social change. Case studies are presented for illustration.

INTRODUCTION

Acute psychosis is a distinctive feature of African psychiatry. Diagnosing and classifying it according to Western criteria has been difficult. In hospital practice, up to half of the patients admitted each year have acute psychosis. If the large number of cases due to organic causes, alcohol, and epilepsy are excluded, what is the nature of the remaining disorder?

- Is it a form of atypical schizophrenia with a good prognosis?
- Is it a culture-bound stress reaction?
- Is it a new phenomenon related to the rapid social change?
- Why is it so prevalent in Africa?
- Has it ever been prevalent elsewhere in the world?

Until recently, most of the work on acute transient psychosis in Africa has been purely descriptive.

French psychiatry has developed the concept of bouffe´e de´lirante. This syndrome has a sudden onset, often is related to stress, and lasts from 3 days to 3 weeks. It is characterized by marked psychomotor agitation, delusions of influence of strong cultural or magicoreligious content, visual and auditory hallucinations, transient thought disorders and some degree of confusion, and inaccessibility followed by complete recovery and often amnesia or denial of the illness. Prodromal restlessness, anxiety, depression, sleep disturbance, and self-neglect are often detected.

British colonial psychiatrists wrote of transient insanity akin to acute mania. Carothers (1947) described a twilight state lasting a few hours or a few weeks and characterized by panic, emotional lability, and psychomotor over activity often leading to violence to self or others. This state remitted spontaneously but occasionally left a Ganser syndrome or other hysterical features. Repeat attacks were related to recurrence of stress.

Other workers attempted classification. Smartt (1964), in what was then Rhodesia, offered a clinical classification into simple delirium, confusion with schizophreniform features, manic confusion, and depressive confusion.The latter three are similar to the ICD-9 category 298.

Jakovljevic (1964) suggested a division into impulsive and fugue types of reactive psychosis, corresponding to the fight-or-flight reaction. The impulsive type was a pathological aggression precipitated by stress, and the fugue type was a frenzied escape into the bush in response to delusions of possession.

In West Africa, Field (1962) gave an account of fear psychosis in response to terrifying cultural beliefs in bewitchment. This would remit in a week at traditional healing shrines, although a few cases might slip into unequivocal schizophrenia a few months later.

Lambo (1962) in Nigeria proposed a psychotic-psychoneurotic symptom complex characterized by frenzied anxiety, short-lived psychotic confusion, automatism, and absences. He suggested that these states may occur as part of schizophrenia or may have a hysterical, epileptic, or migrainous etiology. He emphasizes the importance of cultural precipitates. In his view, this malignant anxiety is more frequently seen in marginal Africans, who are in the process of renouncing their age-old culture and have failed to assimilate the new. This suggests the effects of rapid social change.

German (1972), in Uganda, stressed the importance of toxic and infective agents, marginal nutritional states, and previous cerebral insults.He indicated that malnutrition at critical stages of development of the young child may leave deficits in the higher centers of the brain. Being phylogenetically younger, these are more vulnerable to such nutritional injury. The result is a tendency to heightened emotionality. He cited nutritional experiments on pigs and rats that had this effect.The importance of the organic component is undeniable. Alcohol, herbal drugs (including cannabis), and delirious states related to infection and parasitemia are all contributing causes. One must distinguish phenomena related to epilepsy, not only the postepileptic confusional state so common in uncontrolled epilepsy but also temporal lobe epilepsy. This is much more common in Africa than in the West. It can mimic acute transient psychosis and must be distinguished, through careful history taking, by its episodic course unrelated to stress.

To what extent do these common, recurrent biological factors—i.e., the greater physical morbidity of an impoverished tropical environment—alter the biological substrate and predispose it to psychotic reactions to stress? This is an unexplored area. Prevailing Western opinion is that transient reactive psychosis is a form of schizophrenia with good prognosis. However, psychiatrists in Africa, confronted with this dilemma daily, see at least some acute psychosis as distinct from schizophrenia and primarily a culturally prescribed reaction to stress. The above review indicates the importance of hysterical features and the pathogenic effect of cultural transition.

With the development of more precise diagnostic instruments, such as the Present State Examination (PSE) and more refined methodology, as in the World Health Organization's International Pilot Study of Schizophrenia, it is now possible to explore the nature of acute transient psychosis in Africa and define its relationship to schizophrenia.

German has suggested a useful subdivision of schizophrenia in Africa for research purposes. He suggested that unequivocal nuclear process schizophrenia satisfying diagnostic criteria be regarded as idiopathic schizophrenia of as yet unknown etiology. Schizophrenia-like syndromes associated with identifiable organic, epileptic, affective, or psychogenic factors should be known as symptomatic schizophrenia. The latter would include acute transient psychosis. He stressed that, as investigating techniques become more available, more apparent idiopathic schizophrenia would have to be redefined as symptomatic.

SYMPTOMATIC SCHIZOPHRENIA

The affective and psychogenic types of symptomatic schizophrenia are the subjects of this study. Its purpose is to explore the clinical, psychosocial, and demographic features of acute reactive psychosis and comment on the nature of the syndrome and its relationship with other syndromes; indicate a relationship between rapid social change and a prevalent anxiety state, which can become complicated and develop into acute reactive psychosis; and consider the historical perspective of acute psychosis.

Swaziland is appropriate for such a study because the sociocultural issues are relatively simple. It is a small country of one tribe and has retained much of its traditional culture, yet it is undergoing the industrialization and urbanization similar to that elsewhere in Africa. It lacks the massive conurbations that complicate the issue. Much of its population is in the first generation to be exposed to education.

Figure 1
DISTRIBUTION OF DIAGNOSES AMONG 650 ANNUAL HOSPITAL ADMISSIONS IN SWAZILAND

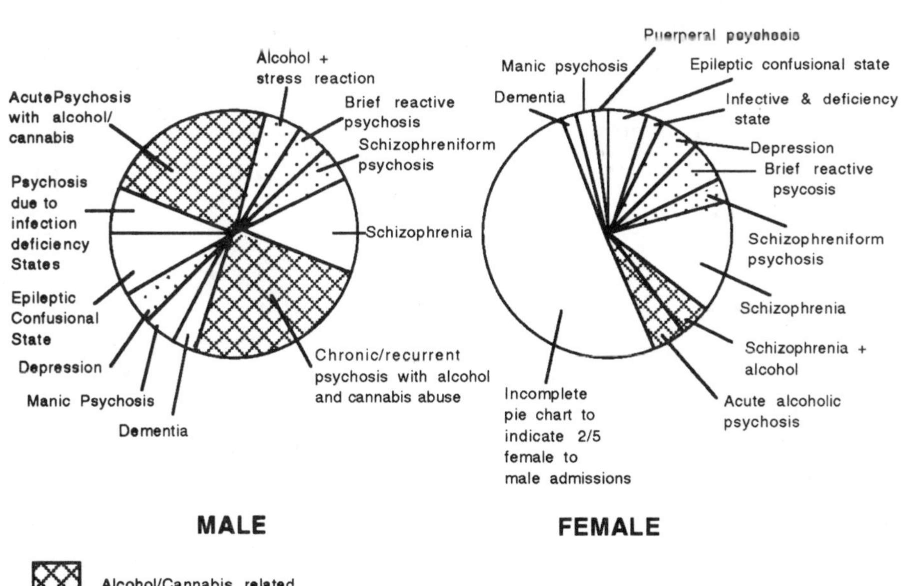

METHOD I

The cases selected for study were equivalent to those defined by DMS-III as brief reactive psychosis—i.e., as having a clear relation to stress and onset within 2 weeks. All possible organic causes were excluded. The group selected is shown in Figure 1, a pie chart of annual hospital admissions.

Over two and one-half years, between 1984 and 1986, 101 cases were collected. Psychiatric histories were taken from the relatives by psychiatric nurses, who then acted as translators for the psychiatrist during clinical examination. Very few investigative facilities were available. Organic or epileptic factors had to be defined on clinical grounds alone--e.g., a history of alcohol or cannabis abuse was based on the relatives' history.

It was essentially a descriptive and qualitative study in the context of a developing African country with typical limitation of resources. Use of precise diagnostic instruments was not feasible.

The cases selected for the study involved brief reactive psychosis. Nearly all of the 650 annual admissions were for psychosis, and half the cases were acute. Many had organic components, however, especially among men; 10% had postepileptic confusion, 2% were in infective or deficiency states, and 35% had disorders related to alcohol or cannabis abuse. Many men had to be excluded from this study because of the contribution of alcohol or cannabis to a stress reaction.

RESULTS I

Of the 101 patients with brief reactive psychosis, 50 were male and 51 were female. The age distribution reflected the predominance of young people in the population: 66 patients were young adults, 27 were adolescents, and eight were over 40 years of age.

The phenomena of brief reactive psychosis are variable (see illustrative case histories). A symptom pattern emerged that was similar to Smartt's classification of psychoses as manic, depressive, and schizophreniform confusional states. It can best be classified according to ICD-9 category 298, as shown in Table I. Men were more likely to show the manic type.

Table I
SYMPTOMATIC TYPES OF REACTIVE PSYCHOSIS IN 101 CASES IN SWAZILAND

ICD-9 CODE	MALE	FEMALE
298.0 - Depressive	4	5
298.1 - Excitative	16	8
298.2 - Reactive confusion	28	30
Hysterical dissociative state	2	8

Table II
SYMPTOM PROFILE OF BRIEF REACTIVE PSYCHOSIS IN 101 CASES IN SWAZILAND

TYPE OF SYMPTOM	NUMBER OF CASES
Hallucinations	
Visual (often animal spirits)	70
Auditory (often ancestral voices)	65
Delusions	
Overvalued cultural beliefs	24
Paranoid delusions	10
Depressive delusions	9
Ideas of influence (modern, e.g., TV, radio, electricity)	9
Grandiose delusions	7
Speech	
Incoherent shouting	52
Flight of ideas	17
Mutism	9
Behavior	
Aggression	44
Bizarre behavior, running away, stripping off clothes	42
Mood	
Excitement, restlessness	52
Panic, fear	17
Agitated depression, suicidal thinking	12

Table II shows the symptom profile. The overall picture is of sudden onset of restlessness and excitement with fleeting, changeable visual and auditory hallucinations and delusions that have a strong cultural context—e.g., the patient sees animal spirits sent by a bewitcher or hears ancestral voices. Speech may be pressured, a flight of ideas. More often it pours forth in an incoherent stream. Sometimes repetitive shouting leads to exhaustion, and the patient becomes unreachable. The patient's overall behavior is characterized by either flight or fight; he either becomes aggressive and destructive or runs away and strips off his clothes. Mood becomes volatile rather than flat.

Table III shows the duration of psychosis. Most cases resolved in 2 weeks or less.

Table III

DURATION OF PSYCHOSIS IN 101 CASES OF BRIEF REACTIVE PSYCHOSIS IN SWAZILAND

DURATION	PERCENT OF CASES
Hours	12
Days	33
2 weeks	3
3 weeks	13
4 weeks	10
6 weeks	1

The patients tended to relapse if the stresses were repeated or prolonged—e.g., if the patient ran away and returned home or if the relatives brought bad news (see Case 8). This longer, intermittent course might suggest underlying schizophrenia.

In 12% of the cases, the psychotic experience lasted only a few hours and occurred in direct response to stress—e.g., exams faced by anxious students. These would seem to be hysterical dissociative states yet were similar in form to the typical reactive psychosis, although milder. Some patients experienced both (Case 6).

Table IV presents the numbers of previous episodes in these

patients. The only indication of prognosis was readmission to the hospital. Over half the patients had no previous episodes. Of 42 with previous episodes, 20 had relapsed within the two and one-half year period. Five showed a pattern of recurrent brief psychosis in response to stress. These were depressed women with personality disorders who had very difficult home situations. Five patients had initial typical but brief psychotic stress reactions, followed by unequivocal schizophrenia within a year (see Cases 10 and 11). Hospital statistics suggest that about 10% of the cases of schizophrenia initially appear as brief reactive psychosis.

Table IV

NUMBER OF PREVIOUS PSYCHOTIC EPISODES IN 101 PATIENTS WITH BRIEF REACTIVE PSYCHOSIS IN SWAZILAND

EPISODE/COURSE	CASES
Number of previous episodes	
None	58%
One	20%
Two	8%
Three	5%
Illness Pattern	
Brief recurrence; depression	5 cases
First episode; brief reactive psychosis heralding schizophrenia	5 cases

Only 25% of the cases appeared to be pure stress reactions; 52% had been preceded by depression, and 24% were preceded by anxiety. Depression is not recognized by the community as an illness. The withdrawn, retarded depressive person attracts little attention. Thus, a common presentation of depression to the hospital is brief psychosis, which clears in a few days, revealing the underlying depression. Such psychosis seems to be a form of culturally sanctioned illness behavior that secures attention. It is typically seen in low-status groups, such as women, and adolescents. Yet the depressed patient's reactive psychosis is usually accompanied not by depressive phenomena (ICD-9 category 298.0) but by manic or schizophreniform confusion (category 298.1 or 298.2).

The 24 patients in whom anxiety had preceded the psychosis were nearly all students suffering from school anxiety, or the brain fag syndrome.

Table V shows the precipitating psychosocial stresses. Fifty percent of the patients had financial problems, often in addition to others. These patients included the only educated member of an extended family, a migrant laborer returning from the mines to find his remittance misused, a student harassed for school fees, and an unsupported mother struggling to rear many children with a negligent husband.

In 36%, fears or accusations of bewitchment or over involvement in religious rituals was the stress. The syncretic Zionist sects are particularly prone to this. When the early missionaries banned the witch doctor without realizing the multiple roles he played, a vacuum was created. This was filled by the numerous syncretic Christian sects. They represent the need of Christians for the expression of cultural beliefs. Their services are often intensely arousing and combine traditional and Christian rituals.

Table V
PSYCHOSOCIAL STRESSES ASSOCIATED WITH 101 CASES OF BRIEF REACTIVE PSYCHOSIS IN SWAZILAND

PSYCHOSOCIAL STRESSES	PERCENT OF CASES
Financial stress	50
Fear of bewitchment or religious over involvement	36
Examinations	29
Marital stress	28
Job stress	23
Family disputes	20
Alcoholism in family	10
Death or illness in family	10
Refugee status	5

The high proportion of patients whose school exams were the precipitating stress demonstrates the importance of education as a new and disturbing factor in the culture.

Marital problems were a major stress for 28% and included a husband's desertion and a delay in marriage settlement (payment of bride price).

Table VI shows demographic factors. The patients' socioeconomic status and education were compared with those of their parents. A difference between the generations in these respects might indicate that social change was contributing to acute psychosis.

Table VI

COMPARISON OF PARENTAL AND PATIENT SOCIOECONOMIC STATUS AND EDUCATION IN 101 CASES OF BRIEF REACTIVE PSYCHOSIS IN SWAZILAND

Socioeconomic status		
Peasant	67	46
Artisan	20	18
Professional	7	6
Student	---	27
Education level reached		
No schooling	58	12
Primary plus	34	42
Secondary	--	47

The proportions of peasants and artisans (miners, drivers, police, clerks) and professionals (teachers, nurses, administrators) were similar in spite of a considerable difference in education.

The proportion of parents without education (58%) is similar to the national average for that age group (55%) (1976 census), whereas the proportion of the patient group with secondary education (47%) is significantly higher than the national average for the younger age group (21%).

Secondary education is definitely a stress factor and does not necessarily lead to rise in social status. Studies based on hospital admissions in Africa are known to be misleading, but resources for community surveys are limited.

A particular population group—i.e., anxious students in secondary education—was selected for a field study to further explore the significance of the psychosocial factors outlined above. Since an association had been found between brief reactive psychosis, anxiety in students, and the stress of secondary education, it seemed relevant to attempt a field survey of this group. Moreover, school populations are a captive audience, which makes limited epidemiological studies feasible.

SCHOOL ANXIETY (BRAIN FAG SYNDROME)

The underlying anxiety state found in students with brief reactive psychosis was, in fact, the brain fag syndrome, originally described by Prince in Nigeria (1962). It was later found to be common in East Africa (German, 1986; Minde, 1974) and is also well recognized in southern Africa. It is much more common in Africa than elsewhere in the world. Significantly, it has recently been reported as prevalent in New Guinea, which is also undergoing rapid social change from traditional tribal lifestyles to twentieth century industrialization.

School anxiety is a form of somatized anxiety and has hysterical features. There are headaches, eye pain, watering or blurring of the eyes unrelated to optical problems, poor concentration, inability to stay awake in class, irritability and fatigue, and various abdominal and chest pains.

Morakinyo (1980) in Nigeria demonstrated that the syndrome is not related to intelligence but that a high neuroticism score is common. It usually occurs in adolescent students but can develop in any group when financial and social advancement of the extended family is contingent on the academic success of the individual. Minde (1974) in Uganda indicated the importance of the generation gap between parents and students and the over expectations about education. It is hypothesized that school anxiety is a widespread, low-grade stress syndrome associated with the dislocating effect of Western education on traditional life styles.

The prevalence and complex sociological etiology of school anxiety was explored in a school survey in Swaziland. Possible psychiatric sequelae, including brief reactive psychosis, were demonstrated.

METHOD II

The syndrome of school anxiety as it occurs in Swaziland was defined by means of a collection of cases from district clinics between 1982 and 1984. Ninety cases were examined. Half of the subjects were still at school, and half had histories of school anxiety and presented with further psychiatric morbidity within a year of leaving school.

Common psychosocial stresses were identified. On the basis of these findings, a self-report fact-finding questionnaire was designed and administered by psychiatric nurses to 1,200 students in nine secondary schools in May 1984. A cross-section of schools was chosen to include rural, urban, and elite schools. The questionnaire elicited symptoms by the simple open-ended question, "Do you have any problems with your health at school?" Any of the previously identified symptoms was regarded as a positive response. However, to detect the syndrome more accurately, two groups of students were defined: those who volunteered one symptom and those with two or more.

The questionnaire went on to inquire about family composition, early rearing, parental occupation, parental attitude to schooling, any problems with school fees, any fears of jealousy or bewitchment, and so on. It was important to define family breakdown, but to do this in an extended family context was difficult.. Finally, family instability was defined as "father dead, deserted, or unknown," "mother with more than two extramarital children," or "child reared by stepmother." Assessment of academic performance was based on class position and teachers' reports.

From the questionnaires, the prevalence of school anxiety in each school was estimated as the percentage of the class admitting to symptoms. The anxious group was then compared to the healthy group using chi-square tests on the various psychosocial and demographic factors.

RESULTS II

Table VI, the symptom profile of school anxiety in Swaziland, shows it to be very similar to that reported elsewhere in Africa. The somatic and cognitive aspects of anxiety are prominent. There are also definite hysterical features. These include tendencies toward stress-related hysterical fits that do not respond to phenobarbital, epidemic hysteria, and spasm of the hands, which prevents writing at exams.

The most common hysterical features are the eye-related complaints of pain, watering, and blurring of vision, which do not in most students seem to be related to optical problems. The secondary gain from these symptoms is clear. The family is convinced that the student is bewitched or ill. When the burden of education becomes intolerable, the symptoms excuse him from study and earn sympathy rather than scolding from the family.

Table VII

SYMPTOM PATTERN OF BRAIN FAG SYNDROME IN STUDENTS IN SWAZILAND SECONDARY SCHOOLS

SYMPTOM	PERCENT OF CASES
Headache or crawling feelings in scalp	70.0
Sore eyes, lack of vision, blurred or clouded vision, inability to see blackboard, twisting of printed figures	41.0
Poor concentration, inability to learn, mind goes blank	29.0
Falling asleep in class	21.0
Fear, nervousness, irritability, "thinking too much"	15.0
Constant fatigue	10.0
Fainting, dizziness	6.0
Abdominal or chest pain	6.0
Premonition of bad news, weeping, sinking heart	5.0
Palpitations, shaking hands	5.0
Poor appetite	2.5
Nosebleeds	2.5

Leaving school creates particular vulnerability. Anxious students can develop acute psychosis at exams, become depressed because of school or job failure, or develop various anxiety symptoms related to job or marriage. Forty-five cases were studied, and the results are shown in Table VIII.

Table VIII
SEQUELAE OF SCHOOL ANXIETY DEVELOPED BY 45 SWAZILAND STUDENTS LEAVING SCHOOL

SEQUELA	NUMBER OF CASES		
Syndrome	**Male**	**Female**	**Total**
Anxiety states, panic attacks, hysterical fits (ICD-9 300.0)	9	9	18
Depression (ICD-9 300.4)	5	4	9
Acute transient psychosis (ICD-9 298.0)	11	7	18

The prevalence of school anxiety was 70-80% in rural schools, 60-70% in urban schools, and only 20% in schools patronized by the professional elite. This represents students admitting to at least one symptom. The two-symptom prevalence were lower but of the same profile. The pattern of psychosocial factors did not, however, significantly differentiate the two groups. This prevalence is similar to that found by Prince in Nigeria (1962).

Figure 2 shows the relationship between school anxiety, location, and parental status. The correlation with parental status indicates that students from peasant homes are more at risk for anxiety than those from professional homes. This factor is multifactorial, of course. Poverty and peasant status can produce biological disadvantage in terms of malnutrition and physical morbidity. Rural schools are often poor, with high teacher turnover, etc. These factors would produce lower academic performance, but why anxiety? It relates to the urgent demand for and high expectations of education in the population. Education holds a very important place in the community.

Figure 2

RELATIONSHIP BETWEEN SCHOOL ANXIETY, PATRONAGE OF SCHOOL, AND PARENTAL STATUS FOR 1,200 STUDENTS IN NINE SWAZILAND SECONDARY SCHOOLS

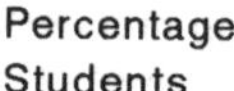

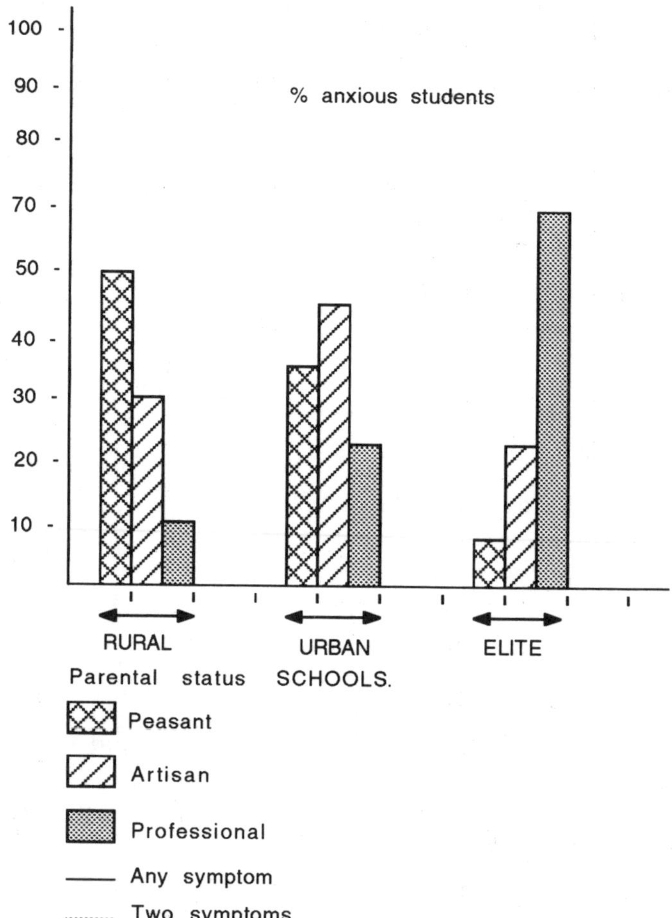

Academic achievement—passing exams and winning certificates—is seen to open all doors, to be the key to good jobs, to be the way to escape from the stagnation of the rural areas. Families invest money and hope in educating their children. As soon as they have completed school, students must start earning and contributing to family finances. Indeed, in large families, younger children cannot start school until older ones start earning. There is much jealousy of those who have educational opportunities and success.

Children from professional homes enjoy an education similar to that of their parents, have fewer problems with school fees, and are envied less by relatives who would like to have similar opportunities. In contrast, the first generation in a peasant family receiving an education is in a particularly vulnerable position. Offspring grow up into a lifestyle different from that of the traditional subsistence farmer, to whom the whole cultural ethos is geared. Their parents may have many misconceptions about this process and cannot guide them. Cultural beliefs that provided a working explanation of threatening stresses are no longer appropriate. Time-honored customs for guiding adolescents are discarded in favor of schooling.

An example is the way a rural community handles epidemic hysteria in its schools. The high level of anxiety in schools, particularly at exam time, provides ideal conditions for epidemic hysteria. It is most common among girls, who start screaming, running around, seeing visions, and hearing voices. It is regarded as a peculiarly African disease (umhayizo) and is attributed to bewitchment of the girls by a man who desires them. A boy in the school is then identified as the bewitcher and expelled.

An opportunity arose for me to examine the girls in such an epidemic (Dhadphale, 1983). Four out of five had been suffering from typical school anxiety and had many problems at home—such as strife, jealousy, or alcoholism—and great fear of exams. Their parents could not understand why they should have any problems since they were enjoying the coveted and expensive advantages of schooling. The parents' cultural beliefs had made good psychological sense in the past, when the chief preoccupation of adolescent girls was their relationship with boys, but was no longer appropriate when the girls were struggling with the demands of an alien education system.

Several of the key psychosocial factors listed in TABLE VIII proved to be highly significant in the survey of schools.

Table VIII

SIGNIFICANCE OF PSYCHOSOCIAL VARIABLES IN RELATION TO SCHOOL ANXIETY IN 1,200 STUDENTS IN NINE SWAZILAND SECONDARY SCHOOLS

	SIGNIFICANCE ON CHI-SQUARE TEST (healthy group, N = 548)	
PSYCHOSOCIAL VARIABLES	One-Symptom Group, N = 441	Two-Symptom Group, N = 245
Family instability	$p<0.0005$	$p<0.0005$
Threat to school fees	$p<0.0005$	$p<0.0005$
Fear of jealousy and bewitchment	$p<0.0005$	$p<0.0005$
Academic ability		
Good	$p<0.025$	$p<0.025$
Bad	$p<0.025$	n.s.
Parental anger at failure	$p<0.025$	n.s.

"Threat to school fees" represents the financial investment in the student, which he must justify. "Family instability" indicates that children reared by a single parent or by stepparents are at risk, despite the valuable effect of the extended family in mitigating parental failure. Fear of jealousy and bewitchment is a potent factor. Jealousy generates anxiety, for instance, in the child of a jealous stepmother who resents her husband's paying fees for another woman's child. Successful students are often suspected of using bewitchment to obtain success. Indeed, the intensity of anxiety at exam time may undermine the validity of exams as a means of assessment. Students obtain spells and muti to ensure that they pass and others fail. Some become so terrified that a brief psychotic reaction supervenes.

Academic ability, although only estimated approximately, was not highly significant. This confirms other workers' findings. Indeed, the more able student is slightly more at risk for anxiety. Parental anger about failure was apparently not significant.

In Table IX, the significance of parental status is demonstrated again, showing no difference between peasant and artisan status but a highly significant difference between professional and either peasant or artisan status.

Table IX

SIGNIFICANCE OF DEMOGRAPHIC VARIABLES IN RELATION TO SCHOOL ANXIETY IN 1,200 STUDENTS IN NINE SWAZILAND SECONDARY SCHOOLS

DEMOGRAPHIC VARIABLES	SIGNIFICANCE ON CHI-SQUARE TEST (healthy group, N = 548) One-Symptom Group, N = 441	Two-Symptom Group, N = 245
Parental status ratio		
Peasant: professional	p<0.0005	p<0.0005
Peasant: artisan	n.s.	n.s.
Artisan: professional	p<0.0005	p<0.0005
Preschool rearing by grandmother	p<0.0005	p<0.0005
Father absent due to migrant labor	p<0.0005	p<0.0005

The factor "preschool rearing by grandmother" was also highly significant. This does not necessarily mean that being reared by a grandmother is predictive of anxiety. It reflects the custom of sending preschool children to the rural areas while the parents and older children remain in town at work or at school. In the past, grandmothers had a valuable place in training the girls of the family, but they were not left alone to do all the heavy farm work as well. This present situation is an example of the overstrained resources of the extended family. Many children are born out of marriage and are sent home to the grandmother to rear. Such overburdened old women cannot feed, train, protect, and immunize so many young children.

The father's absence due to his migrant labor is also weakening the extended family, removing parental influence, damaging marriages, and creating illegitimate children.

Adolescents from extended families belonging to a group-oriented culture contend with the demands of a Western, examination-based educational system, where individual achievement is necessary and lessons are conducted in a foreign language. This educational system, introduced by British colonials, was originally designed to produce candidates for the professions in the nineteenth century. It was most democratic, and it enabled a peasant's son to rise to the heights of the professions or academic achievement. But imagine the stresses involved in such a change of life style between father and son, the jealousy incurred, the frustration and disappointment of the many compared with the success of the few. The defense mechanisms of the cultural belief system become distorted. Moreover, the student is not simply striving for his own personal benefit. His whole extended family has invested money and hope in him. At the same time, the cohesion of the extended family is being eroded by the effects of rapid social change on family ties and marriage.

DISCUSSION

Transient reactive psychosis in Africa is probably a composite syndrome best considered in relation to other syndromes rather than as a single entity. This can be shown by a Venn diagram (see Figure 5). Many cases (75%) are associated with preexisting anxiety or depression. Further stress precipitates the acute psychosis, which seems to be a reaction to acute-on-chronic stress, a culturally acceptable form of illness behavior that takes the form of extreme affective disinhibition approaching psychotic dimensions. Prognosis is good, although the psychosis can recur if the stress is repeated or prolonged.

Another group of patients seem to show a hysterical dissociative state. Further study of the underlying anxiety supports this. The low-grade stress syndrome, related to the stresses of education in Africa, has definite features of hysterical conversion and dissociation. These features are the non-optical difficulties in vision, spasm of the hands, hysterical fits, and epidemic hysteria. If the stresses on the student were to increase suddenly, it is understandable that a state of hysterical dissociation might supervene and, given the auto-suggestibility of the hysterical state, might take a culturally prescribed course.

Here is an example. A person under sudden stress will suspect that he is bewitched; he might experience visual and auditory hallucinations that take the form of the evil spirits he dreads or the ancestral displeasure he fears he has incurred. The frequency of genuine toxic confusional states in the community lends credence to this. The visual hallucinations, especially of alcoholic confusional states, are taken as evidence of the evil spirits. Believing himself possessed and controlled, he experiences mounting terror, and his bizarre and aggressive behavior results in a state of frenzied excitement.

This form of psychosis may represent the ultimate defense mechanisms—discrete brief ego disruption followed by amnesia and denial. But is it truly psychotic?

In any case, the distinction between it and schizophrenia is not clear-cut. In some cases, typical belief reactive psychosis can herald the onset of nuclear schizophrenia. Moreover, there seems to be a gradation between brief reactive psychosis and schizophreniform psychosis in terms of speed of recovery, but there is very little difference in phenomena.

African transient psychosis has been compared to the concept of hysterical psychosis of nineteenth century Europe. Although the concept has been discarded, many psychiatrists in Africa have felt the need for such a category. Smartt (1956), Carothers (1951), and Lambo (1965) all suggested a hysterical etiology. Hollender and Hirsch (1964), in New Guinea, a comparable environment, observed hysterical psychosis, and they described it as a form of ego disruption marked by sudden and dramatic onset, temporarily related to a profoundly upsetting event. Its manifestations include hallucinations, delusions, depersonalizations, and grossly unusual behavior. Thought disorders, when they occur, are sharply circumscribed and very transient.

Affectivity, if altered, is changed in the direction of volatility, not flatness. The acute episode seldom lasts longer than three weeks and the eruption is sealed off so that there is practically no residue.

This could stand as a general phenomenological definition of brief reactive psychosis. Hollender and Hirsch identified three processes that may produce the clinical picture of hysterical psychosis. The processes are culturally sanctioned behavior, appropriation of psychotic behavior in conversion and dissociation reactions, true psychosis.

This reflects the complex picture described in this study. Of relevance to the question of the validity of hysterical psychosis is Leff's concept of the evolution of psychiatric symptoms in parallel with linguistic sophistication (Leff, 1981). He traced the decline in hysteria in Europe from the nineteenth century, when it was a major form of mental illness, through two world wars, between which the ratio of hysteria to anxiety became reversed, to the virtual disappearance of hysteria in postwar Britain.

Leff related this change to two factors. As the oral tradition of earlier cultures becomes replaced by the literary tradition of modern civilization, hysterical manifestations of distress are replaced by more overtly psychological symptoms. People verbalize their psychological suffering rather than somaticizing it. The second factor is the change in family structure from the extended to nuclear family, from group to individual orientation. In the former, relationships are determined by role and status rather than by choice and emotion. As kin behavior becomes more permissive, relationships are explored and evaluated, emotions become refined, and the language for expressing them develops. With this develops the patient's concept of disorders treatable by doctors. There is no longer the need for hysterical stress reactions.

In brief, reactive psychosis is a culture-bound hysterical psychosis superimposed on a dysthymic state. One is tempted to look for its equivalent in the West. What happens to an anxious adolescent who suffers a sudden stressful life event, the equivalent of an anxious student in Africa who becomes briefly psychotic after exams? His Western counterpart would probably make a parasuicidal attempt. Interestingly, one patient in this study, in Case 7, did just this. He presented with brief psychosis at exams one year, and the next year he took on overdose of the chlorpromazine with which we had conveniently supplied him. He subsequently responded to antidepressants. The psychosis was irrelevant; depression was the essential problem.

In Zululand, Wessels (1982) showed that hysterical manifestations are more common among rural, traditional people than among urban. He also showed that belief in witchcraft is associated with hysterical phenomena. A person in distress presents what he thinks is acceptable to the doctor. These brief hysterical psychoses are eminently acceptable and treatable by African traditional healers.

Wessels has worked clinically with Zulu healers and correlated their classification of mental illness with Western diagnostic categories. They recognize the major functional psychoses, epilepsy, and mental retardation as distinct entities. The brief reactive psychoses they regard as peculiarly African diseases requiring traditional treatment. Wessels considered them culture-bound hysterical psychoses, preferably treated by healers rather than with powerful neuroleptics.

Zulu healers consider these disorders to be new in this century, particularly since the advent of the mines, where they occurred in epidemics in the 1920s. The cause is attributed by the healers to spirit possession or bewitchment by invading tribes or to the influence of alien spirits of other racial groups.This could be interpreted as a cultural expression of the impact of industrialization and urbanization on traditional people.

Other workers have noticed the increase in acute psychosis in Africa during this century. The Mayers, anthropologist/psychiatrist couple, worked among the Tallensi, a tribe in Northern Ghana, in the 1930s and again in the 1960s. They noticed an increase in psychosis, which they attributed to cultural change. Ammar (1964) commented on an apparent increase in pseudoschizophrenic reactions during the sociocultural upheavals in Tunisia after independence.

In this study an attempt was made to show a relationship between brief reactive psychosis and acculturative stress by means of a field study of the underlying anxiety state. Adolescents in secondary education are at the interface of two cultures. They suffer a form of somatic anxiety with hysterical features in which brief reactive psychosis can occur if the stresses are exacerbated. The psychosocial precipitants found to be highly significant were those related to the traditional African culture under stress:

- The change from peasant status to cash economy, represented by the financial investment in the student.

- The wide difference in world view and ethnic stance between school and home.
- The breakdown of extended family support systems—45% of the anxious students came from unstable homes, compared with 23% of the healthy students.

These observations suggest that these psychoses may not only be due to the pathoplastic effect of culture but also to the pathogenic effect of cultural change. If acute psychosis is a relatively new phenomenon in Africa and if it is increasing and is related to rapid social change, it is important to look elsewhere for similar conditions.

Psychosis must be viewed from a historical perspective. Consider the nineteenth century literature. The plethora of psychoses confronting nineteenth-century psychiatrists seem to be more reminiscent of modern African than modern Western psychiatry. In Vienna, Meynert (1889) described psychotic confusional states with frenzied anxiety void of delusions and a good prognosis, which he called transient amentia. This term is derived from the Hippocratic description amnesia cum tristi spirito, or amnesia with a sad spirit. Meynert separated etiology into psychogenic, nutritional, and epileptic and resulting from intoxication or infection. How reminiscent of the current African debate! Stransky (1904) differentiated hallucinatory confusion with good outcome, amentia, from what he called the affective dementia and intrapsychic ataxia of dementia praecox. Later, in 1907, he commented on the apparent decrease in amentia due, he thought, to change in either medical care or ethnic structure of the population.

Several other great nineteenth century psychiatrists wrote of the hysterical nature of acute transient psychosis. Some were: Morel (1860), Folie hysterique; Charcot (1892), Delire hysterique; Kraepelin (1983), Hysterisches Irresin; Freud (1895), Hysterisches Psychosen.

Later this concept was discarded in favor of Kraepelin's dementia praecox. Was this because it was not valid or because as a clinical entity it had ceased to be important by the early twentieth century, when the concept of nuclear-process schizophrenia was being developed?

However, such brief reactive psychosis has not entirely disappeared in Europe. Among isolated rural groups living relatively primitively, tradition-directed life styles involving acute hallucinatory states with frenzied excitement and delusions of bewitchment have been described. Risso and Baker (1964) described this state among migratory Italian workers in Switzerland. These brief psychotic states had a good prognosis and were associated with magical archaic thinking.

At the time hysterical psychosis was being described in nineteenth century Europe, the conditions were comparable in many ways with those in modern Africa. There was a high level of physical morbidity, infections, disease, malnutrition, alcoholism, and poverty. People were uneducated and superstitious. In the wake of the Industrial Revolution, rapid social change was taking place, from a traditional agricultural economy to urbanization and industrialization, with a concomitant breakup of extended family support systems. For instance, the large number of illegitimate children, orphans, abandoned children, and homeless children living in the gutters so reminiscent of nineteenth century London, the London of Dickens and Barnado is now becoming a new feature of African society. It was the age of the great orphanages, which is, of course, a measure of family failure.

Quantitative measures of the complex social conditions of those days are, of course, hard to find in retrospect. Alcohol is indirectly related to the present discussion in that it increases the vulnerability of the biological substrate to psychosis. It certainly is a major factor in African mental hospitals today.

The information contained in Figure 4 below was taken from customs and excise statistics (Royal College of Psychiatrists Special Committee, 1979). It indicates that alcohol consumption per capita was much higher in Great Britain at the turn of the century than in 1975. It was also higher than in any modern European country. Howarth has made an approximate projectional estimate of a vulnerable population group in Swaziland (1982)—i.e., the wage-earning men with access to bottled beer. It may be as high as 20 liters of pure alcohol per person per year.

Do these social upheavals following the European Industrial Revolution bear any relation to the explosive increase in mental asylum populations that occurred in Europe 100 or 200 years ago? It is not clear whether this represented a true increase in the prevalence of psychosis or simply the housing of psychotics who would formerly have been vagrant or short-lived. Torrey (1980) reviewed historical data and thought it indicated a real increase in insanity in the nineteenth century. He even postulated schizophrenia as a disease of industrialized society. Hare (1983) reviewed the statistics of the mental asylums in nineteenth century Great Britain and concluded that the steady increase was not accounted for by increased detection of cases or by admission of patients with milder cases but was a real increase. He postulated a viral etiology to account for this apparent epidemic of schizophrenia, which leveled off at the turn of the century.

Figure 4
ALCOHOL CONSUMPTION IN GREAT BRITAIN OVER 100 YEARS

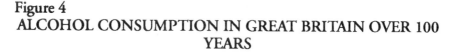

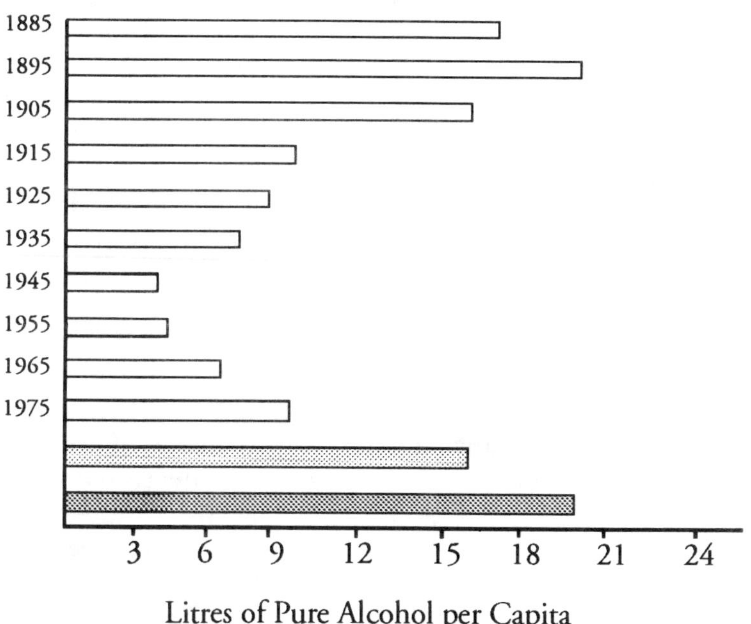

FRANCE 1975

PROJECTED ESTIMATE FOR SWAZILAND (at risk commercial alcohol consumption group)

This medical model seems oversimplified. Schizophrenia is a complex disturbance of biological, psychological, and social integration. A state of sociocultural flux, together with a high organic component, such as occurs in a society during industrial development, might increase the vulnerability to schizophrenia. Is it possible that an equivalent state in the evolution of psychiatric morbidity is occurring in Africa? Certainly, the few mental institutions began to fill up alarmingly until the trend was reversed by modern drugs and decentralization policies. This is illustrated in miniature by developments in mental health services in Swaziland (Figure 5). It, of course, says nothing about prevalence. It simply illustrates a trend. It is not hard to see how a nineteenth century situation could have developed.

Figure 5

MENTAL HEALTH PATIENTS AND SERVICES IN SWAZILAND, 1970-1985

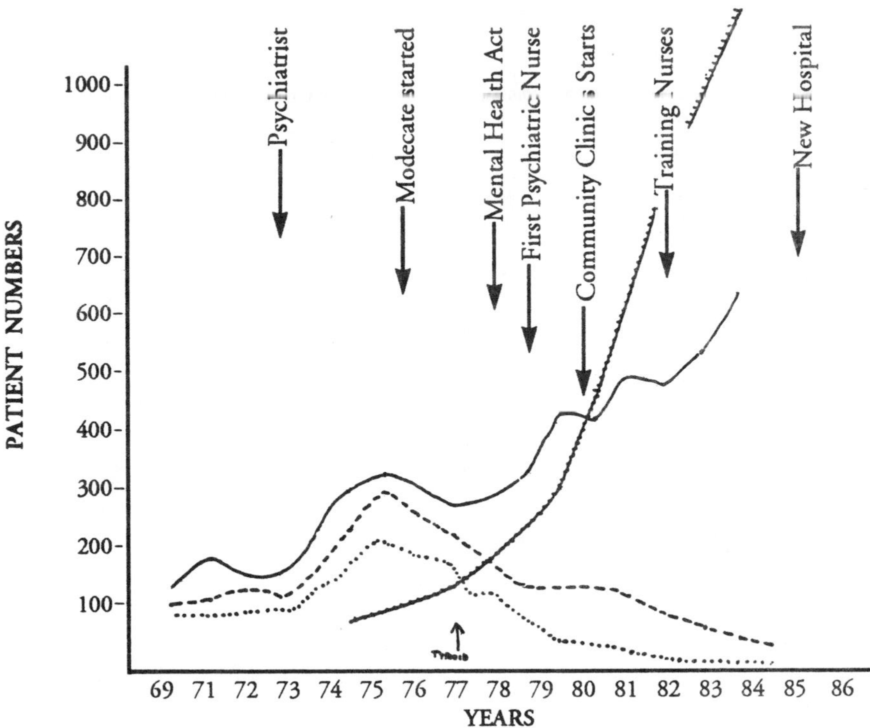

— Admissions
---- Bed Occupancy
Registered Patients at Matsapa Mental Hospital since 1969 and Yearly Total Registered of Clinic Patients
···· Chronicity Over a Year

Current developments can be seen in the context of the trends illustrated in Figure 6. These show a steady evolution from custodial care to the beginnings of community involvement.

SUMMARY

In this paper I have indicated a relationship between acute transient psychosis and rapid social change. Acute transient psychosis is distinct from, yet related to, schizophrenia. It can recur or can become prolonged if the stress persists. It can also herald nuclear schizophrenia. Furthermore, acute transient psychosis in Africa is equivalent to the hysterical psychosis or transient amentia as described in the nineteenth century; also, these syndromes may be temporary phenomena occurring in a transitional society as part of the evolution of psychiatric manifestations.

This view poses a number of interesting questions. Is a person in a state of cultural flux more at risk for psychosis? What is the relationship between hysterical psychosis and schizophrenia? Given a certain biological vulnerability, does destabilization of internal psychological milieu by rapid social change and cultural and family fragmentation predispose a person to schizophrenia? Can one postulate a continuum of increasing severity so that, above a certain threshold, hysterical psychosis becomes functional?

The strictly medical model of psychosis, particularly schizophrenia, has considerable limitations in accounting for this diversity and historical change. The model put forward by Ciompi (1985) is a most useful conceptual framework. In this framework, schizophrenia is seen not as a disease entity so much as the critical overtaxing of a vulnerable hierarchy of integrated systems for processing complex affective and cognitive information. Such a vulnerability is seen as developing from a complex interaction between the biological substrate (genetic predisposition and acquired organic factors, such as minimal brain damage) and the total input of psychosocial life experience.

Unstable, contradictory social experiences during personality development produce unstable, contradictory frames of reference, which produce inadequate coping systems and reduced stress tolerance, predisposing an individual to psychotic breakdown.

Ciompi postulated three phases:

- a premorbid vulnerability, with low tolerance of cognitive and emotional stress;
- a second phase, in which stressful life events lead to unique or repeated acute psychotic episodes; and
- a third phase, in which there is the most vulnerability, under unfavorable conditions, to chronic schizophrenia.

He suggested that this chronic course could be psychosocial artifact related to society's expectations, the patient himself, his caretakers, and his family.

This model makes good sense in the African situation.The high level of physical morbidity would increase organic vulnerability, and the cultural fragmentation would destabilize frames of reference, while the higher threshold for incapacity in African society (as Lambo phrased it) would protect the patient from the chronic state.

This would account for the greater prevalence of acute transient psychosis. The episodes of brief hysterical dissociation presenting a transient psychotic picture can be understood as discrete, circumscribed events of loss of ego boundary in response to stress whereas more vulnerable patients would proceed to a longer psychotic episode more closely resembling schizophrenia.

We must maintain the fundamental consistency of expression of mental illness in human beings, modified, albeit, by culture, environment, and history. If psychiatry is viewed in three dimensions—i.e., with the dimension of time—the current classification debate can be resolved. We certainly do not need different classifications for Africa and Western society. We need to recognize that conditions once common in Europe, such as acute psychosis, have declined but are currently common in Africa. After all, this is taken for granted in general medicine and obstetrics. At the time of the European transition, there was no framework for understanding psychiatric illness, nor was there an infrastructure for collecting data. In modern Africa, we have both and can, by studying the current status, view the evolution of psychiatric morbidity.

ILLUSTRATIVE CASE HISTORIES

Case 1:
DEPRESSION WITH ACUTE PSYCHOSIS FOLLOWING RELIGIOUS EXCITEMENT

A 28-year-old clerk at a sugar mill. He was the only one of his family to be educated and employed. His extended family pressured him for money. His wife had left him 6 months previously, and he became depressed. He could not sleep or eat well. The healer gave him muti to cause the wife to return. He put it under his pillow and developed terrifying dreams of his drunken father spearing him. He was convinced his father was bewitching him. He developed overvalued religious ideas. During a Zionist service, he became overexcited; he shouted and wailed that he could see animal spirits attacking him. He ran away, stripped off his clothes, and attacked the family. He was manneristic and incoherent. His family took him to the inyanga, where was given the vomiting rituals to expel the evil. He became dehydrated and exhausted and collapsed. Two days after admission to the hospital, the psychosis had cleared, revealing the underlying depression. He explained the pressure on him, his lost wife, and his alcoholic father.

Case 2:
ACUTE REACTIVE PSYCHOSIS, DEPRESSIVE TYPE, IN RESPONSE TO FINANCIAL DEMANDS

A 25-year-old teacher, the son of a peasant farmer. He had obtained his education with difficulty, receiving help from his maternal uncle. At school, he had had a brief psychosis in response to exams. Now, he was preparing for his marriage and trying to collect the lobola (bride price). Being the only educated one in his family, he encountered many demands on his salary. Two weeks before the wedding, the in-laws demanded the lobola.

He became acutely agitated and had to stop teaching. He could not sleep, refused food, and believed that he was dead and buried and that he had committed great crimes. He continually begged his relatives and the hospital staff to forgive him for all the wrongs he had done them, and he apologized constantly. He was suicidal and disoriented and had hallucinations.

The psychosis cleared completely in 2 weeks with chlorpromazine treatment. Then he was able to describe his financial problems, but he denied any previous depressive symptoms.

Case 3:
ACUTE PSYCHOSIS AS A CULTURALLY PRESCRIBED REACTION TO A LABOR DISPUTE

A 35-year-old laborer in the sugar-milling company. He was elected by his mates to lodge a complaint with the manager about the unpopular supervisor. He procrastinated for 6 months and became mildly anxious and depressed. All the workers feared this supervisor and were convinced he was bewitching them, causing the deaths of their children and the infertility of their wives.

Finally, his mates insisted that he lodge the complaint and held a prayer meeting, during which it was revealed to him that the supervisor was bewitching him. That night he awoke from a nightmare shouting that he could see the man on a television screen telling him to cut his throat. He proceeded to do it, damaging his larynx. For 3 days he remained in a manic state, restless, excited, and acting destructive and aggressive. A year later, this supervisor sued him for the accusation of bewitchment. He did not relapse but sought medical evidence, after which the charge was dropped.

Case 4:
ACUTE PSYCHOSIS ASSOCIATED WITH DEPRESSION AND DIFFICULT MARRIAGE

A 35-year-old married woman with six children from a poor peasant family. Her husband was an alcoholic, beat her, and spent the money on drink. There was very little food. After giving birth to her youngest child she had become depressed, had difficulty sleeping, and lost weight, but she continued to care for the baby. Four months after delivery, she became psychotic for one week, talking continuously and incoherently, heard voices, and saw cows chasing her and people putting lice on her. She felt strangled and suffocated. The psychosis resolved at once after admission to the hospital, and her underlying depression and malnutrition were revealed.

Two years later, she had a similar recurrence, again with a very transient psychosis that drew attention to her depression and difficult marital situation.

Case 5:
RECURRENT PSYCHOTIC EPISODES IN AN UNATTACHED WOMAN

A 32-year-old unmarried woman who took temporary laboring jobs. She had three children, fathered by different men. She had many family conflicts, jealousies, and problems. All three of the children had been taken by the boyfriends' relatives. Over 11 years, she had had four brief psychotic episodes associated with depression. She would complain of palpitations, weakness, and seeing dead spirits. Then she would shout, strip off her clothes, and run away. She feared bewitchment intensely. Some of these episodes followed stressful events, such as the death of the brother who was supporting her or attending a wedding ceremony. One episode followed an illness (pleural effusion). She was a lonely, poorly functioning, and unsupported woman.

Case 6:
DISCORD IN THE EXTENDED FAMILY LEADING TO DEPRESSION WITH ACUTE PSYCHOSIS

A 20 year old, married and expecting a baby. Her husband was away, working as a migrant laborer at mines in South Africa. He was the eldest son and would inherit his family's cattle and homestead. There was much jealousy. When his father died, his younger brother supplanted him in his absence. She was accused of bewitching her father-in-law in order to obtain the property. She became depressed, isolated herself, could not eat or sleep, and complained of a sore heart and a mind that could not think. After 3 months, she became acutely disturbed and was admitted to the hospital. She rapidly calmed down and explained her fears of this witch hunt but then ran away from the hospital. She was readmitted a month later, however; since coming home she had been restless and destructive, had been behaving bizarrely, and had had visual and auditory hallucinations. Once again, she calmed down immediately when she was removed from stress. She was advised to wait until her husband could visit from the mines and make a separate home for her.

Case 7:
SCHOOL ANXIETY WITH HYSTERICAL PSYCHOSIS

A 20-year-old student in form four, was the eldest of six children, whose mother was struggling to rear them singlehandedly. The father had deserted them for another wife. The mother was desperate for funds to start sending the younger children to school. She often urged her daughter to do well. This student became anxious about her studies, developed headaches and pain in her eyes, and could not stay awake in class. At the start of the term she was euphoric for a week; then she became intensely restless and destructive, hallucinated, saw "spooks," and heard voices. She sang and shouted. She was inaccessible, and her consciousness was clouded. This state resolved in two weeks with chlorpromazine treatment.. She reported a similar episode three years before, when she had begun secondary school.

For the next year, she had many somatic anxiety symptoms in class. A week before final exams, she became psychotic again. However, this time the condition was intermittent. She recovered enough to write the exams but relapsed between exams and afterward. This suggests a hysterical dissociative state.

Case 8:
DEPRESSION ASSOCIATED WITH SCHOOL ANXIETY, ACUTE PSYCHOSIS AND PARASUICIDE

A 14 year old, was the second son of a laborer who had two wives and nine children. He was approaching the exams for leaving primary school and developed school anxiety, headaches, flickering vision, and sleepiness in class. He failed the trial exams and then became acutely disturbed, cried incoherently, burned his clothes, saw small creatures squeezing him, and ran away. He recovered in the hospital in a week but remained very anxious, convinced he had been bewitched. His headaches continued all year.

The following year, at exam time, he took an overdose of chlorpromazine. He was sent back to school and began to show recurrent aggressive behavior and ran away. He had difficulty sleeping, lost weight, and felt miserable. He finally responded to antidepressants.

Case 9:
SCHOOL ANXIETY LEADING TO ACUTE PSYCHOSIS

A 17-year-old son of an ambitious teacher became intensely anxious about his studies. His anxiety was focused on the theft of his books at boarding school. He believed he would be bewitched through them: the spells would be put into the pages and would enter his eyes when he read. In the next 3 months, he had three brief florid psychotic episodes, during which he was violent, disoriented, and inaccessible. He experienced visual and auditory hallucinations and frightening ideas of reference. He believed that voices on the radio spoke about him and that the television showed his brothers on the screen. He ran away and mutilated himself. Each episode lasted 2 weeks. He relapsed when he returned to school and again when his brothers returned home and spoke of school. He had little memory of the episodes and remained intensely uneasy about the stolen books.

REFERENCES

Ammar, S.: Les de´sordres psychiques dans la socie´te´ Tunisienne: leur evolution et frequence en fonction des transformations socio-economiques et culturelles dupis l'independance. Tunisie Medicale 42:37-53, 1964.

Carothers, J. C.: A study of mental dreangement in Africans, and an attempt to explain its peculiarities, more especially in relation to the African attitude to life. Journal of Mental Science 93:548-596, 1947.

Carothers, J. C.: Frontal lobe function and the African. Journal of Mental Science 97:12-48, 1951.

Charcot, M.: Lecáons du mardi a′ la Salpeàtrieäre Policlinique, 1887-1888. Paris, France, Battaille, 1892.

Ciompi, L.: Toward a coherent multidimensional understanding and therapy of schizophrenia: converging new concepts. Presented at the International Symposium of Psychosocial Management of Schizophrenia, Berne, Switzerland, 1985.

Dhadphale, M.: Epidemic hysteria in a Zambia school. British Journal of Psychiatry 142:85-88, 1983.

Field, M.: Search for Security: An Ethno-Psychiatric Study of Rural Ghana. Chicago, U.S.A., Northwestern University Press, 1962.

Freud, S.: The Origins of Psychoanalysis: Letters of Wilhelm Fliess, Drafts, and Notes, 1887-1902. Edited by Bonaparte, M., Freud, A., Kris, E. London, England, Imago, 1954.

German, G. A.: Aspects of clinical psychiatry in sub-Saharan Africa British Journal of Psychiatry 121:461-479, 1972

German, G. A.: The Extent and Nature of Mental Health Problems in Africa Today: A Review of Epidemiological Knowledge. Geneva, Switzerland, World Health Organization, 1986.

Hare, E.: Was Insanity on the Increase? British Journal of Psychiatry 142:439-455, 1983

Hollender, M. H., Hirsh, S. J.: Hysterical psychosis: clarification of the concept. American Journal of Psychiatry 120:1066-1074, 1964

Jakovljevic, V.: Transcultural psychiatric experiences from African New Guinea. Transcultural Psychiatric Research Review 1:55-88, 1964.

Kraepelin, E.: Psychiatrie: ein kurzes Lehrbuchfu"r Studierende und Aerzte. (A. Abel) 4. Leipzig, Germany, 1893.

Lambo, T. A.: Malignant anxiety, a syndrome associated with criminal conduct. African Journal of Mental Science 108:256-264, 1962

Lambo, T. A.: Schizophrenic and borderline states, in Transcultural Psychiatry. Edited by DeReuck, A. V. S., Porter, R., London, England, Churchill, 1965.

Leff, J.: Psychiatry Round the Globe: A Transcultural View. New York, U.S.A., Marcel Dekker, 1981.

Meynert, T.: Amentia, die Verwirrheit. JB Psychiatrie 9:1-112, 1889

Minde, K. K.: Study problems in Ugandan secondary school students: a controlled evaluation. British Journal of Psychiatry 125:131-137, 1974

Morakinyo, V. O.: Personality variables in psychiatric illness associated with study among Africans. African Journal of Psychiatry 6(e,4):1-5, 1980.

Morel, B. A.: Traite des maladies mentales. Paris, France, Masson Paris, 1860

Prince, R. A.: Functional symptoms associated with study in Nigerian students. West Africa Medical Journal 11:198-206, 1962

Risso, M., Baker, W.: Ein Beitrag zum Verstanduis von Wahnerkrankurgen Siiditalienischer Arbeiter in de Schweiz. Basel, Switzerland, Karger, 1964.

Royal College of Psychiatrists Special Committee: Alcohol and Alcoholism, London. London, England,Tavistock, 1979

Smartt, C. G. F.: Mental maladjustment in East Africa. Journal of Mental Science 102:441-466, 1956

Smartt, C. G.: Short-term treatment of the African psychotic. Central African Journal of Medicine 10(suppl 10):1-12, 1964.

Stransky, E.: Zurlehre von der Dementia Praecox Cbl. Nervenheilk Psychiatrie 15:1-19, 1904

Stransky, E.: Zurlehre von der Dementia Praecox Cbl. Nervenheilk Psychiatrie 18:809-816, 1907

Torrey, E. F.: Schizophrenia and Civilization. New York, U.S.A., Jason Aronson, 1980, Chap. 2

Wessels, W. H.: Conversion disorders among Zulu Patients. South African Medical Journal 62:97-99, 1982

Chapter 5

Psychiatry in Libya's Eastern Region

by

Selim M. Elbadri, MD,
Registrar in Psychiatry,
Psychiatric Hospital,
Benghazi, Libya

ABSTRACT

The first sanatorium for mental disorders in Jamahiriya, Libya's eastern region, was established in 1950, and the first formal psychiatric hospital was built in 1974. The new Hawari psychiatric hospital outside Benghazi is part of a multi-hospital medical center and includes other mental health and medical specialties. Outpatient and emergency services are available. Psychiatric instruction has been provided for physicians in general medicine, students in nonpsychiatric mental health disciplines, and primary health care givers. Benghazi Psychiatric Hospital is a teaching hospital affiliated with the Al-Arab Medical University. Emphasis is currently being placed on construction of new psychiatric facilities and development of primary health care centers that can provide psychiatric services.

HISTORICAL INTRODUCTION

Jamahiriya occupies approximately 1.8 million square kilometers in northern Africa and has a population of 3.5 million. Tripoli, situated on the west coast, is the capital of Libya. Benghazi is the second largest city and is situated on the eastern coast of the country. The distance between the two cities is about 1,000 kilometers.

The first sanatorium for mental disorders was established in 1950 at Al-Marj Khadim, a small town 100 kilometers from Benghazi, under the supervision of one foreign doctor and a small number of unqualified nurses.

In 1963, the town of Al-Marj was demolished in a severe earthquake. As a result, the majority of patients were transferred to the Tripoli Psychiatric Hospital, and a small number were shifted to the Central Hospital in Benghazi. Jamahiriya Hospital's psychiatric ward operated with two foreign doctors, a number of Arab nurses, and limited facilities for 11 years. Traditional faith healers also took an active role in the management of the mentally ill.

LIBYAN PSYCHIATRIC HOSPITALS

In 1974, the first formal psychiatric hospitaL in Jamahiriya was built in the village of Gwarsha, about 15 kilometers west of Benghazi. It was named Dar Al-Shafa and had 200 beds. In the beginning, owing to a shortage of trained personnel and the stigma associated with mental illness, admission to the hospital was considered a social disgrace. Not until 1980 was a serious attempt made to provide modern facilities for the mentally ill.

HAWARI HOSPITAL

The site chosen for the new hospital was in Hawari, one of the suburbs of Benghazi, where the Al-Arab Medical University, Children's Hospital, and the 7th-of-April Hospital are situated. The hospital was completed and opened in 1982, and it gave psychiatry a new look and status in Benghazi. Whereas the old psychiatric hospital at Gwarsha was isolated, the new psychiatric hospital was rightly placed in a medical center with other hospitals. However, the old Gwarsha hospital was kept open for 125 long-term psychiatric patients. In the new hospital, there are departments of clinical psychology, neurophysiology (EEG), and psychiatric social services. There are also ancillary services, such as radiology, hematology, and biochemistry.

INPATIENT STATISTICS

A summary of inpatient admissions and discharges for 1985 is shown in Table I. The table also indicates the need for several state-of-the-art psychiatric facilities in Libya and in North Africa in general.

Table 1

1985 Inpatient Admissions and Discharges at the Hawari, Libya, Psychiatric Hospital

	ADMISSIONS			DISCHARGES		
MONTH	Male	Female	Total	Male	Female	Total
January	79	49	128	72	43	115
February	85	40	125	68	39	107
March	75	39	114	74	47	121
April	102	47	149	65	30	95
May	87	49	136	103	51	154
June	73	35	108	73	47	120
July	108	50	158	84	40	124
August	92	46	138	74	38	112
September	81	43	124	69	27	96
October	84	47	131	76	41	117
November	96	36	132	82	43	125
December	103	45	148	98	69	167
Total	1,065	526	1,591	937	495	1,433

OUTPATIENT CARE

The outpatient services are provided at the El-Keish Polyclinic, which is in the city center. Sessions are held four full days a week by a specialist in psychiatry, with the help of two registrars. The average number of outpatients per day is about 50, of whom 10 are new patients. Outpatient services for children are given once a week at the Children's Hospital.

COMMUNITY SERVICES

Besides the outpatient facilities at the clinic, the psychiatric hospital provides 24-hour emergency services, where referred and unreferred patients can come for advice. This provides a kind of crisis-intervention service for the management of patients within the community. Community services are still not well developed, but serious efforts are being made to provide community psychiatric help and guidance to geriatric homes, child welfare centers, and special schools for the mentally retarded.

TEACHING PROGRAMS

To provide a comprehensive teaching program, distinguished professors in special areas of psychiatry are invited for 2-4 weeks to provide supplementary sessions for the undergraduates and to give postgraduate lectures to the doctors in general medicine. Besides medical students, students in the Department of Psychology at Garyounis University and the Institute of Social Studies come for training in clinical psychology and clinical psychiatric social work.

To improve primary health care, a basic course in psychiatry was held in December 1985 at the new psychiatric hospital, where a large number of general practitioners and medical officers from all over Libya participated in a special 1-week seminar.

This seminar was a complete success, and there is a demand for more meetings like this in the future. There is not yet a department of psychiatry at Al- Arab Medical University, but psychiatry is under the Department of Medicine, which provides the hospital with a well-qualified teaching staff.

The Benghazi Psychiatric Hospital is affiliated with the Al-Arab Medical University as a teaching hospital. Psychiatric education is one of the important subjects in medicine, and fourth-year undergraduate students attend psychiatric training and education programs. Lectures are given by specialists once a week at the university and cover the whole field of psychiatry. Medical students spend a month at the hospital in groups of eight to twelve. They study a case fully and present it for discussion. Examinations are held at the end of each month, and the marks and attendance count toward the final examinations.

PROJECTED DEVELOPMENT

Plans for the future call for new university Hospitals with a capacity of 1,200 beds. Some of those under construction have psychiatric wings with 50-bed capacities. Other modern and fully equipped psychiatric hospitals, with capacities of 400 each, are to be built in Benghazi and other places in accordance with the latest world standards.

Multipurpose primary health care centers will be developed to enable primary health care givers to provide prophylactic and therapeutic psychiatric medicine.

RESEARCH

Three academic and clinical research projects have been completed, including a study on hysteria that was published in the British Journal of Psychiatry (Pu et al., 1986).

CONCLUSION

The mental health services of Libya's eastern region are developing slowly but in the right direction. They are following the guidelines and recommendations of the World Health Organization and those set forth by the Scientific Panel of O.A.U. in 1975.

REFERENCES

Pu, T., Mohamed, E., Imam, K., et al.: One hundred cases of hysteria in eastern Libya: a socio-demographic study. British Journal of Psychiatry 148:606-609, 1986

Chapter 6

Monosymptomatic Delusions of Smell: Are These New Symptoms In East Africa?

by

M. A. Fazal, MD, MB, BS, DPM
Specialist Psychiatrist

and

A. M. Shah, MD
Mathari Hospital
Nairobi, Kenya,

ABSTRACT

The authors describe four cases of monosymptomatic delusions of smell in Kenya. One patient became psychotic, killed two of his children, then tried to kill himself; he was convicted and sentenced to prison. The other three patients were treated with behavioral therapy; in the two cases followed up, the patients experienced improvements and disappearance of symptoms, respectively. The authors discuss the psychodynamic and treatment aspects of monosymptomatic delusions of smell. Such delusions have not previously been reported from East Africa, and their recent occurrence may be due to developments in the mass media and the influence of advertisements for such products as perfumes and deodorants.

INTRODUCTION

Patients with monosymptomatic olfactory delusions relating to personal odor have been described in the literature. Bebbington (1976) reviewed the literature and concluded that these patients tend to be resistant to any form of treatment; he also noted that one of his patients committed suicide.

These patients usually present with the complaint that unpleasant odors are emanating from their bodies. Such odors are not necessarily experienced as coming from the mouth or perineum in particular, but from themselves. Commonly patients are only referred to psychiatrists after all other medical investigations of the cause of the problem have proved fruitless. Beary and Cobb (1981) described three patients who complained of foul odors coming from the anus and mouth. Pryse-Phillips (1971) suggested that the syndrome be referred to as the olfactory reference syndrome and pointed out that, in the differential diagnosis, it is important to exclude temporal lobe epilepsy, schizophrenia, and severe depressive illness. The only successful treatment of the olfactory reference syndrome appears to be behavioral therapy (Milton et al., 1978; Watt et al., 1973).

In this paper we will describe three patients, all indigenous of East Africa and all showing clear-cut symptoms of the olfactory reference syndrome. In each case, the premorbid personality appeared to be relatively intact and the olfactory delusion appeared without other signs of psychotic disorder. These cases occurred in a culture quite different from that usually described in the Western literature. In Western and Eastern cultures, personal smell (or the lack of it) is important; this is shown clearly by, among other things, the preoccupation of the commercial world with the sale of perfumes, deodorants, and other substances intended to minimize odor. Perfumes and sweet- smelling substances have been used from time immemorial in the East, the Middle East, and the Far East. In sharp contrast is the fact that, to our knowledge, there are no references to smell in the traditional literature, folklore, or customs of East and Central Africa. Personal inquiries have revealed nothing of significance in this respect. The traditional foods are also bland and devoid of any herbs, condiments, or spices. Smell emanating either from food or from persons appears to have played an insignificant role in cultural thought. Viewed in this way, the concept of smell might be regarded as a new one. Recent changes in concern about it may be the result of rapidly developing mass media, which might be influencing people to purchase products designed to make them smell better.

In East and Central Africa a relationship between smell and the self may be a new concept, and, therefore, the development of any related delusion might also be new in this part of the world. This is not to say that monosymptomatic delusions themselves are new; however, the content of these delusions has rarely if ever been concerned with odor.

DESCRIPTION OF CASES

The patients to be described came directly to the psychiatric service at Mathari Hospital in Nairobi. All four were men. Their demographic and clinical characteristics are shown in Table I. In three cases, the premorbid personality appeared to be intact and there were no other psychotic signs; one of the three had a history of psychotic breakdown, but it had not been characterized by olfactory delusions. One patient had previously been treated with psychotherapy and two with neuroleptics, without improvement in their conditions.

CASE 1

The first patient was admitted after he had attempted suicide and killed two of his children with organophosphate poison. Before that time he had consulted a dermatologist, complaining of an unpleasant body odor. Thorough investigations of this complaint had been undertaken without result. After his crime, he was convicted and imprisoned, and follow-up was not attempted. His case should be reviewed again after his punishment, and it should be determined whether his delusions have changed or disappeared.

Table I
CHARACTERISTICS OF FOUR EAST AFRICAN PATIENTS WITH MONOSYMPTOMATIC DELUSIONS OF SMELL

FEATURE	1	2	3	4
Age (years)	31	45	24	29
Sex	M	M	M	M
Social class	4	1	4	4
Length of illness (years)	11	6	3	6
Marital status	M	M	M	M
Previous psychotic symptoms	No	No	No	Yes
Previous suicide attempt	No	No	No	No
Previous antidepressant or phenothiazine therapy	Yes	Yes	No	Yes
Previous nondrug therapy	Yes	Yes	No	Yes
Previous behavior therapy	No	No	No	No
Improvement at follow-up	—			

CASE 2

This man was referred by a general practitioner who had investigated every possible physical aspect of the case. The man held a responsible job as a marketing manager and had been with his company for 16 years. He was married and had several children. For 6 years he had believed that an unpleasant odor came from his body. As a result, he would leave rooms or places when he thought he was responsible for producing this unpleasant smell. The smell he experienced was not always the same. He described it as coming from his body as a whole and referred to its quality as "like burning food, like petrol" or even a rather sweetish smell. He was extremely self-conscious in the presence of other people and had ideas of reference about their gestures, etc. He was convinced that his employers were aware of his smell but were polite enough not to mention it to him. In other cases, he believed that senior members of the staff did not mention the smell to him because they were aware that he already knew of it. He did not experience this odor when he was with his wife. Nothing of significance emerged from the examination or following investigation. In particular, there was no evidence of schizophrenia or depressive illness, and his history was not at all consistent with temporal lobe epilepsy (an EEG was not carried out). He was diagnosed as suffering from a monosymptomatic delusion of smell (olfactory reference syndrome).

CASE 3

This patient was 24 years old, was unmarried, and had experienced delusions of smell for 3 years. He believed that a foul odor emanated from his armpits and genitals. His juniors at his workplace did not like him, he said, and told him that he smelled bad. He said that pregnant women avoided him. During the examination he showed no evidence of odor but was obsessed with his smell. In addition, he showed a marked lack of self-confidence and somewhat diminished concentration, apart from his preoccupation with his delusion. There were no other signs of schizophrenia, depression, or temporal lobe epilepsy. He continued to avoid social situations, believing that the people around him indicated in various ways that he produced a bad odor. They might demonstrate this by coughing, scratching their noses, or lighting up cigarettes. He avoided dating women because of fear of rejection.

CASE 4

This patient was referred from a general hospital, where he had been treated for symptoms of depression. He had suffered from an olfactory delusion of personal smell for 6 years. It had begun after what he described as a severe cold followed by severe pain all over his body. Later these pains disappeared and, as he began to feel better, he suddenly began to experience a bad smell coming from his body. Since then he would remove himself from the company of friends and avoid social contacts. He had functioned well in his work situation but was afflicted by occasional suicidal thoughts related to his smell. The examination revealed no other psychotic features, no evidence on which to base a diagnosis of primary depression, and no evidence of temporal lobe epilepsy. It should be noted that this patient, like those described by Pryse-Phillips (1971), had some symptoms suggestive of secondary depression. Such depression may be common in patients with monosymptomatic delusions and must be distinguished from a primary affective disorder. Since this patient was referred only recently, he has not yet been followed up.

TREATMENT

A treatment program was developed for each patient, and attention was paid to the various aspects of their individual cases. Patients 2, 3, and 4 were asked to keep records of the frequency and the time of the thoughts concerning their odors. Each of these instances was recorded and discussed with the therapist. The patients were asked to be aware of their own reactions and fantasize the reactions of other people when they were aware of the smell. Other aspects of the behavior program involved role playing and graded exposure to social situations. Reverse role playing was undertaken: the therapist assumed the role of a person who emitted an unpleasant odor. In this situation, whenever there was any evidence of movement by the patient, the therapist would claim that the patient was indicating by his movements that the therapist was emitting an unpleasant odor. In all three cases, after no more than six sessions, the patients became more relaxed and began to find such accusations humorous.

Patient 3 was also exposed to a treatment session with junior nurses at Mathari Hospital. These nurses were not aware of the patients' complaints. After a period of time, the supervising therapist asked the nurses if they were aware of a smell. When they answered in the negative, the nurses left the room and discussion with the patient continued. Indirect behavioral sessions involved endeavors to improve the patient's self-image, self-confidence, and ability to concentrate on issues other than his delusion. The patients were asked to list the positive and negative aspects of their personal relationships. Throughout these sessions, positive statements made by the patients were strongly reinforced.

During all treatment sessions, pulse rate and respiration rate were regularly recorded. These measures were taken as rough indications of arousal levels. They showed a steady decline throughout the period of therapy.

Progress was assessed with the self rating scale of Beary and Cobb (1981). In addition, patients 2 and 3 were reassessed by another psychiatrist after 3 months and 6 months, respectively.

FOLLOW-UP

Patient 2, reassessed at 3 months, reported that his surroundings were now pleasant to work in. He believed that the smell might be coming from someone else and not from himself. On occasions, however, he attributed the smell to his cigarette smoking and asked if he should stop smoking. Thus, his delusion of smell was still present, but his tendency to refer it to his body appeared to have vanished. With this change had come increased self-esteem and self-confidence and an improvement in his working relationships.

Patient 3, assessed at 6 months, made no mention of odors. Instead, he talked of his inability to find another job. Jobs for those who leave school are exceedingly difficult to obtain in Kenya, and this patient's difficulty appeared to be related to real factors and not to avoidance due to delusions of smell. He had still not been able to date a woman. He did not attribute this to smells but, rather, to his impoverished state and his financial dependence on other members of his family.

DISCUSSION

Of the four cases described here, only two were both actively treated and followed up. In both these cases, after behavioral treatment, the delusions of smell either changed (patient 2, who lost the self-referential quality of the delusion) or disappeared (patient 3). Although both men continued to have some doubts about themselves, they both began to function normally in social and occupational situations.

Viewed psychodynamically, this delusion may have been a defensive mechanism to prevent close contact with the environment, particularly the social environment. Not all these patients related their smell to a specific area of the body; for most, the whole person was offensive. The patient with a well-preserved personality takes specific steps to overcome this problem. He either avoids contact with other people or removes himself from their company. Certain universal aspects of human behavior are demonstrated by these patients. It appeared that some experienced substantial aggression and hostility toward the world in general, and the elaboration of an unpleasant personal odor could be seen as a mechanism to permit the removal of oneself from contact with the offending object. Schilder (1950) wrote.

These functions are familiar from a large number of experiences of the child; and these experiences themselves are organized in the image of the body, one of the apparatus of the ego. Further, the symptom can portray a conflict between the desire to express hostility and defiance towards the parent by the passage of gas from the body and the desire to please her by not flatulating. The conflict has been displaced from the lower end of the gastrointestinal tract of its upper end . (Stream, 1971)

Beary and Cobb believed that simple exposure to behavioral therapy enables the patient to alter his behavior pattern fundamentally. They stated, "Avoidance behavior may reinforce delusional thinking, as often happens in obsessive compulsive and phobic neuroses. Once the link between behavior and ideation has been challenged, and the abnormal behavior reduced, it is possible that the delusions may gradually wane."

In this Kenyan experience, behavioral therapy appears to have been more successful than previous therapies in changing the nature of the pathological experience and permitting the resumption of normal social and occupational functioning.

Apart from psychodynamic and behavioral formulations and treatment, drugs have been used in this syndrome, and pimozide has been reported to be particularly useful (Riding et al., 1975; Reily et al., 1978). Pimozide was not tried in these cases, so its efficacy for these patients is unknown. However, previous treatment with phenothiazines and antidepressants had involved adequate doses and adequate periods of time but had produced no significant change. Further treatment trials, including behavior therapy, dynamic psychotherapy, and pimozide should be conducted in the future. Unnecessary extensive medical and surgical intervention and investigation, which may reinforce the delusions, should be avoided.

As far as we are aware, no cases of this type have previously been reported in East and Central Africa. It may be that under the influence of modern mass communications new ideas about what is offensive have emerged. This might at least alter the content of delusions if not the form of psychopathology. Monosymptomatic delusions of an olfactory sort have been previously reported only in Western cultures. In Africa, it may be that the advertisers of perfumes, deodorants, etc., are now beginning to have an impact on these cultures that is markedly changing the phenomenology of psychopathology. Such changes in symptom content may be expected to occur in other psychiatric syndromes.

Chapter 7

Notes on the History of Blacks In American Psychiatry

by

Jeanne Spurlock, MD,
Deputy Medical Director,
American Psychiatric Association,
Washington, D.C.,
U.S.A.

ABSTRACT

Drawing on the literature, colleagues, and broader historical events, the author identifies Blacks who have been influential in American psychiatry. Many trained and worked at Tuskegee, other Veterans Administration hospitals, state hospitals, and Black medical schools. Their accomplishments are described in the context of the social, legal, and medical discrimination prevalent during their careers, specific group efforts to attain racial equality during this century, and achievements growing out of the confrontations in the 1960s. Since the formation of Black Psychiatrists of America and other group actions in the 1960s, Black psychiatrists have achieved recognition and leadership roles in many U.S. medical and psychiatric organizations.

INTRODUCTION

Several years ago, my latent interest in the history of Blacks in psychiatry was rekindled by a specific assignment. I was asked to participate in a panel discussion and to speak about Black psychiatrists in mental health administration. A literature search turned up relatively little. In making use of the African tradition of oral history, I turned to several colleagues in my effort to obtain historical facts. Subsequently, I expanded my focus and broadened my contacts. However, it is likely that I have barely scratched the surface. In developing this paper, I drew on some of the works of historian John Hope Franklin in order to identify some of the broader historical events that paralleled the history of Afro-American psychiatrists. It should be noted that this paper is not a complete historical review. The sketches focus on the periods before the 1970s. However, there are some glimpses of the events of the 1970s and 1980s.

AMERICAN PSYCHIATRISTS

SOLOMON CARTER FULLER: Solomon Carter Fuller has been identified as the first Black psychiatrist in the United States. A native of Liberia, he received his undergraduate education at Livingston College, Salisbury, North Carolina, and medical education at Boston University, from which he graduated in 1897. The fact that Fuller had graduated from a prestigious medical school, even though he had been turned down by Harvard, would lead a casual observer to conclude that racial discrimination was at least on the decline. This conclusion might be reinforced by the information that 2 years previously, sociologist W. E. B. Dubois earned his Ph.D. from Harvard. This was an era in which selected Negro leaders gained considerable visibility and acceptance by some Caucasians in significant policy-making arenas. Two years before Fuller's graduation, Booker T. Washington, founder of the Tuskegee Institute, delivered a well-known speech, accepting segregation and disfranchisement and advocating a policy of conciliation and gradualism. This was the same year, 1893, that Dr. Daniel Hale Williams made news by performing the first open-heart surgical procedure at Chicago's Provident Hospital. However, expressions of doubt that such a procedure could have been performed by a Negro physician serve to illustrate the absence of a radically equal society at that time. Racial discrimination was alive and actively operating in spite of the significant contributions Blacks had made that benefit the country as a whole. It is interesting that an account of the early contributions of Blacks was included in a two-volume 1883 publication, History of the Negro Race in America from 1619 to 1880, by George Washington Williams (1968). Parenthetically, it should be noted that historian John Hope Franklin's biography of Williams has been published recently (Franklin, 1985).

Several historical highlights will illustrate the racist practices operating around the time of Fuller's graduation from Boston University. A Supreme Court decision handed down in 1890 gave segregationists a boost. The case, Plessy v. Ferguson, was rooted in action related to a Louisiana law that stated: "All railroad companies carrying passengers in their coaches . . . shall provide separate but equal accommodation for the white and colored races."

Speaking for the court, Mr. Justice Bradley interpreted the statute as allowing for the enforcement of absolute equality of the two races before the law. The very same year, 1890, Blacks were disfranchised in Mississippi. The legislative bodies in South Carolina, Virginia, Georgia, Alabama, and Oklahoma enacted similar laws within the next decade. Discriminatory practices were also prevalent in organized medicine and led to the organization of the National Medical Association in 1897. Some years later, the Section on Neurology and Psychiatry was established. In the early 1950s, new life was infused into the section under the leadership of Pittsburgh-based Eugene Youngue. Reorganization of the section took place in the early 1980s with the establishment of an autonomous section for neurologists and neurosurgeons and the identification of the Section on Psychiatry and Behavioral Sciences.

The route Fuller took for postgraduate training reflects some of the discrimination he experienced. It has been reported that he pursued pathology and neuropathology training because of the difficulties Blacks had in entering private practice and obtaining training in clinical neurology and psychiatry. However, Fuller was able to arrange to study psychiatry under Emil Kraepelin and neuropathology with Alois Alzheimer at the University of Munich. Upon his return to the United States, he gained recognition and acceptance as a neuropathologist. At the 62nd annual meeting of the

American Psychiatric Association (APA) in June 1906, he presented a summary report, "A Study of the Neurofibrils in Dementia Paralytica, Dementia Senilis, Chronic Alcoholism, Cerebral Lues, and Microcephalic Idiocy." A fuller account was published in the American Journal of Insanity (1907), now known as the American Journal of Psychiatry.

Charles Pinderhughes, who knew Fuller fairly well, reported that he served as a clinical psychiatrist and neurologist at Westborough State Hospital in Westborough, Massachusetts, for 45 years, during 22 of which he was also pathologist. Fuller taught at Boston University, where he rose to rank of Associate Professor, and on his retirement in 1933, he was given the rank of Professor Emeritus in neurology. He edited the Westborough State Hospital Papers, a journal developed through his initiative, and did clinical work at the Massachusetts General, Allentown (A Pennsylvania state hospital), Massachusetts Memorial, and Framingham Hospitals.

Pinderhughes also reported that Fuller was always alert to and looking for situational and psychological factors that might be playing a role in psychiatric disorders, even though his medical and psychiatric training stressed biological factors. He spent much time discussing psychoanalytic theory and method . . .., and in his later years of blindness he procured recorded books about psychoanalysis to which he would listen. His long-standing interest in psychoanalysis has been documented earlier by his appearance in the group photograph of the psychiatrists who met with Freud at Clark University . . . during Freud's first visit to the United States.

The early 1900s were critical years for Black Americans. In 1903, opposition of Blacks to Booker T. Washington's accommodation philosophy took an organized form. Two years later, W. E. B. Dubois took on a leadership role in the Niagara movement, a drive to ensure full citizenship for Negroes. Although Dubois earned his doctorate before the formal recognition of sociology as a discipline, he identified and worked as a sociologist. Partial preparation for this role was rooted in some academic work in the social sciences. Early in his career he believed that research findings would lead to a racially equalitarian society. An opportunity to test his hypothesis came in 1896, a year before Fuller's graduation from medical school and the period in which activists in the Philadelphia settlement house movement invited him to study the participation of Afro-Americans in local politics and other social institutions. Many of his findings parallel those of contemporary researchers and suggest that the more things change, the more they remain the same. The work of Dubois foreshadowed the interests of sociologists E. Franklin Frazier and Charles S. Johnson and of social anthropologist Allison Davis, who studied the impact of segregation and discrimination on Blacks. Historical accounts provide more than a hint that Dubois' patience dwindled with the passage of time and he determined an action-oriented approach was needed. The Niagara movement was virtually ignored by the dominant group and undermined by Booker T. Washington, who, as previously mentioned, was a firm believer in gradualism. It should be noted that Dubois was not alone in advocating direct action to achieve racial equality at that time in history. A vivid example is the organization of the National Association for the Advancement of Colored People (NAACP) in 1909. Although it was considered radical by opponents, the NAACP's strategy was to work within the system and use the professed ideals and legal institutions of the system to obtain civil rights for Afro-Americans. Parallels between the two approaches can be seen in accounts of the struggles of Black physicians and other professional and occupational Black groups in their respective struggles for equal opportunities in the workplace.

The following excerpts from psychiatric publications of the early 1900s illustrate the biases that had become incorporated into psychiatric concepts and practices:

During its years of savagery the Negro race has learned no lessons in emotional control, and what they attained during their few generations of striving left them unstable. For this reason we find deterioration in the emotional sphere most often an early and persistent manifestation. (Evarts, 1914)

The student of psychology working in the United States has access to a people [Negroes] the average level of whose development is lower than the white race and which furnishes numerous individuals showing psychological aspects quite similar to most of the savages . . .

This being the case, it is to be expected that their dream life would enjoy a relative freedom from the endo-psychic censor, exactly as that of the child does. (Lind, 1914)

CHARLES PRUDHOMME: In the era of the struggles of Dubois and Washington, Blacks in various local communities made specific demands of the policy makers. So it was with the leadership of the Tuskegee community in the early 1920s. The protests and demands were related to the absence of Black psychiatrists in the segregated Veterans Administration Hospital. Fuller was contacted and asked to identify Black psychiatrists for staff appointments to the Tuskegee Veterans Administration Hospital. According to reports from Charles Prudhomme, the first psychoanalytically trained Black psychiatrist and the first Black to be elected to a national APA office, Fuller recruited and provided some elementary psychiatry training for medical students George Branch, S. (Simon) O. Johnson, and Touissaint Tilden, all of whom graduated from medical school in 1923.

S. O. JOHNSON: According to APA files, Johnson pursued formal training at the Boston Psychopathic and Montefiore Hospitals in the United States and received additional training at the London National Hospital and in La Salpetriere in Paris. During his professional career, he served as Superintendent of Larkin State Hospital in West Virginia.

TOUISSAINT TILDEN: Four years after medical school graduation in 1923, Tilden served an internship at Kansas City General Hospital and then returned to Tuskegee for additional clinical training prior to a year of training in administrative psychiatry at Walter Reed Hospital. Most of Tilden's career was spent at Tuskegee in the areas of clinical and administrative psychiatry.

GEORGE BRANCH: Branch pursued formal training in neuropsychiatry in the Veterans Administration hospital system in New York. He, too, held a number of clinical posts at Tuskegee Veterans Administration Hospital, where he was appointed Chief of Clinical Services in 1946.

I have not yet located records regarding other early recruitment efforts for the Tuskegee facility, but I have identified a contemporary of Branch, Johnson, and Tilden.

E. PENTOKA HENRY: E Pentoka Henry completed his undergraduate medical education at the University of West Tennessee in 1921. According to APA biographical directories, the greater percentage of Henry's career was spent as Medical Superintendent of Taft State Hospital, originally known as the State Hospital for the Negro Insane, in Taft, Oklahoma.

EUGENE YOUNGUE: Larkin State Hospital in Larkin, West

Virginia, played an integral role in the professional careers of many of the Black pioneers in American psychiatry. Eugene Youngue, trained and certified in psychiatry and neurology, recently informed me that his father, a neurologist, served as the Superintendent. Gene, recently brought out of retirement to serve as the Clinical Director of a public psychiatric hospital in the Pittsburgh area, was a member of Larkin's clinical staff for a year following his army discharge after World War II.

MILDRED MITHCELL-BATEMAN: Mildred Mitchell-Bateman, a former Commissioner of Mental Health of West Virginia, Kathryn Rainbow- Earhart, now in Topeka, Kansas, and Robert Walden, now in Toledo, Ohio, also served as Superintendents of this facility. Their respective years of superintendency occurred between 1958 and 1965.

DOROTHEA SIMMONS AND LUTHER ROBINSON: Other peers I know to have been appointed to the clinical staff of Larkin Hospital during the postWorld-War-II period include child psychiatrist Dorothea Simmons, now based at Worchester, Massachusetts, child psychiatry facility, and Luther Robinson, currently the acting head of Howard University's Department of Psychiatry.

ERNEST Y. WILLIAMS: The development of psychiatry departments and training programs in the predominantly Black medical schools is another integral part of the history of Black psychiatrists in America. Ernest Y. Williams, a 1930 graduate of Howard University College of Medicine, was the first head of the Psychiatry- Neurology Service at Freedman's Hospital, Howard's original teaching hospital, from 1939 to 1970. With the assistance of several benefactors, he was accepted for postgraduate training at New York University from 1931 to 1933 and at Cornell from 1933 to 1936.

RAPHAEL HERNANDEZ AND LLOYD ELAM: Raphael Hernandez, a 1928 graduate of Meharry Medical College, was appointed Clinical Professor of Psychiatry, Neurology, and Legal Medicine Services at Meharry in 1955. Hernandez, who was multilingual (Spanish, English, French, Italian, and Portuguese) and held a law degree from Kent College of Law (1944), had received postgraduate training in neuropsychiatry and encephalography in New York and Illinois. The department and training program were developed and headed by Lloyd Elam in the early sixties.

ELIZABETH DAVIS, ALFRED CANNON, AND HERBERT (RED) ERWIN: During this period, Elizabeth Davis, the first Director of the Department of Psychiatry at Harlem Hospital, and Alfred Cannon, the first Director of the Psychiatry Department at the Drew-King Medical Center in Los Angeles, also made significant contributions in the training of Black psychiatrists. The contributions of Herbert (Red) Erwin must also be highlighted in the context of psychiatric training for Blacks before the 1960s. Erwin, who had pursued postgraduate training in St. Louis and at Columbia University, held the posts of Acting Director and Director of Psychiatry at Homer G. Phillips Hospital in St. Louis.

DISCRIMINATORY PRACTICES

In the context of the theme of this presentation, the discriminatory practices in the 1930s of the broader society and within the medical profession must be noted. Many Blacks and probably more than a few physicians of the dominant group were yet smarting from the psychological blows delivered by the Flexner Report of 1925. A few statements may refresh the memories of those who have forgotten the content of the part of the report labelled "The Medical Education of the Negro,"

The practice of the negro [sic] doctor will be limited to his own race, which in its turn will be cared for better by good negro physicians than by poor white ones. But the physical well-being of the negro is not only of moment to the negro himself. Ten million of them live in close contact with six million whites. Not only does the negro himself suffer from hookworm and tuberculosis; he communicates them to his white neighbors, precisely as the ignorant and unfortunate white contaminates him. Self- protection not less than humanity offers weighty counsel in this matter; self-interest seconds philanthropy. The negro must be educated not only for his sake, but for ours. He is, as far as human eye can see, a permanent factor in the nation. He has his rights and due and value as an individual; but he has, besides, the tremendous importance that belongs to a potential source of infection and contagion. . . . The pioneer work in educating the race to know and to practice fundamental hygienic principles must be done largely by the negro doctor and the negro nurse. It is important that they both be sensibly and effectively trained at the level at which their services are now important.

Certainly, the recommendations did not provide any encouragement for specialty training.

In the 1930s, Afro-Americans were actively protesting racial discrimination at home and abroad. Boycotts were directed against white-owned businesses that had large Negro trades but no Negro employees. The efforts of various groups, such as the Colored Merchants Association, Jobs for Negroes, and the Citizens' League for Fair Play, were applauded by large numbers of Blacks, although a sizeable number followed more drastic measures and became involved in Marcus Garvey's back-to-Africa movement. Regarding protests against racism beyond the borders of United States, Blacks were among the first Americans to agitate for intervention against fascist aggression and loudly protested the Italian invasion of Ethiopia.

During a recent videotaping conducted by Black Psychiatrists of America President, Richard Fields, E.Y. Williams, now retired, spoke of a number of experiences of discrimination, both subtle and overt, during his postgraduate training in the 1930s. Charles Prudhomme has recalled similar experiences related to his efforts to obtain a training post at St. Elizabeths Hospital. In view of Prudhomme's experiences, it is of particular significance that more Black psychiatrists have been trained at St. Elizabeths than any other single program. I have no hard data to offer as an explanation for this finding. No doubt, there are multiple reasons; one is the large number of training slots compared to the small number of positions at the predominantly Black training programs. Integration is another and probably more obvious reason. As Prudhomme noted, "The laws under which St. Elizabeths [once] operated specifically prevented any . . . possibility of an integrated staff."

MARY McCLEOD BETHUME: The name of educator Mary McLeod Bethune must be invoked in any reference to historical accounts of Afro-Americans in the 1930s. A segment of her biographical sketch, which appeared in The Negro Almanac, provides confirmation of these observations:

Herbert Hoover was the first American president to utilize her abilities when, in 1930, he invited her to a White House Conference on Child Health and Protection. Franklin D. Roosevelt was quick to follow his predecessor's lead by asking her to serve on the Advisory Committee of one of the organizations he helped establish, the National Youth Administration (NYA). In 1935. . .her work had so impressed the President that he was persuaded to set up an Office of Minority Affairs, with Mrs. Bethune as administrator. During the 1930s she was one of the leading figures (and the only woman) in the unofficial "Black Cabinet" which had begun the fight for advanced integration in U.S. Government. (Ploski and Marr, 1976)

Charles Prudhomme recalled that a visit to St. Elizabeths Hospital by Mrs. Bethune and Mrs. Roosevelt resulted in improvement of the facilities set aside for Black patients. Another plus was their support of a plan, initially proposed by Dr. Prudhomme, to develop a cosmetology unit for the Black female patients.

EFFECTIVENESS OF PSYCHIATRIC ORGANIZATIONS

A history of Black psychiatrists must necessarily include the formation and development of Black Psychiatrists of America (BPA), a national organization that grew out of the confrontations of the 1960s. A detailed account can be found in Racism and Mental Health (Pierce, 1974).

Although the BPA has multiple roots, a major one is the efforts of a small group of Black psychiatrists brought together in the early 1960s by Charles Wilkinson, currently the Executive Director of the Greater Kansas City Mental Health Foundation and Associate Dean at the University of Missouri Kansas City School of Medicine. Others in the group included Elizabeth Davis, Hugh Butts, Lloyd Elam, Calvin Calhoun (a neurologist), Alfred Cannon, Chester Pierce, James Comer, Alvin Poussaint, William Tompkins, and myself. Wilkinson was successful in obtaining a small grant from the National Institute of Mental Health (NIMH) for a study to identify the roots of the then growing racial conflicts. At that time (1968), Wilkinson was a member of an NIMH review committee, and the respect for his work was probably an enabling factor in the subsequent entree of BPA executives to NIMH. Another large BPA root was the efforts of a Washington-based group of Black psychiatrists, the Alliance for Psychiatric Progress.

Black psychiatrists who attended the 1969 APA annual meeting met to discuss concerns of Black members and to develop a list of demands for presentation to the APA Board of Trustees. The caucus elected Chester Pierce and Alfred Cannon to the respective posts of chairman and vice-chairman. An executive committee was established to present the demands, which were drawn up by James Comer, Hiawatha Harris, Cannon, and Pierce and were approved by the members of the caucus.

The APA board did not consider it possible to implement all 10 demands. For example, the APA constitution did not allow appointments to the Board of Trustees; all positions were filled by election rather than appointment. A task force of Black psychiatrists was immediately established; that component is now a standing committee. The caucus mobilized considerable political steam, which led to the placement of Charles Prudhomme's name on the slate for APA Vice President. He was subsequently elected to the post but not without considerable resistance by a number of members of the Washington Psychiatric Society. Pierce pointed out the irony of the situation: many who signed the petition to place a white man on the ballot to oppose Prudhomme were teaching at Howard. A combination of pressures and events caused the rival candidate to withdraw.

In its early history, BPA initiated the following significant actions:

- Appointed James Comer to head the negotiations that yielded the establishment of the Center for Minority Group Mental Health Programs at NIMH; James Ralph was appointed Chief of the center.
- Negotiated with the American Board of Psychiatry and Neurology (ABPN) and brought about the recommendation for consideration of Chester Pierce as a director of ABPN; he was subsequently elected.
- Spearheaded the establishment of the Solomon Carter Fuller Institute, which was to serve as a conduit through which funding for Black-oriented projects, from government or private sources, could be funneled.

- Advocated the appointments of Black psychiatrists to editorial boards of psychiatry journals. Before any negotiations with any editors-in-chief, Comer and Pierce were invited to serve on the board of the American Journal of Orthopsychiatry. Subsequently, Pierce and, more recently, Wilkinson were appointed to the editorial board of the American Journal of Psychiatry.

Since the 1960's, Black psychiatrists have been appointed or elected to top posts, as illustrated by the following:

- June Jackson Christmas's appointment to President Carter's transition cabinet as Secretary of the Department of Health, Education, and Welfare, and her election to the presidency of the American Public Health Association and the vice-presidency of APA.
- Chester Pierce's election to the presidency of the American Orthopsychiatric Association and Charles Wilkinson's two-time election to the post of Treasurer of APA.
- Encouragement of two Black psychiatrists to run for APA president—i.e., Mildred Mitchell-Bateman, the first woman to be nominated for the post, and Charles Wilkinson.

TRIBUTES TO BLACK PSYCHIATRISTS

There must be scores of unsung leaders and significant contributors among Afro-American psychiatrists. Fortunately, tribute has been paid to some.

The Solomon Carter Fuller Lecture and Award was established by APA's Committee of Black Psychiatrists in 1969. Obviously, the award is a tribute to the late Solomon Carter Fuller. It is given to a Black citizen who has pioneered in an area that has benefitted significantly the quality of life for Black people. Three of our psychiatry colleagues have been recipients: Charles Pinderhughes, Luther Robinson, and Chester Pierce.

The Annual E. Y. Williams, M.D., Scholars of Distinction Awards commemorate the contributions of Dr. Williams. The awards program, administered through the Section on Psychiatry and Behavioral Science of the National Medical Association, also recognizes the achievements of the recipients. To date, the recipients in the Distinguished Senior Psychiatrists category have included Jesse Barber, Margaret Morgan Lawrence, Charles Pinderhughes, Chester Pierce, and Eugene Youngue.

- Michele Reid, Detroit Psychiatric Institute, Freda Lewish-Hall, Howard, Robert Phillips, Yale, and Janet Williams, Yale, have received the Resident of Distinction Award in the four successive years since the award was established. George Mallory, during his tenure as chairperson of the National Medical Association Section on Psychiatry and Behavioral Science, initiated the efforts that led to the development of the program.
- At the 1986 APA annual meeting, the Committee of Black Psychiatrists hosted a reception to pay public tribute to 14 Black psychiatrists who had served in significant leadership roles before 1960: .

    - Frances Jones Bonner
    - Robert Bragg
    - June Jackson Christmas
    - James Curtis
    - Elizabeth Davis
    - Hiawatha Harris
    - Mildred Mitchell-Bateman
    - Chester Pierce
    - Charles Pinderhughes
    - Charles Prudhomme
    - Luther Robinson
    - Jeanne Spurlock
    - Ernest Y. Williams
    - Eugene Youngue

- APA recognized the contributions of James Comer in 1985 by naming him the recipient of the Ittleson

Research Award. This award is given to an individual child psychiatrist or group of investigators for the published results of research pertaining to the mental health of children. The findings of such research will have led, or strongly promise to lead, to a significant improvement of the mental health of children.

- The most monumental tribute to Chester Pierce has been the naming of Pierce Peak near Filchner Ice Shelf, Antarctica Pantuxet Mountain Range.

GOALS

Of course, history is being continuously developed. New issues warrant attention, and old issues have to be addressed again. Contemporary Black psychiatrists share the responsibilities, to varying degrees, for

- Recruiting in order to increase the small pool of 871 Afro-American psychiatrists in the United States;
- Effecting curriculum changes that will allow for the inclusion of pertinent cultural materials in required courses with well-supervised clinical experiences with minority patients;
- Developing and carrying out research that specifically pertains to mental health and mental illness of the Afro-American populations;
- Ongoing collaboration with colleagues of the dominant group to effect the delivery of competent psychiatric services to the underserved populations in a variety of settings.

The achievement of these goals will surely have many positive ripple effects on the community at large.

REFERENCES

Evarts, A. B.: Dementia praecox in the colored race. The Psychoanalytic Review 1:388-403, 1914

Franklin, J. H.: George Washington Williams: A Biography. Chicago, U.S.A., University of Chicago Press, 1985

Fuller, S. C.: A study of the neurofibrils in dementia paralytica, dementia senilis, chronic alcoholism, cerebral Ives and microcephalic idiocy. American Journal of Insanity 63:415-468, 1907

Lind, J. E.: The dream as a simple wish-fulfillment in the Negro. The Psychoanalytic Review 1:295-300, 1914

Pierce, C.: The formation of the Black Psychiatrists of America, in Racism and Mental Health: Essays. Edited by Willia, C. V., Kramer, B. M., Brown, B. S. Pittsburgh, U.S.A., University of Pittsburgh Press, 1974

Ploski, H. A., Marr, W. III: Negro Almanac: A Reference Work on the Afro-American. New York, U.S.A., Bellweather Publications, 1976, p. 1000

Williams, G. W.: History of the Negro Race in America from 1619 to 1880, 2 vols. (1883). Salem, N.H., U.S.A., Ayer Company Publications, 1968

Chapter 8

Psychiatric Care Of The AIDS Patient In Africa And The Americas

by

Joyce M. Johnson, MA, DO
St. Elizabeths Hospital
Washington, D.C
U.S.A.

ABSTRACT

The acquired immunodeficiency syndrome (AIDS) was first recognized in the United States in the spring of 1981.

It was later found to be endemic in parts of Central Africa.

AIDS patients are at special risk for psychiatric illness because of the complex pathophysiology, often sudden onset, poor prognosis, and social implications of the disease.

As the number of identified cases continues to increase throughout the world, mental health professionals should be aware of the neuropsychiatric consequences of AIDS, the high prevalence of intravenous drug use among AIDS patients in the United States, and the relationship of AIDS to preexisting psychiatric illnesses.

Psychiatric treatment of the AIDS patient should focus on providing supportive, culturally sensitive care.

Psychiatrists can also play a large role in AIDS education and policy making because of their unique medical-psychosocial perspective.

INTRODUCTION

The acquired immunodeficiency syndrome (AIDS) was first recognized in the United States in the spring of 1981 through an increase in the number of cases of Kaposi's sarcoma and Pneumocystis carinii pneumonia in otherwise healthy persons (CDC, 1981a & 1981b). Later, similar syndromes were recognized in other parts of the world, including Europe, South America, the Caribbean, and Africa (WHO, 1986; Pape et al., 1983; Biggar, 1986; Brunet and Ancelle, 1985). At first, AIDS was recognized as primarily a medical problem. Now, however, the many neuropsychiatric and psychosocial problems associated with the disease are becoming known (Johnson, 1987).

AIDS is caused by a retrovirus, variously known as lymphadenopathy virus (LAV), human T-cell lymphotropic virus, type III (HTLV-III), and human immunodeficiency virus (HIV). In this presentation, the virus will be referred to as HIV. The virus invades the imune system and leaves the patient susceptible to any of a number of opportunistic infections and tumors (Gallo et al., 1984; Barre-Sinoussi et al., 1983).

DISEASE PRESENTATION :

OPPORTUNISTIC INFECTIONS

The opportunistic infections and tumors associated with AIDS include selected protozoal, fungal, bacterial, and viral infections. Kaposi's sarcoma is the most common AIDS-related tumor. When one develops these infections or tumors, one fulfills the definition of an AIDS case if there is no other known cause for the immune deficiency-e.g., immune suppressive therapy or cancer (CDC, 1985c).

Many of the opportunistic infections are common, such as Candida albicans and herpes. The case definition for AIDS requires an unusually serious presentation. For example, Candida in AIDS presents as esophageal disease and herpes presents as a severe ulcerating lesion lasting a month or more. These contrast with the minor diaper rash and vaginal infections caused by Candida albicans and simple recurrent self-limited herpetic blisters.

OTHER HIV PRESENTATIONS

Not all HIV infections develop into AIDS. The range of presentations can be thought of as an iceberg. AIDS is the tip of the iceberg. The other presentations of HIV infection are less serious illnesses and can be considered the less obvious, underwater parts of the iceberg.

In the United States, longitudinal studies have shown that about one-third of those infected with HIV remain asymptomatic. One-third or more develop less serious symptoms, which have been called pre-AIDS or AIDS- related complex (ARC). These symptoms include lymphadenopathy, fever, diarrhea, weight loss, and lethargy. Up to one-third of these individuals develop AIDS, which is the immune deficiency with an opportunisitc infection or tumor (Jaffe et al., 1986). All of those infected with the virus, no matter how mild or serious their symptoms, should be viewed as potentially infectious and able to spread the disease to others. Epidemiological data strongly indicate that the virus is transmitted by blood, sexual, and perinatal contact and that it is not transmitted by casual contact (Sher, 1985; CDC, 1985b).

EPIDEMIOLOGY:

UNITED STATES

In the United States, the number of AIDS cases has continued to increase since 1981. As of July 28, 1986, 22,792 adult and 323 pediatric cases had been reported. Nearly half of the patients (47%) were 30-39 years old; 88% were 20-49 years old. Of the adult patients, 93% were male and 7% were female. The racial distribution of the adult patients was as follows: 60% white, 24% black, 14% Hispanic, and 2% other or unknown (CDC, 1986). It was estimated that one to two million persons were infected with the virus. In the United States, many patients die within 6 months of AIDS diagnosis; over 90% die within 2 years (Barnes, 1986).

AFRICA

In Africa, the epidemiology of HIV infection is less well known, although there are similarities to the United States. In both places, sexual, blood and perinatal contact are the primary routes of transmission, although the specifics of these routes vary. In Africa, sexual transmission is more often heterosexual, whereas in the United States it is homosexual.

In Africa, blood contact can result from the use of contaminated or improperly sterilized needles and medical instruments. In the United States, blood contact is frequently through sharing of needles by intravenous drug users. Transfusion of blood and blood products is linked to the disease on both continents, although as the HIV antibody test is used more, this route of transmission should decrease.

Perinatal spread is an important route of transmission for the pediatric cases. In Africa, however, the diagnosis of AIDS in infants is difficult on clinical grounds because of the high prevalence of gastroenteritis due to other causes (Clumeck et al., 1984, 1985a, & 1985b; Mann et al., 1986; Kreiss et al., 1986; Van de Perre et al., 1984 & 1985; Colebunders et al., 1985; Biggar et al., 1985; Katlama et al., 1984; Saxinger et al., 1985; Hunsmann et al., 1985; Norman, 1985).

As of Aug. 4, 1986, the World Health Organization (WHO) had received AIDS surveillance data from 13 African countries, including five nations that reported no cases. The remaining eight countries reported 703, as shown in Table I (WHO, 1986a).

The AIDS case definition for surveillance purposes in the United States is very similar to the WHO case definition. Additionally, WHO developed an alternative clinical case definition for the African nations that is more sensitive to their medical practice. Serologic and other expensive diagnostic tools are not needed. A case may be identified solely on clinical grounds (WHO, 1986B).

In Africa, AIDS generally presents as severe diarrhea, oral thrush, and weight loss. The weight loss can be so extreme that in rural Uganda it has been called slim disease (Serwadda, et al., 1985).

TABLE I
AFRICAN COUNTRIES REPORTING AIDS CASES TO WHO AS OF AUG. 4, 1986[1]

COUNTRY	NUMBER OF CASES
Central African Republic	150
Ghana	7
Kenya	26
South Africa	21
Tanzania	462
Tunisia	2
Uganda	2
Zimbabwe	6
Total	703

1. Comores, Ethiopia, Gambia, Mauritius, and Nigeria reported no cases.

PSYCHIATRIC

Unlike most infectious diseases, HIV disease results in significant neuropsychiatric problems. HIV has been isolated from the brain, cerebrospinal fluid, spinal cord, and peripheral nerves (Black, 1985; Resnick et al., 1985; Ho et al., 1985).

The psychiatric illnesses of patients with HIV disease include those directly related to HIV and the AIDS- associated opportunistic infections and tumors, psychosocial complications, and psychiatric problems unrelated to and frequently predating the HIV infection.

Direct central nervous system invasion by HIV and the AIDS-related opportunistic infections and tumors results in organic mental disorders meeting DSM-III criteria (APA, 1980). These organic mental disorders are caused by various mechanisms, including anoxia, metabolic disturbances, and space-occupying lesions, such as brain abscesses, calcifications, and tumors. The specific signs and symptoms vary widely and include depression, dementia, delirium, amnesia, hallucinations, delusions, and personality changes. About 30% to 40% of adults with AIDS have neurologic signs and symptoms. HIV infection causes acute and chronic meningitis, myelopathy, peripheral neuropathy, spinal cord degeneration, encephalopathy, and chronic progressive dementia (Snider et al., 1983; Hoffman, 1984; Lowenstein and Sharfstein, 1984; Navia and Prince, 1986). Nearly 80% of children with AIDS show some neurologic sequelae. These include encephalopathies, acquired microcephaly, pyramidal tract signs, cognitive impairment, developmental delays and regressions, and seizure disorders (Belman et al., 1985; Fox, 1986).

In the United States, patients with HIV disease face a myriad of psychosocial problems. Prejudices against the groups at high risk, particularly homosexual men and intravenous drug users, and misconceptions about the transmission of HIV have resulted in undue social isolation and discrimination. Many patients are abandoned by their families and friends. Others may be afraid that the illness will be transmitted to them. Patients who are physically able to work may lose their jobs because of the unjustified fears of others. Children with AIDS have been barred entry to schools.

In addition to social discrimination from the outside world, these patients also experience debilitating psychosocial stresses from within themselves. When a patient is told that he or she is infected with HIV, he or she must deal with the uncertainty of the prognosis unless AIDS has already been diagnosed. The patient must accept a changing body image and uncertain health. Relationships with family and friends change markedly. He or she may feel guilty about the life- style that placed him or her at risk. Questions are raised about transmission of the disease to others. Issues of death and dying surface.

Patients with HIV infections may also have psychiatric illnesses etiologically unrelated to HIV. These include the range of DSM-III Axis I and Axis II diagnoses and the psychiatric diagnoses of the International Classification of Diseases (ICD-9). In the United States, the most significant are the illnesses related to substance use. Approximately one-fourth of the AIDS patients in the United States have histories of intravenous drug use (Des Jarlais et al., New York

State Division of Substance Abuse Serivces data, reported by CDC, 1985a). In parts of the United States, the prevalence of HIV antibodies among selected intravenous drug users exceeds 80% (Fox, 1986).

In Africa, the psychiatric aspects of AIDS and other forms of HIV disease are less well documented. However, as the disease becomes better characterized, the neuropsychiatric aspects, those caused by the virus' direct invasion of the central nervous system, will likely resemble those identified in the United States. However, since AIDS in Africa is primarily transmitted through heterosexual contact, the psychosocial issues related to homosexuality and drug abuse are less relevant.

PSYCHIATRIC CARE

First, there is no medical cure for AIDS, although some of the opportunisitc infections and tumors can be treated. The patient's overall 2-year prognosis, no matter what the treatment, remains very poor. However, this makes the role of the psychiatrist critically important to the patient. For the AIDS patient with a terminal disease, mental health care can be invaluable.

As psychiatrists, we would like to provide care to these patients on several levels. We would like to treat the causes of the organic mental disorders. We have no treatment for the direct central nervous system invasion by HIV. However, we can provide at least limited treatment for anoxia, seizures, and some other related problems. Even with the most sophisticated treatment, though, the long-term outcome has probably changed little. Once the patient is diagnosed as having AIDS, he or she has a terminal disease, which the psychiatrist should recognize.

Psychiatric treatment, then, should focus on providing care in the most comfortable cultural context for the patient. In the United States this usually means a hospital liaison psychiatry, referral or outpatient treatment, either individual or group therapy, depending on the patient's condition and needs and the availability of services in the community. In San Francisco and other U.S. cities, a number of gay volunteer organizations are providing lay supportive care to these patients. In New York City, Mother Theresa recently opened an

AIDS hospice that provides both hospice and home care services. These help the patient to cope with the numerous psychosocial stresses, so the patient feels less helpless, isolated, and alone.

In Africa, the psychiatric care of AIDS patients should also be sensitive to the cultural aspects of the patient's needs. For some patients, particularly the more educated in the cities, formal psychiatric treatment may be indicated. For patients who have traditional cultural and religious beliefs, traditional healers are able to help them cope with their psychosocial stresses, including issues related to death and dying.

Since no particular type of mental health care has been clearly shown to be superior to others in the care of AIDS patients, a culturally sensitive approach is indicated. Primarily, these patients require caring and supportive environments that encourage them to openly discuss the various issues which concern them.

THE PSYCHIATRIST'S ROLE

Psychiatrists in Africa and America share a public health role in helping persons with concerns about AIDS and helping to reduce the spread of disease. Psychiatrists should become well informed about the psychiatric, medical, and epidemiologic aspects of AIDS so that they can provide optimum care to patients. We should also help those in other health professions with their own emotional responses to the care of these patients. Caring for AIDS patients is difficult for all health care providers because of the often unjustified fear of disease transmission and the significant emotional toll these patients take.

The psychiatric profession should assume a leadership role in helping to educate others, both health professionals and the lay public, about AIDS. Psychiatrists should provide consultation to the media, community organizations, and employers to help dispel the myths about the disease. Undoubtedly, some of the unjustified AIDS-related fears and discrimination are due to a general misunderstanding about transmission and lack of awareness about the disease's significant emotional effects.

The psychiatric profession should work with public officials to develop the most appropriate AIDS policies, which should reflect sensitivity to the individual patient's humanity and a concern for the public's health.

We, as psychiatrists, have a responsibility to our individual patients, as well as to the community, to help combat the AIDS epidemic. We have a unique perspective to offer through our understanding of the emotional aspects of the disease. We have a crucial role to play in both Africa and the Americas.

REFERENCES

American Psychiatric Association: Diagnostic and Statistical Manual of Mental Disorders, 3rd ed. (DSM- III). Washgton, D.C., U.S.A., APA, 1980

Barnes, D. H.: Grim projections for AIDS epidemic. Science 232:1589-1590, 1986

Barre-Sinoussi, F., Chaerman, J. C., Rey, F., et al.: Isolation of T-lymphotropic retroviruses from a patient at risk for acquired immunodeficiency syndrome (AIDS). Science 220:868-871, 1983

Belman, A. L., Ultmann, M. D., Horoupian, D., et al.: Neurological complications in infants and children with acquired immune deficiency syndrome. Annals of Neurology 18:560-566, 1985

Biggar, R. J.: The AIDS problem in Africa. Lancet 2:79- 82, 1986

Biggar, R. J., Melbye, M., Kestens, L., et al.: Seroepidemiology of HTLV-III antibodies in a remote population of Eastern Zaire. British Medical Journal 290:808-811, 1985

Black, P.: HTLV-III, AIDS, and the brain. New England Journal of Medicine 313:1538-1540, 1985

Brunet, J. B., Ancelle, R. A.: The international occurrence of the acquired immunodeficiency syndrome. Annals of Internal Medicine 103:670-674, 1985

Centers for Disease Control: Followup on Kaposi's sarcoma and Pneumosystis pneumonia, Mortality and Morbidity Weekly Review, 30:409-140, 1981a

Centers for Disease Control: Pneumocystis pneumonia. Mortality and Morbidity Weekly Review 30:250-252, 1981b

Centers for Disease Control: The Epidemiology of AIDS. Atlanta, U.S.A., CDC, April 15, 1985a

Centers for Disease Control: Recommendations for presenting transmission of infection with human T- lymphotropic virus type III/lymphadenopathy-associated virus in he workplace. Mortality and Morbidity Weekly Review 34:681-696, 1985b

Centers for Disease Control: Revision of the case definition of acquired immunodeficiency syndrome for national reporting - United States. Mortality and Morbidity Weekly Review 34:373-375, 1985c

Centers for Disease Control: Weekly Surveillance Report - United States. Atlanta, U.S.A., CDC, July 28, 1986

Clumeck, N., Sonnet, J., Taelman, H.: Acquired immunodeficiency syndrome in African patients. New England Journal of Medicine 310:492-497, 1984

Clumeck, N., Robert-Guroff, M., Van de Perre, P., et al.: Seroepidemiological studies of HTLV-III antibody prevalence among selected groups of heterosexual Africans. Journal of the American Medical Association 254:2599-2602, 1985a

Clumeck, N., Van de Perre, P., Carael, M., et al.: Heterosexual promiscuity among African patients with AIDS (letter). New England Journal of Medicine 313:182, 1985b

Colebunders, R., Taelman, H., Piot, P.: Acquired immunodeficiency syndrome (AIDS) in Africa, a review. Tropical Doctor 15:9-12, 1985

Fox, J. E.: Gamma globulin injections may slow HTLV-III infection. U.S. Medicine, July 1986

Gallo, R. C., Salahuddin, S. Z., Popovic, M., et al.: Frequent detection and isolation of cytopathic retroviruses (HTLV-III) from patients at risk for acquired immunodeficiency syndrome (AIDS). Science 224:550-503, 1984

Ho, D. D., Rota, T. R., Schooley, R. T., et al.: Isolation of HTLV-III from cerebrospinal fluid and neural tissues of patients with neurologic syndromes related to acquired immunodeficiency syndrome. New England Journal of Medicine 313:1493-1497, 1985

Hoffman, R. S.: Neuropsychiatric complications of AIDS. Psychosomatics 25:393-400, 1984

Hunsmann, G., Schneider, J., Wendler, I., et al.: HTLV positivity in Africans (letter). Lancet 2:952-953, 1985

Jaffe, H. W., O'Malley, P. M., Darrow, W. W., et al.: Outcome of HTLV-III/LAV infection in a cohort of gay men. Presented at the NIH Consensus Development Conference, Washington, D.C., U.S.A., July 7, 1986

Johnson, J.: Psychiatric aspects of AIDS: overview for the general practitioner. Journal of the American Osteopathic Association 87:99-102, 1987

Katlama, C., Leport, C., Materon, S., et al.: Acquired immunodeficiency syndrome (AIDS) in Africans. Annales de la Societe` Belge de Medecine Tropcale 64:379-389, 1984

Kreiss, J. K., Koech, D., Plummer, F. A., et al.: AIDS virus infection in Nairobi prostitutes: spread of the epidemic to East Africa. New England Journal of Medicine 314:414-418, 1986

Lowenstein, R. J., Sharfstein, S. A.: Neuropsychiatric aspects of acquired immune deficiency syndrome. International Journal of Psychiatry in Medicine 13:255-260, 1984

Mann, J. M., Francies, H., Quinn, T., et al.: Surveillance for AIDS in a Central African city (Kinshasa, Zaire). Journal of the American Medical Association 255:3255- 3259, 1986

Navia, V. A., Price R. S.: Demintia complicating AIDS. Psychiatric Annals 16:158-167, 1986

Norman, C.: Politics and science clash on African AIDS. Science 230:1140-1142, 1985

Pape, J. W., Liautaud, B., Thomas, F., et al.: Characteristics of the acquired immunodeficiency syndrome (AIDS) in Haiti. New England Journal of Medicine 309:945-950, 1983

Resnick, L., diMarzo-Veronese, F., Schupbach, J., et al.: Intra-blood-brain-barrier synthesis of HTLV-III-- specific IgG in patients with neurologic symptoms associated with AIDS or Aids-related complex. New England Journal of Medicine 313:1498-1504, 1985

Saxinger, W. C., Levine, P. H., Dean, A. G., et al.: Evidence for exposure to HTLV-III in Uganda before 1983. Science 227:1036-1038, 1985

Serwadda, D., Mugerwa, R. D., Sweankambo, N. K., et al.: Slim disease: a new disease in Uganda and its association with HTLV-III infection. Lancet 2:849-852, 1985

Sher, R.: AIDS and related conditions - infection control. South African Medical Journal 68:843-848, 1985

Snider, W. D., Simpson, D. M., Nielson, S.: Neurological complications of acquired immune deficiency syndrome: analysis of 50 patients. Annals of Neurology 14:403- 418, 1983

Van de Perre, P., Rouvroy, D., Lepage, P., et al.: Acquired immunodeficiency syndrome in Rwanda. Lancet 2:62-65, 1984

Van de Perre, P., Clumeck, N., Carael, M., et al.: Female prostitutes: a risk group for infection with human T- cell lymphotropic virus type III. Lancet 2:524-527, 1985

World Health Organization: Surveillance data (personal communication). Geneva, Switzerland, WHO, August 4, 1986a

World Health Organization: Weekly Epidemiological Record 61(17):1, 1986b

SECTION II:

Adult and General Psychiatry

Chapter 9

Biological Approaches to Mental Health Problems in Africa Today

by

A.O. Odejide, M.D.,
Department of Psychiatry,
University College Hospital,
Ibadan, Nigeria.

and

S.W. Acuda, M.D.
Department of Psychiatry
University of Nairobi
Kenyatta National Hospital
Nairobi, Kenya.

INTRODUCTION

The definition of biological psychiatry favored in this paper is based on that referred to in the aims of a WHO-sponsored long-term training programme[1], namely: the application of contemporary biological methods in psychiatric diagnosis and treatment. This involves psychophysiologic (neurophysiological) instrumentation, neuro-radiology and biochemical (pharmacokinetic) techniques.

The thinking that biological mechanisms underlie psychiatric symptoms is not new in psychiatry. Griesinger in the 19th century wrote that "mental diseases are brain diseases. Psychiatry and Neuropathology are not merely two closely related fields: they are but one field in which only one language is spoken and the same laws rule"[2]. This was central to Freud's thinking, as shown in his "project"[3], though psychoanalysis did not try to uncover these mechanisms by use of the methods outlined above. Through psychoanalysis, psychiatric aetiology and management shifted from demoniacal possession and exorcism to psychodynamic conflicts and psycho therapy. As a result, interest in psychosocial factors held sway in psychiatry until recently. At the turn of this century when developed countries of today had problems of wars, epidemics coupled with the relatively poor state of knowledge in science and technology, the emphasis laid on psychosocial factors among workers in psychiatry was not surprising. Interest in biological factors became renewed with the knowledge that infections by bacteria (e.g. General paralysis of the insane) and viruses (e.g. Von Economo's disease) could lead to manifestation of psychiatric symptoms. This interest has been given added impetus with the description of the principle of neurohumoral transmission at nerve endings by Loewi in 1921, and Dale and Feldberg in 1934[4]. The fantastic success of science and technology has given man new tools and methods to probe the body, so that, in the past twenty-five years or so, psychiatric literature from the western world has become dominated by interest in biological factors.

According to Woods[5] (1986), "laboratory methods are now available to help confirm clinical diagnostic impressions, to predict response to treatment, to regulate dosage of medication, to improve the efficiency of therapeutic interventions and to help in the estimation of prognosis. The sensitivity, specifity and confidence level of these laboratory tests now approach that which obtains for many of the routine tests regularly employed in medicine. The use of laboratory testing and diagnostic procedures in psychiatry is becoming an integral part of the evaluation and treatment of psychiatric patients. Some examples are computerized axial tomography (CAT), nuclear magnetic resonance (NMR), positron emission transaxial tomography (PET), biological markers (Dexathasone suppression test, DST, diurnal cortisol tests, DCT etc.) and trait markers (platelet monamine oxidase inhibitor, platelet imipramine binding etc).

In Africa, the situation today is in many ways like that of Europe and America at the turn of the century. In fact, Bean (quoted in German, 1972)[6] noted that : "In a world where far more than half the inhabitants live under the menace of hunger, serious disease and early death, where small-pox, malaria, plague, cholera and malnutrition affect many hundreds of millions, the situation of psychiatry is not unlike that of public health in the pre-pasteur period...". Again, the majority of African countries currently do not possess the complex expensive technological equipment and specialized staff necessary for research in biological psychiatry. It was therefore not surprising that when in 1975, Herding, a WHO scientist, sent out questionnaires to all African psychiatrists in Africa, seeking information on research in mental health which had been done in their countries, an overwhelming majority of them named epidemiological studies, followed by research on health service provision[7]. The only aspect of biological psychiatry mentioned were research on drug and alcoholism, but here also the respondents were more interested in the epidemiological aspects. At the College of Medicine of the University of Ibadan, the only studies in biological psychiatry meeting our operational definition after three decades of research were those of Akindele et al.[8, 9, 10] and Osuntokun[11]. It was absolutely vital to establish the prevalence and characteristics of mental disorders on the continent, not only for comparison with similar data from developed countries but also to help convince African Governments that mental health problems indeed existed in their countries and require more attention.

Epidemiological studies on mental illness have now been done in several African countries, and though more needs to be done, it has now been shown that the prevalence and nature of psychiatric disorders are on the whole similar in both African and developed countries[12,13,14]. We cannot assume, however, that the same biological mechanisms underlie all mental disorders in the two worlds. As one African medical scientist pointed out in a lecture, we have G6PD deficiency and malaria, and they don't. After following up 104 maniac patients of Yoruba origin, Makanjuola[15] found that in the Yoruba, maniac disorder occurs predominantly as a recurrent unipolar disorder whereas in Western European society it occurs predominantly as part of a bipolar disorder. He, like Odejide (1986)[16], pointed out that a common biological basis may predispose to episodes of affective disorder, while the actual nature of the episodes could be culturally determined. Again, whereas there seems to be a consensus of opinion among workers from Europe and America that Type II Schizophrenia is associated with increased ventricular brain ratio (VBR)[17, 18], the one study from Japan does not support this finding among the Japanese[19].

The above considerations, coupled with the fact that a few countries in Africa now have both the necessary staff and equipment, make it imperative that research in mental health be diversified to include biological psychiatry .

The possible effects of biological approaches to mental health problems in present day Africa shall be discussed under aetiology of major psychiatric disorders, psychiatric misdiagnosis, effective treatment methods, training, and research.

AETIOLOGY OF PSYCHIATRIC DISORDERS

Contrary to Szasz' (1961)[20] hypothesis, it is now widely accepted that psychiatric disorders cut across the various cultures, but the pattern of presentation of symptoms may be influenced by culture. What remains uncertain are the possible aetiological factors across cultures, especially with the functional psychoses such as schizophrenia and affective disorders. As Osuntokun (1985)[21] observed, most of the biological factors associated with functional psychoses in developed countries are of relevance to mental health care delivery in Africa.

SCHIZOPHRENIA

The DSM III definition of schizophrenia implies 'that the disease is an idiopathic syndrome with heterogeneous causes such as heredity, familial and environmental causes'. Genetic studies indicate that the risk of the illness increases with the degree of biological relatedness to an affected family member[22]. Though there are evidences to support this observation yet the mode of transmission remains unclear. The two main hypotheses put forward to explain the mode of transmission are monogenic (autosomal dominance with reduced penetrance) and polygenic theory as exemplified by results of adaptive studies[23]. These theories can still not explain why a large number of schizophrenic patients have no family history of the illness or why the concordance rate of schizophrenia in monozygotic twins is as low as 30 to 58%.

There is increasing evidence that environmental factors contribute to the development of schizophrenia[24-28]. These include psychosocial and physical factors which are prevalent in most of the African countries. This viewpoint gave rise to Crow's[29] division of schizophrenic illnesses into Type I and Type II similar to Leonhard's[30] (1936) schizophrenic subdivision into nonsystematic and systematic. Type I (nonsystematic) schizophrenia presents with acute onset, positive symptoms such as hallucinations, delusions, thinking disorders and good response to treatment whereas Type II (systematic) is characterized by negative symptoms such as apathy, poverty of thought, flattening of affect, negativism, and social withdrawal. In the International Pilot Study of Schizophrenia by the WHO[31], a large percentage of the schizophrenics included in the study from the developing countries with acute onset and good prognosis would be classified as Type I schizophrenia.

It is widely believed now, that Type I schizophrenia may be viral induced including incorporation of viral nuclear matter into dopaminergic neurones with enhanced dopaminergic transmission hence good prognosis on treatment with dopamine receptor blockade[21]. Bacterial infections, use of psychoactive drugs, can also manifest with schizophrenia-like[27, 28] features. Unlike the Type I schizophrenics, Type II respond poorly to antipsychotic drug treatment and may show progressive intellectual deterioration with CAT scan demonstration of enlarged cerebral ventricles with statistically significant increase in ventricular brain ratio[34, 35].

In the genesis of both types, biochemical (dopamine hypothesis), neurobiological (neurobiology of dopamine receptors) and environmental factors have been incriminated. Modern techniques in biological psychiatry tend to produce further evidence that schizophrenia is an organic brain disease. In Lishman's (1983) review, few shizoprenic patients showed presence of abnormal dominant hemispheric dysfunction, abnormal inter-hemispheric transfer as revealed by neuropsychologlcal tests, cognitive deficiency or impairment, the presence of non-specific neurological 'soft' signs such as dysarthria, right-left confusion etc,.

The extensive aetiological factors and polymorphous presentation of schizophrenia call for detailed diagnostic and laboratory investigations of clinically diagnosed cases of schizophrenia. This is even more so in the African sub-region where malnutrition and infections compete with psychosocial factors.

AFFECTIVE DISORDER

As in schizophrenia, genetic and environmental factors have been found to be associated with the onset of unipolar and bipolar affective disorders. These factors may be causative, precipitating, exacerbating, or coexistent. Disturbances in cholinergic-catecholeminergic equilibrium in the central mechanism have been postulated as a neurochemical basis of affective disorders. In mania for example, increased noradrenaline metabolite (3-methoxy-4-phenoxy hydroxylglykol, MPHG) has been reported in the cerebro-spinal fluid. Apart from the cathecolamines, abnormalities of the hypothalamic hypophyseal endocrine system have also been incriminated in the aetiology of affective disorders.

Some of the above observations have shed light on a number of neuroendocrine and other biological markers associated with major depressive disorders and given birth to diagnostic tests such as dexamethasone suppression test (DST)[34], diurnal cortisol test (DCT), and thyrothropin releasing hormone (TRH)[35]. These tests help to confirm the diagnosis of primary psychiatric major depression and help to identify candidates for psychopharmacological treatment or electroconvulsive therapy.

Since most of the studies cited above were carried out in the developed countries, in order to have a better perspective of the causes of major psychiatric disorders in the African countries, neuropsychiatric evaluation is urgently needed.

MISDIAGNOSIS AND TREATMENT OF PSYCHIATRIC DISORDERS.

It is necessary to remind ourselves that most psychiatric and behavioural symptoms are non-specific[36, 37, 38]. Therefore other causes must first be ruled out before any psychiatric treatment begins. For example catatonia, which for many years was considered peculiar to catatonic schizophrenia, has now been found as a symptom in both psychological and physical illnesses[39, 40, 41, 42]. Gelenberg[41] listed myriads of physical illnesses which could present with catatonia. We also know that symptoms such as delusions, auditory hallucinations, depersonalization, and elevation of mood can be caused by physical and/or psychological illnesses. Subclinical hypothyroidism may present as depression. These observations confirm the need to carry out a thorough neuropsychiatric evaluation of psychiatric patients in order to make correct diagnosis and offer appropriate treatment.

Misdiagnosis may result in protracted treatment of psychiatric patients. In a follow up study of 200 new patients attending the psychiatric outpatient clinic of Ibadan University Teaching Hospital, Nigeria, the patients diagnosed as having depression or anxiety states showed less tendency to improve than the psychotics exemplified by schizophrenia[43]. With the high prevalence of infections, vitamin deficiency diseases, and drug abuse problems, a thorough neuropsychiatric evaluation of the resistant cases in essential similar situations exist in most of the African countries.

Development in the use of state and trait markers have advanced to the extent that they can be used to confirm the diagnosis of psychiatric illnesses and help to determine the effectiveness of pharmacological treatment. State markers detect the presence of the active neurobiological disease state and may assist to identify patients with high relapse potential. Examples of these are DST, DCT and TRH which are currently being used in the evaluation and treatment of patients suffering from affective disorders. Unlike state markers, trait markers identify patients with abnormal genes which may or may not be expressed as an illness. A few examples of this are platelet serotonin tests and receptor studies. Tuomisto et al (1979)[44] and Paul et al (1981)[45] reported that in major depression of unipolar type, there is a decrease in serotonin receptors and a decrease in serotonin uptake. These authors observed a highly significant decrease in the number of (3H) impramine binding sites in platelets from depressed patients compared with controls. This observation suggests that an inherited deficiency of the serotonin transport mechanism may be involved in the pathogenesis of depression. A few centers should be developed in the sub-region of the continent of Africa to contribute to these studies, especially for cross-cultural comparisons.

An even more relevant area where clinical diagnosis needs to be confirmed by laboratory tests is drug abuse. Psychotic symptoms have been identified with the abuse of drugs like alcohol, amphetamine, cannabis, phencyclidine (PCP), cocaine, and lysergic-acid diethylamide (LSD). Such drug-induced psychoses have a different prognosis and must be treated differently from psychosis attributed to endogenous psychoses. As pointed out by Verebey et al (1986)[46], the treatment of drug abusers is extremely handicapped if drug abuse monitoring is not provided or not accurate. Therefore, comprehensive drug testing to distinguish the presence and or absence of drugs is now important for psychiatrists in making the precise evaluation and appropriate treatment of any patient. For example, cannabis has been reported in different parts of Africa to cause transient panic attacks, anxiety reactions, acute toxic psychoses with or without clouding of consciousness that clear within a few weeks. and amotivational syndrome[47, 48] . It is therefore important to exclude the abuse of such a drug in several neuropsychiatric disorders.

The presence of commonly abused drugs in Africa (alcohol, cannabis, CNS stimulants etc) can be confirmed in body fluids (saliva, CSF, urine, blood) with laboratory tests such as thin layer chromatography (TLC), enzyme/radio immunoassay (EIA/RIA) and Gas chromatography/mass spectroscopy (GC/MS). These tests have not been used to any appreciable extent in Africa.

CHOICE OF PHARMACOLOGICAL TREATMENT

Biological psychiatry has improved our knowledge of drug effects on neurotransmitters and the receptors. Hence, clinicians selectively determine the appropriate chemotherapeutic agents for clearly defined psychiatric disorders. For example, bipolar depressives respond better to lithium carbonate treatment than the unipolar types. Even in the use of tricyclic antidepressants consideration must be given to the extent to which such selected drugs can produce disturbing side effects such as sedation, (H_1 histamine receptor blockade[49]), anticholinergic effects (blockade of muscarinic acetylcholine receptors), and orthostatic hypotension (adrenergic receptor blockade). Similarly, the mechanism by which the tricyclic antidepressants produce their effects differ.

RESEARCH AND TRAINING

As previously discussed, African psychiatrists need to utilize available diagnostic and laboratory tests available in biological psychiatry to unravel some of the myths about psychiatric disorders in Africa. Some of the important areas of research that we urgently need are the establishment of biological norms for the African population, investigation of psychiatric disorders supposedly peculiar to Africa (e.g. brain fag syndrome), and biological studies in drug free populations. Biological norms are needed in psychopharmacology and electroencephalography. Reports claiming that African patients require much lower doses of psychotropic drugs than their caucasian counterparts have been based on personal or clinical impressions . The situation regarding standardization of serum lithium levels needs special mention because lithium metabolism is influenced by such factors as dehydration and salt intake which occur more frequently in Africa as a result of its climate. The therapeutic dose-range and toxicity levels therefore need to be determined for Africans.

As for electroencephalography (EEG), if much reliance is to be put on EEG reports, then there is the urgent need for an extensive data collection on EEG norms as well as its variation with age, sex, ethnic groups, etc.

Though it may be difficult, if not impossible, for many African psychiatrists to acquaint themselves with recent advances in biological psychiatry, it is however, necessary for psychiatrists at the university teaching centers to update their knowledge in these areas. A new generation of psychiatrists must be created in order to bring psychiatry into the tradition of medicine. In agreement with Gold and Pottash (1986)[50], "dramatic changes in the self-identity of psychiatrists and the perception of psychiatrists are likely to follow the reintegration of psychiatry into medicine and incorporation of technological advances into the practice of psychiatry." Biological psychiatry should serve as adjuncts to the practice of clinical psychiatry in Africa.

REFERENCES

1. Ban, T.A. & OdeJide, A.O. (19801: Training in Biological Psychiatry: a WHO-sponsored long term program Health Community Information, 6 (2) 96-100.

2. Lishman, W.A. (1983). The apparatus of mind: brain structure, and function in mental disorder. Psychosomatics 24:699-726.

3. Freedman & Kaplan: Comprehensive Textbook of Psychiatry, second edition. Vol. 1. p. 489

4. Editorial Comment on: Neurotransmitters - their role in Neurological disorders. Hexagon (Roche) 7, No. 2 (1983).

5. Woods, S.M. (1986) In diagnosis and Laboratory testing in Psychiatry (eds). Mark S. Gold and A.L.C. Pottash p. vii.

6. German, A.G, (1972). Aspects of Clinical psychiatry in subsaharan Africa. Br. J. Psychiatry, 121, 461

7. Harding, T.W. (1977). Mental health research in Africa: Preliminary results of a questionnaire survey. Afr. J. Psychiatry 1, 2, 31-37.

8. Akindele, M.O. et al (1970): Mono-amine oxidase inhibitors and sleep. Electro enceph Clin. Neurophysiology 29:47-56.

9. Lewis, S.A. - and Akindele, M.O. et al (1970): Heroin ar~ human sleep. Electro enceph Clin. Neurophysiology. 28:374-381.

10. Akindele, M.O. Adeniyi, F.A. & Olatunbosun, D.A. (1976) . Serum Zinc in Schizophrenia in Nigerians. Afric. J. Psychiatry: 3: 379 380.

11. Osuntokun, B.0. (1969): Anticonvulsant therapy, folic acid deficiency and neuropsychiatric disorders. Br. Med. J. 2: 636-637.

12. Dhadphale, M. (1985). me frequency and distribution of psychiatric morbidity among patients attending district hospital out-patient clinics in Kenya., M.D. Thesis ,University of Nairobi.

13. Odejide, A.O., Olatawura, M.O. and Makanjuola, R.O. (1978): A psychiatric service in a Nigerian general hospital. Afr. J. of Psychiatry. 4(3 &4), 97-102.

14. Odejide, A.O. (1979). Cross-cultural Psychiatry: A myth or reality. Comprehensive Psychiatry 20(2), 103-109.

15. Makanjuola, R.A. (1985) Recurrent unipolar manic disorder in the Yoruba Nigerian: Further evidence. Brit. J. Psychiatry 147, 434-437.

16. Odejide, A.O. (1986) Standard Instruments used in the Assessment of Depression in Africa. A chapter in "Assessment of Depression" (eds.) Nbr~an Sartorius and Thomas A. Ban Springer-Verlag pp.55-59.

17. Johnstone, E.C., Crow, T.J., Frlth, C.D., Husband, J. and Kreel, L. (1976). Cerebral Ventricular Size and Cognitive impairment in Chronic Schizophrenia. Lancet, 11, 924-926.

18 . Reverley, M.A. (1985): Ventricular enlargement in Schizophrenia: The Validity of computerized Tomographic Findings. Br. J. Psychiatry 147, 233-240.

19. Kolakowska, T.A.O., Williams et al (1985): Schizophrenia with good and poor outcome I. British J. Psychiatry 146, 229-339.

20. Szasz, T. (1961): The Myth of Mental illness. New York, Hoeber-Herper;

21. Osuntokun, B.0. (1985) Biological factors in mental health in Nigerians. The Anumonye memorial Lecture, April, 1985. College of Medicine, University of Lagos, Nigeria.

22. Menschreck, T.C. (1981). Current concepts in Psychiatry: Schizophrenic disorders. New England J. Med. 305, 1628-16~2.

23. Wynne, L.C. and Singer, W.T. (1963 a & b): Thought disorder and family relations of schizophrenics. Archives cf General Psychiatry 9, 191-206.

24. Reveley, A.M., Reveley, M.A., Murray, R.M. (1984). Cerebral Ventricular enlargement in non-genetic schizophrenia: a controlled twin study. Br. J. Psychiatry. 144, 89-93.

25. Crow, T.J. (1984) A re-evaluation of the viral hypothesis: is psychosis the result of retroviral integration at a site close to the cerebral dominance gene? Br. J. Psychiatry. 145: 243-253.

26. Crow, T.J., Ferrier, I.M. Jobinstone, C.E. et al. (1979) Characteristics of patients with schizophrenia or neurological disorder and virus agent in cerebrospinal fluid. Lancet 1:842-4.

27. Osuntokun, B.O., Bademosi O., Ogunremi, K. and Wright, S.G. (1972) . The neuropsychiatric manifestations of typhoid fever in 959 Nigerians. Arch. Neurol., 27:9-13.

28. Muhangi, J.R. (1972). Functional or organic psychosis. 4 cases of typhoid fever initially presenting as various forms of psychiatric disorders. Afri. J. Med. Sci. 3:319-326

29. Crow, T.J. (1982). Two syndromes in schizophrenia? Trends in Neurosciences 351:4.

30. Leonhard, K: (1936). The classification of endogenous psychoses. 5th ed. (Irvington Press, New York, 1979).

31. The Report of the International Pilot study of Schizophrenia, (1973). Vol. I. W.H.o. Geneva.

32. Lishman, W.A. (1983). The apparatus of mind: brain structure and function in mental disorder. Psychosomatics, 24, 699-726.

33. Gold, M.S., Pottash, A.L.C., Exteian, L. (1981): Diagnosis of depression in the 1980s. JAMA 245:1562-1564.

34. Caroll, B.J., Feinberg M., Gredon JF, et al (1981): A s F cific laboratory test for the diagnosis of melancholia. Arch. Gen. Psychiatry 38:15122.

35. Extein, I, Pottash A.L.C., Gold, M.S. (1981): The thyrothropin-releasing hormone tegt in the diagnosis of unipolar depression. Psychiatry Res. 5: 311-316.

36. Hall, R.C.W., Popkin, M.K., Devaul R.A. et al (1978). Physical illness presenting as psychiatric disease. Arch. Gen. Psychiatry 35:1315.

37. Hall, R.C.W., Gardner, E.R., Popkin, M.K. et al (1981): Unrecognized physical illness prompting psychiatric admission: A prospective study. Am. J. Psychiatry 138:629.

38. Koranyi, E.K., (1979). Morbidity and rate of undiagnosed physical illness in a psychiatric clinic population. arch. Gen. Psychiatry 36: 414-419.

39. Abrams, R., Taylor M.A. (1976): Catatonia, a prospective clinical study. Arch. Gen. Psychiatry 33:579-581.

40. Abrams, R., Taylor, M.A. (1976):Catatonia, a prospective clinical study: Arch. Gen. Psychiatry. 33:579 81.

41. Gelenberg A (1976): The catatonlc syndrome. Lancet 1: 1339-1341.

42. Weddington, W.W., Marks R.C., Verghese. JP (1980) Disulfrian encephalopathy as a cause of catatonia syndrome. Am. J. Psychiatry. 137:1217-1219.

43. Odejide, A.O., Olatawura, N.O, and Makanjuola, R.O. (1978). A F psychiatric service in a Nigerian general Hospital. Afr. J. of Psychiatry. Vol 4 (3 & 4): 97-102.

44. Tuomisto. J. Tukiainan E. (1979): Decreased uptake of 5-droxytryptamine in blood platelets from patients with endogenous depression. Psychopharmacology 65:141-147.

45. Paul, S.M., Reharl, M. Skolnick, P, et al. (1981): Depressed patients have decreased binding of tritilated imipramine to platelet serotinin 'transporter'. Arch. Gen. Psychiatry 3&:1315-1321.

46. Verebey, K., Martin D. and Gold M.S. (1986): Drug Abuse. Interpretation of Laboratory Tests In Diagnostic and Laboratory Testing in Psychiatry (Eds) Mark S. Gold and A.L.C. Pottash, pp. 155-167.

47. Ogunremi, O.O. and Okonofua, F.E. (1977) Abuse of drugs among Nigerian youths; A University Experience. African Journal of Psychiatry, 3:107.

48. Odejide A.O. (1982) Problems of drug abuse in Nigeria: A review of the existing literature and suggestions on preventive measure. Nigerian Med. J. Vol. lo (1 & 2); 5-11.

49. Odejide, A.O. and Ban, T.A. (1982). Psychotropic drug prescription pattern in a developing country (Nigeria): The need for an essential psychotherapeutic drug list. Intenational Pharmacopsychiatry 17(3): 163-169.

50. Gold, M.S. and Pottash, A.L.C. (1986). Diagnostic and Laboratory Testing in Psychiatry. Plenum Medical Book Company p.7.

Chapter 10

Possible Cultural Variations in Adult Development

by

Samuel O. Okpaku, M.B.,Ch.B., Ph.D., M.R.C.P.(I), F.R.C.P.(C)
Associate Research Professor of Public Policy
and
Associate Clinical Professor of Psychiatry
Vanderbilt University,
Nashville, Tennessee
U.S.A.

INTRODUCTION

Previous ethnocentrism has given rise to attempts to identify similarities between different cultures. Simultaneously perhaps, following on the successful publication and television serialization of Roots by Alex Haley, there has been an increasing interest in individuals yearning for their roots. Concurrently there has been an upsurge of theories and studies on adult development. These theories may heuristically be classified into two categories. The first category applies to those that emphasize the uniqueness of the individual as he or she grows through the adult phase of life and the second category emphasizes the chronological significance of adult life. This paper is an attempt to contribute to this debate. I will point out contextual and structural cultural factors that are likely to influence adult life and hence result in possible cultural variations in adult development.

This will be done by (1) African ethnographic material largely drawing upon the work by LeVine amongst the Gusii of Kenya, (2) examples of common human conflicts, and (3) a brief description of an African funeral ceremony.

The following objectives will be attempted.

1. Attention will be drawn to the limitations of those theories that postulate, at least, implicitly, a "universal pathway" to adulthood.
2. It will be emphasized that superficial analogues of human experiences, behavior and conflicts with their solutions, while parallel, may differ in intensity and meaning in different cultural contexts.
3. It will be pointed out that with modernity, there are significant shifts in traditional behaviors, but that apparent contradictions are sometimes made intelligible in the light of the historical cultural backgrounds of the peoples involved in terms of their values, morals, beliefs, and traditional concepts.
4. Some cultural elements such as childbirth, childrearing, marriage, and old age are universal occurrences. It will be emphasized that the relative significance of the above elements for individuals vary from culture to culture, and sometimes within the same cultural context, the social meanings and implications of these elements may change significantly.
5. It will be demonstrated that while age, sex, and status factors occur in all cultures, their significances are relative to the social organization of the people concerned and the context of their social interactions.
6. It will be shown that domestic organizations change over time. Therefore the history of a people, together with the use of their resources and their social security systems, are important elements in adult development.

Different societies are likely to provide different opportunities for adult development, and hence they may define adulthood differently.

7. Lastly it will be argued that the above elements of adulthood are transmitted intergenerationally in a non-genetic sense. These transmissions can be discerned by individual self-examination and evaluation, observable public behavior, and major persistent preoccupations. The combination of all these elements sometimes shows only limited explicit rationales as in rituals and ceremonies. Hence the insights into these cultural factors are sometimes derived only from an analysis of intimate contact with the individuals, their families, and a working knowledge of the culture of those concerned. Also, these insights are more fully appreciated, either as an individual grows older and/or increases his or her knowledge of his or her cultural roots and heritage.

BACKGROUND ON ETHNOGRAPHIC MATERIAL

LeVine and the Gusii of Kenya: A Synopsis

LeVine has published extensively on the Gusii of Kenya based on his field research amongst those people. Some of his important observations can be found in his essay on "Adulthood Among the Gusii of Kenya." Briefly, he defined life span as "a people's collective representation of the life course viewed as an organized system of shared ideals about how life should be lived and shared expectancies about how lives are lived." He described the life course for Gusii males as consisting of the following stages: infant (ekenwerere), uncircumcised boy (omoisca), circumcised boy warrior (omomura), and a male elder (omogaaka). For females there is a parallel course. The infant phase (ekenwerere) is identical to that for the Gusii males. Then there are four additional phases (instead of the three phases for the men). These are as follows: uncircumcised girl (egesagaane), circumcised girl (omoiseke), married woman (omosubaati), and female elder (omonina). The labels to these stages imply various statuses, roles and expectations. For example, LeVine indicated that the label omoisca (uncircumcised boy), is used to convey the expectation of the boys in this age group to participate in tasks that involve herding the cattle under the supervision and guidance of their elders. According to LeVine, omomura (circumcised boy warrior), is derived from a word that means warrior. He further indicated that transition into this stage is the most important one for a Gusii male. Firstly, it implies the transition from dependency and intimacy with his mother to manhood. This is associated with military and personal responsibilities, as well as the opportunities for marriage. To commemorate this transition, the newly circumcised boy warrior's father takes a public oath not to punish him any more. Also, he is barred from his mother's house until he presents her with a goat and then only in the entrance to the foyer. This young warrior, according to LeVine, is expected to live in his own house in the homestead. The life stage of omomura terminates only when the man's first child marries. Based on his observations, LeVine has pointed out that depending on the time of marriage of the warrior, the time of birth of his first child, and the marriage of that child, the period of male warriorship may vary from about 15 to 30 years for various individuals. For Gusii females, the corresponding period consists of 2 phases, the circumcised girl (omoiseke), and the married woman (omosubaati). In the former phase the girl is prepared for marriage. According to LeVine, individuals in this phase are treated by their parents with ambivalence and suspicion. On one hand, the parents expect some compensation for their efforts in raising the girl and on the other hand, they fear she might elope, and they may hence lose the bride wealth. For the omosubaati (married woman), marriage is very predictable and occurs at approximately the same age for all Gusii females. This period in the life of a Gusii female, according to LeVine, is believed to be very difficult as she has to adjust to a homestead different from her own. A major event for her, however, is the circumcision of her first child of either sex and she attains the female elder stage (omonina) upon the marriage of her first child.

LeVine assets that the life span, with it's various stages, provides the scaffolding around which the Gusii life course evolves. It provides the statuses, the roles, the expectations, economic and reproductive careers and goals, as well as other life strategies to achieve their spiritual objectives.

At the structural level, LeVine has drawn the picture of a society where the homestead is a virilocal residence, polygamy is an ideal, and women had a good deal of autonomy deriving from their cultivation, their houses and the products of their farming. At the functional level, LeVine has also identified a variety of important tasks and ramifications. He emphasized that transitions during the life stage of the Gusii are not simply based on chronological age, especially after marriage. As an example he cites the fact that the transition from a young warrior to a male elder is determined by the combined factors of the age of his first marriage, and the age of the marriage of his first child. LeVine draws attention to the fact that these two events depend on the availability of cattle and their accumulation by the young warrior as bride wealth. Also, if his first child is a son or daughter, the factors that determine their marriage will therefore be different and provide variation in the life course of the adult warrior. Thus, LeVine identified a status hierarchy which in ascending order is as follows: "circumcised adults of each sex, those married with children, grandparents, grandparents with no living seniors of the same sex in the homestead." Here seniority is based on birth order and within each homestead it is then based on generational age.

According to LeVine, getting older is cherished, provided the different life stages are occurring approximately as expected. He states further that deviations from the time sequence, can be a source of concern. He cites the occurrence of the death of a male without a living son. In this instance his post-menopausal wife is allowed to "marry" a young woman who will have sexual relations with a local man in the hope that sons will be provided to continue the lineage. This is particularly necessary since daughters move away at marriage.

LeVine cites other important deviations from the age and time sequences and their potential consequences for the individual. He indicated that these deviations may be a source of psychological distress and may in fact result in public scorn. Examples of these deviations include delayed marriage, childbirth, lack of adequate proportion of daughters and sons, infertility and monogamy.

In addition to the age-time constraints, LeVine also cites the significance of sex constraints. He emphasizes the obligations imposed on the sons by the virilocal nature of the homesteads, eg. the sons continue to reside locally and the daughters move out of the homestead at marriage. This implies that often men have to carry the burden of ritual neglect by their forebears. One example cited by LeVine is that of an individual who for one or another reason did not complete the funeral rites of his parents prior to his own demise. This can provide the ancestral spirits with a motive to impose afflictions on his descendants.

Another important constraint is the birth order/sex constraint in cultures like the Gusii. This birth order/sex constraints indicate certain expectations. In addition to those expectations, they also furnish reference groups which enable the individual to evaluate himself and compare his or her development with other reference group members. According to LeVine, for the men, these are the individuals who were born around the same year and were circumcised together and continue to live in the homestead. For the female, these are initially the girls who were circumcised at the same time, but later, after marriage, the reference group composition will consist of co-wives, sisters-in-law, and other women in their new homestead. LeVine has emphasized the need to move along with one's mates and its significance in relation to "self evaluation, self esteem and life satisfaction."

Another important strand emphasized by LeVine has to do with the more private "goals and strategies" that relate to a spiritual life. He alludes to the energies and significance given to rituals, sacrifices and funeral rites. These may be an attempt to "placate the ancestral spirits, reverse family misfortunes, guard against infertility, sickness, and mental disorder and ensure continuity of the lineage." (Although LeVine rightly calls these activities the spiritual career, this author prefers to call them the healing activities.)

In summary, LeVine has described the structure and context of a cultural entity, the Gusii of Kenya. He has identified specific statuses and roles. He emphasized the fact that the transitions among the life stages are not simply based on chronological age, especially after marriage. He indicated that children confer status after marriage. According to LeVine, for the Gusii, the life plan consists of "marriage, birth and death occurring at the expected times with the expected results." He emphasized that deviations from these may expose the individual unfavorably to public "mockery, disgrace or loss of status." The reference groups of age and status serve as a basis for competition and comparisons. Nevertheless, according to LeVine, the culture provides safeguards for deviation from the normal. LeVine identified three important careers in the life of the Gusii. These are the procreative, the economic and the spiritual. In traditional Gusii culture, childbearing and production is an important life goal which is linked to the economic life goal of cattle rearing and accumulation of bride wealth. LeVine relates the spiritual careers as embodied in the aim to provide "invulnerability to spiritual dangers that may threaten the individual's and family's sanity, health, fertility, and economic welfare."

The structure and context provided by Gusii have analogues in various cultures ranging from Appalachian America, industrialized Japan, to a Swiss canton, or urban Africa. However, the expressions and social meanings of the "careers, goals, strategies and expectations" placed on adult individuals in these varied cultures are likely to differ significantly as to constitute a variation in adult development. This variation can be seen within the context of a transcultural psychiatry practice illustrated by the following very brief clinical vignettes and themes.

1. An Italian woman, in her middle age, who during an interview for social security disability broke down in tears and stated, "A mother can take care of 10 children, but 10 children cannot take care of one mother".
2. A 16 year old who was failing at school and had attempted suicide. Earlier in the year she had asked for a car from her parents. As a condition of buying the car for her, she had agreed to help in transporting her brothers and sisters from school and sport activities. Later on, she felt this commitment was an imposition. She preferred to drive her friends home after Saturday evening parties rather than comply with her parent's wishes. A possible solution was suicide.
3. An African young man with a master's degree. He had an episode of psychosis. After recovery, he expressed intense feelings of guilt for not being at home to take care of his mother. This was in spite of frequent financial contributions to her upkeep as well as the

fact that he had helped support a younger relative through college.

4. A white American who had a history of drug abuse and a jail term. He was in his thirties. The only relationship he had had was with a prostitute who he described as his girlfriend. He was immature and extremely dependent on his mother.

Further examples can be provided by citing some human conflicts with cultural overtones in "everyday psychopathology".

1. A young male Nigerian pilot who was visiting the United States was informed of the recent premature retirement of his aunt from her Civil Service job. His immediate comment was "I must return home immediately".
2. A retired Nigerian who cherishes the fact that for the first time in his life he is living in his own home and the retired Nigerian civil servant whose only preoccupation is to complete his house in his home town.
3. Lord Kitchener, the West Indian Calypso singer in one of his ballads sang, "If your mother and your wife were drowning, I wonder which you will be saving".

The therapeutic management of the clinical cases and the private resolution of the above anecdotes are likely to vary from culture to culture. This realization is very real and graphic for any individual who has spent a significant amount of time away from his/her home and has to return either for a brief visit or during a period of family crisis such as a funeral.

A Critique of LeVine's Ethonograpic Material

LeVine's ethnographic material is excellent in many ways. However, he seems to have paid little attention to what I consider important strands in the Gusii and other related African cultures such as the Dahomeans, the Yorubas and the Oras of West Africa.

Here I am referring to the following features:

1. The coexistence of the sacred and the secular.
2. An extended kinship system.
3. A cosmological representation of terrestrial arrangements.
4. A continuation of lineage.
5. A filial-pietal relationship in which parents are committed to taking care of their children who in turn will respect and take care of their parents in a reciprocal fashion.

Some of the above features, as indicated by Meyer Fortes, contribute to a major moral and social code in relationship to one's parents and kinship groups as well as ancestral spirits. This code also provides the basis for responsibility and hence the relative absence of guilt[2]. But more especially, this author believes that this religious-ethical framework provides a major opportunity for healing. An illustration of this is a funeral rite which I observed a few years ago. The deceased was a prominent Nigerian who died in his early 80's. The family is a Christian family. Just before his burial the family (extended kinship) was assembled at the instruction of the elders. The deceased only surviving brother was then invited to present his side of a dispute that he had with his deceased brother. He defended himself and maintained that his actions were appropriate and right. The elders insisted that he should pay a fine so as to enable the deceased to feel satisfied and depart in peace and harmony. This was no dramatization but was a real and emotionally laden session. Subsequently, the deceased sons and daughters were seen individually at the same meeting. Each one attempted to give an account of his or her relationship to their father. If the elders were aware of any conflict, this was brought to the open for discussion. If there was an apparent conflict, the individual was closely interviewed to the point of setting up a hypothetical conflict and each was asked how he or she took care of their father during his lifetime. This occasion provided resolution of conflicts and opportunity for individual healing, family healing and community healing. Therefore, the influence of the spiritual basis of the aforementioned features cannot be minimized as they together provide the basis and explanation for the understanding of the contextual nature of these cultures.

Illustrations of Common Human Conflicts

1. The Italian woman obviously is lamenting her disappointment at her children not fulfilling some reciprocal expectations. This illustrates an intergenerational conflict.
2. The 16 year old white female in attempting to gain her "autonomy" prefers to invest, in an "external economy" rather than contribute to the family or "internal economy". Another example of conflict in this area is the young woman's contention to stay out as late as she pleased without parental control.
3. The Nigerian professional is conflicted over his responsibility to take care of his mother at all costs and feels he has betrayed his mother by staying abroad.
4. The 30 year old American of Italian or Irish background illustrates a "developmental" arrest which speculatively could have been ameliorated perhaps by some form of participation in a state sanctioned activity such as national service. Here the society may provide opportunities for attaining maturity.
5. The young Nigerian pilot is deeply committed to family relationships beyond the nuclear family.
6. The prominent Nigerian in his 60's who frequently referred to the first time he was living in his own house rather than in official quarters and the retired Nigerian whose remaining life preoccupation was the completion of his house in his home village is an illustration of the significance of having a home to return to before death. Incidentally, for an elder not to have such a home in his village is considered a potentially serious disgrace and a source of mockery and anger. Such an individual, if he happens to be the head of the clan or subclan, may not officiate in the settlement of disputes, etc., unless he owns a house where such meetings can be held. It is unthinkable that such an individual dies prior to the possession of his own house as his funeral rites will be marred by the disgrace.

7. Lord Kitchener continues his ballad - "you can always get another wife, but you can't always get another mother."

SUMMARY

In summary, therefore, between life and death and also possibly beyond, there are different trajectories and different stage expectations in the life plan of a culture, and these factors have contextual implications.

A people's historical antecedent may color their life expectations. The definition of the beginning of adulthood and its end may vary with different cultures. Sometimes these variations may actually be physiological, e.g. the age of menarche is occurring earlier now than before. Such changes may influence the timing of rites of passage, e.g. circumcision or marriage.

The influence of modernity may alter the practice of those rites which previously clearly signal different life stages. Different cultures view different rites of passage differently. There are intergenerational aspects of different cultures that produce different psychological subjectives, e.g. the significance of polygamy in some societies is not the potential opportunity to be permitted to have more than one wife, but rather the paternal responsibility for parenting. In other words out of wedlock children are discouraged, and the culture affirms the right of every child to a father.

Different cultures vary with respect to accessibility to resources which may impact on domestic and social security arrangements. What are the possible consequences of the cultures of overcrowded nations, and what are the consequences of island or mountain dwelling for the respective populations?

Cultures may also vary in terms of the balance between the traditional and non-traditional position. In the traditional situation, the usual relevant question is, "How am I going to carry out this task?" Whilst in the non-traditional situation, the issue is really,"You don't have to do this." The emotional catharsis' in both instances are different.

Lastly, though it may sound redundant, we should bear in mind that the elements of culture are dynamic and may change at different historical and political points. In the United States, we are witnessing a trend towards young adults staying longer at home for financial reasons and also increased single parenthood. All these may influence social interrelationships and hence may change the norms of society.

CONCLUSION

The use of the musical metaphor aptly clarifies the above points. Music essentially consists of tempo, pitch, and tone; these are irrespective of culture. In other words, the essential ingredients of the West Indian calypso, the Nigerian nightlife, the South American samba, and the Viennese classical music are the same in being an aggregate of tempo, pitch and tone. However, the different expressions of those culturally distinct forms are indisputable and in their differences they are capable of producing different psychological effects. My message, therefore, is that individuals from different cultures may have distinctive life goals and hence different life plans in reaching these goals. These life plans are based on value systems, social roles, the resources of the society, the social security system, and the historical antecedents of the society, amongst other factors. For example, in Japanese culture, the emphasis is on interdependence rather than dependence, and resolution of conflicts is, I believe, by consensus. Other examples include the characterizations of children of the American economic depression of the 1920's or the shame and guilt of contemporary Japanese which are traceable to the experiences of the second World War.

The above, therefore, have implications for psychiatry. With respect to training entrants to the disciplines, they should, very early in their career, be exposed to training and education in the areas of cultural psychiatry. This should not be a once and for all phenomenon because we, even as cultural psychiatrists, have our own stereotypes. An important approach, therefore, is to assume that each patient has his or her own "culture" which needs to be understood within the therapeutic context as we work to bring relief to the individual.

REFERENCES

1. LeVine, Robert A. 1980. Adulthood among the Gusii of Kenya in Themes of Work and Love in Adulthood, Smelser, N. J. and Erikson, E. H. Harvard University Press.

2. Fortes, M. 1960. Oedipus and Job in West African Religion in Anthropology of Folk Religion.ed. Leslie C. Vantage Books, New York.

OTHER READINGS

LeVine, Robert A. 1959. Gusii sex offenses: a study in social control. American Anthropologist, 61:12-59.

LeVine, Robert A. and LeVine, Barbara B. 1966. Nyansongo: a Gusii community in Kenya. New York: Wiley; rpt. Kreeger, 1977.

LeVine, Sarah. 1979. Mothers and wives: Gusii women of East Africa. Chicago: University of Chicago Press.

Chapter 11

The Emergence of Psychological Discourse in Kenya

by

Marie Coleman Nelson,
Director of Training,
A*mani Counselling Centre,*
Nairobi, Kenya

ABSTRACT

The author discusses the recent appearance in Kenyan popular culture of a psychological orientation. The evolving complexities of social organization in Kenya compel individuated redefinitions of the self to clarify its transitional nature. Two examples are couples who must consider family planning outside the context of traditional values and patients with new presentations of psychopathology. The popularity of newspaper advice columns attests not only to the need for counseling, but to alterations in the structures of consciousness.

INTRODUCTION

This paper is a condensation of a longer report that discusses the recent appearance in Kenya popular culture of a psychological orientation and a growing tendency toward psychological inquiry by emotionally disturbed members of the relatively literate public and by workers in the mental health field and related professions.

The notable proliferation since 1984 of psychiatric and psychological articles and newspaper advice columns and the ever-increasing patient load in the counseling center where I work not only indicate a felt need in society for education in this area, but, from a civilizational viewpoint, signify profound alterations in the structures of consciousness and conscience. In place of the metaphoric allusions formerly employed to convey inner states or held opinions—enigmatic weavings through parables, maxims, and/or folktales to express a point—one tends to find much less of the ambiguity that must have contributed to Carothers' observation (1953) of a "lack of personal integration which has become the clearest feature of African mentality."

THE KENYAN IN CIVILIZATIONAL TRANSITION

Styles of communication—like styles of courtship and definitions of love (de Rougement, 1956; Leites, 1986)— vary between different historic periods and different cultures. In the West, too, before the twentieth century, slight attention was given to attitudes toward inner states (except in the domains of philosophy, religion, and ethics).

Indeed, just as the physical sciences require an expanding lexicon, the evolving complexities of social organization in Kenya and other parts of Africa compel individuated redefinitions of the self that clarify the contemporary self in transition, a self that cannot remain embedded in or bound by conventions of the traditional past. For, given accelerated change, these archaic precepts lose vitality with each succeeding generation. However, today's Kenyan may cherish his cultural heritage, and his daily experiences confront him with the task of understanding himself and his relationships in a dynamic experimental context and of making his peace with the paradoxical aspects of civilization transition.

Various forces and circumstances precipitate alterations in the self concept and, through such revisions, the emergence of what may be regarded as psychological or introspective thinking. Two examples may suffice.

First, the present intensive government campaign for family planning curbs Kenya's perilously high birth rate and opposes the powerful tradition that accords status to bearing of many children and no status whatsoever to childless women of child-bearing age, be they married or single. Regardless of the religious issues involved, the decision to exercise birth control is ultimately a matter of personal responsibility. Couples targeted by the injunction are obliged to act unilaterally—that is, to isolate themselves psychologically in the immediate present and to experimentally sample how it feels to distance themselves from a traditional norm still actively espoused by family and community elders. Unlike the tangible rewards of upward mobility, husband and wife are obliged to revisualize themselves psychosocially, to link themselves less to the past and more to the future, regardless of their decision in the matter.

Another type of pervasive influence on psychic life may be at work in the process of symptom formation. In a paper in this collection, Fazal and Shah cite four cases of African men with monosymptomatic olfactory delusions, a clinical condition hitherto unreported in Kenyan psychiatry. Observing that the typically bland diet of Kenyans contains no spices or condiments—which might cause bodily odors—the authors note that the current barrage of commercial and television advertising of deodorants and perfumes may well influence the content, albeit not the structure, of delusional phenomena. Given the predisposition in the culture to somatize emotional difficulties, it will be interesting to monitor whether parallel advertising and television campaigns directed toward women encourage narcissistic symptoms associated with body image.

There is considerable criticism in newspaper columns of young Kenyans for attempting to ape their Western counterparts. Such identification with Western models may indeed take place through repeated exposure of Kenyan audiences to certain modes of behavior in films, for instance, and through processes characteristic in the films' countries of origin. More significantly, however, the symbolic structures, which typically inform the viewer's fantasy life, may undergo modification through unconscious incorporation of implicit cultural directives underlying the dramatic film enactments. Thus, the prominent emphasis in American scenarios on psychologically interpretive, self-revelatory data may well contribute indirectly to the development of psychological thought in this country.

AMANI COUNSELING CENTER

When the Amani Counseling Center was founded in 1979, its clients were predominantly expatriates. Today, both our clients and candidates in training are predominantly Kenyan.

In 1983, we offered several workshop courses for the public. In 1984, we initiated a unified training program in psychotherapeutic counseling. In 1985, we pioneered the first newspaper advice column in the nation. Hundreds of communications have been received from all parts of the country, even from readers in Uganda and Tanzania, asking for help with almost every conceivable type of emotional problem and generally describing the condition in great detail. According to some correspondents, the very existence of such columns reduces anxiety for the many persons who privately believe they are mad until they read letters by others with similar pathology and crazy thoughts. This revelation alone, in a community of fellow sufferers, helps them to feel less isolated.

CONCLUSIONS

Modernization poses a variety of inescapable dilemmas, which the individual, unequipped with psychological understanding—the ability to examine, identify, and objectify his psychic processes—will simply endure as confusion, frustration, alienation, feelings of guilt, depression, psychosomatic disorder, or periodic psychotic breakdown.

Whether Carothers' blanket assessment of 1953 of the Africans' lack of personal integration was actually true at that time or whether, as I suspect, he projected his own Western expectations of a corresponding style of communication on to Africans and failed to grasp, much less interpret, their metaphoric mode of discourse, we may never know. Clearly, the present period indicates cross-cultural accommodation between the two forms.

REFERENCES

Carothers, J. C.: The African Mind in Health and Disease: A Study in Ethnopsychiatry. World Health Organization monograph series No. 17. Geneva, Switzerland, WHO, 1953, p. 107

de Rougement, D.: Love in the Western World. Translated by Belgion, M. Princeton, N.J., Princeton University Press, 1983

Leites, E.: The Puritan Conscience and Modern Sexuality. New Haven, Conn., U.S.A., Yale University Press, 1986

Chapter 12

Epidemiology of Medical Disorders in Kenya

by

Manohar Dhadphale, MD, PhD
Senior Lecturer
Department of Psychiatry
Faculty of Medicine
University of Nairobi
Nairobi, Kenya

ABSTRACT

The author describes some of the important findings of a nationwide study on the prevalence of mental disorders in Kenya. Four district hospitals were chosen, and a research team screened randomly selected outpatients who were seeking help for physical problems. Using a two-stage screening procedure that employed locally validated instruments, the author estimated that a quarter of the primary care attenders had psychiatric disorders. By asking questions significantly correlated with psychiatric morbidity, the primary health care worker can identify psychiatric cases, thereby improving mental health care and decreasing visits by chronic psychiatric patients.

INTRODUCTION

Psychiatrists in Kenya have consistently estimated that the prevalence of psychiatric disorders among general outpatients is high (Mustafa, 1974; Muya and Muhangi, 1976), but there are no reliable data on the true magnitude of psychiatric morbidity among patients at primary health care clinics. With the aim of providing such vital information, the author commenced this study in 1980. The following hypotheses were tested:

1. The prevalence of psychiatric morbidity among primary health care attenders at district hospitals is high.

2. Most patients with psychiatric problems present themselves with physical symptoms; only a few report psychological problems. When specifically asked, however, many admit to having such complaints.

3. The majority of mental cases are not recognized as psychiatric disorders (hidden psychiatric morbidity) by primary health care workers, whether they are physicians, clinical officers, medical assistants, or clinic nurses. Accordingly, such patients typically receive only symptomatic treatment for their presenting somatic symptoms or undergo multiple investigations, often expensive and fruitless.

The author also determined variables significantly related to psychiatric morbidity, which can help the primary health care worker identify psychiatric cases and thereby improve delivery of mental health services in Kenya and other developing countries, which share similar problems in both urban and rural health clinics.

METHOD

A two-stage procedure was used to detect and confirm cases of psychiatric disorders among patients attending filter outpatient clinics in the Kenyan district hospitals at Kisii, Kisumu, Meru, and Voi.

A locally validated version of the Self-Rating Questionnaire of Harding et al. (1980) was used to detect potential psychiatric cases. The suspected cases were then confirmed by the author during interviews with the Standardized Psychiatric Interview of Goldberg et al. (1970). A standard severity scale was used to rate the degree of incapacity in the identified psychiatric cases. For psychiatric diagnosis, ICD-8 (WHO, 1965) definitions were followed (see Figure 1).

Figure 1

TWO-STAGE SCREENING PROCEDURE FOR IDENTIFYING PSYCHIATRIC MORBIDITY IN 881 PRIMARY CARE PATIENTS IN KENYA

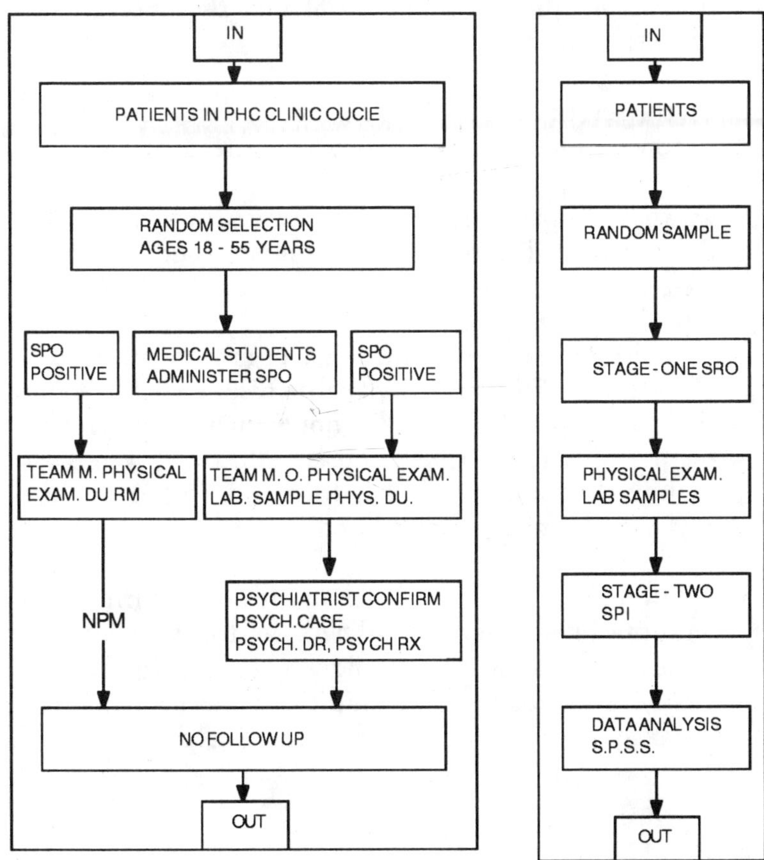

The subjects were 881 primary care patients between 18 and 55 years of age who were selected randomly (nondiagnostic queue-based triage). The entire sample was physically examined by the medical team. Basic laboratory tests (blood count, urine and stool analysis, and malaria smear) were done for all psychiatric cases. The investigators collected data on clinical and demographic variables, history of drug use, and other relevant information for all cases. The data were analyzed with the Statistical Package for the Social Sciences (SPSS) (Nie et al., 1975).

FINDINGS

The significant findings were as follows:

1. Of 881 patients screened in the general medical outpatient queue, 220 (25.0%) met the criteria for psychiatric cases.

2. On the severity scale, 64% of the cases were ruled mild, 28% were moderate, and 8% were severe cases.

3. Of the 220 patients with psychiatric disorders, 85% did not have discernible organic illness, but 15% did have associated physical disorders.

4. Psychoneuroses were the most common group of disorders (58.2% of the psychiatric cases and 14.5% of the total sample). These diagnoses included neurotic depression and anxiety neurosis. Affective psychosis, mainly the manic type, was found in 15.5% of the psychiatric cases (see Table I and Figure 2).

5. A number of indicators were significantly correlated with psychiatric morbidity. The indicators were longer duration of illness, slightly older age group (36 to 55 years), previous visits to traditional healers, longer distance traveled, and more frequent visits to clinics.

The items on the Self-Rating Questionnaire that significantly distinguished the patients with psychiatric disorders from the other patients are listed in Table I, as are items that failed to distinguish the two groups. Sex, marital status, number of children, area of residence (rural or semi-urban), and education did not significantly differ between the psychiatric and nonpsychiatric groups. Fewer than 4% of the patients with psychiatric disorders had been suspected by the primary health care worker to have psychiatric problems (had conspicuous psychiatric morbidity) or were receiving psychotropic medication.

Table I

SQR RESPONSE OF PM PATIENTS

(A) Questions with significant correlation with PM Cases	
I. Do you feel unhappy?	P < 0.00
II. Do you have trouble in thinking?	P < 0.00
III. Do you sleep badly?	P < 0.00
IV. Do your hands shake?	P < 0.00
V. Do you feel nervous, tense and worried?	P < 0.00
VI. Do you cry more than usual?	P < 0.00
VII. Do you find it difficult to enjoy your daily activities?	P < 0.01
VIII. Are you frightened?	P < 0.02
IX. Have you lost interest in things?	P < 0.05
X. Are you unable to play a useful part in life?	P < 0.00
XI. Has the thought of ending your life been in your mind?	P < 0.00

(B) Questions with no significant correlation with PM cases	
I. Do you often have headaches?	N.S
II. Is your appetite poor?	N.S
III. Is your indigestion poor?	N.S
IV. Do you find it difficult to make decisions?	N.S
V. Do you feel you are a worthless person?	N.S
VI. Do you feel tired all the time?	N.S
VII. Do you have an uncomfortable feeling in the stomach?	N.S
VIII. Are you easily tired?	N.S
IX. Is your daily work suffering?	N.S

Table II

PSYCHIATRIC DIAGNOSES OF ICD-8

HOSPITAL	295	296	300.0 300.2	300.1	300.4	301	291/303	Other	TOTAL PM
KISII	3	8	12	1	12	2	8	2	48
KISUMU	3	9	15	2	22	2	7	1	61
MERU	6	8	14	1	23	3	8	2	65
VOI	2	9	12	1	13	3	5	1	46
ALL	14(6.3)	34(15.4)	53(24)	5(2.2)	70(31.8)	10(4.5)	28(12.7)	6(2.7)	220(100)
TOTAL SAMPLE	1.5	3.8	6.0	0.5	7.9	1.1	3.1	0.6	24.9
Contribution	1.33	0.99	0.28	included with "other"	1.4 9	0.63	0.79	0.21	5.71

Note: (1) No significant difference was noted on any diagnosis. (11) Figures in brackets are % of PM.

Legend:
- 291 Alcoholic psychosis
- 295 Schizophrenia
- 296 Affective psychosis (MDP)
- 300.0 Anxiety neurosis
- 300.1 Hysteria
- 300.2 Phobic neurosis
- 300.4 Depressive neurosis
- 301 Personality disorder
- 303 Alcoholism

Other - suspected drug dependence & organic psychosis

Figure 2
PROFILE OF PSYCHIATRIC DIAGNOSES AMONG 881 PRIMARY CARE PATIENTS IN KENYA

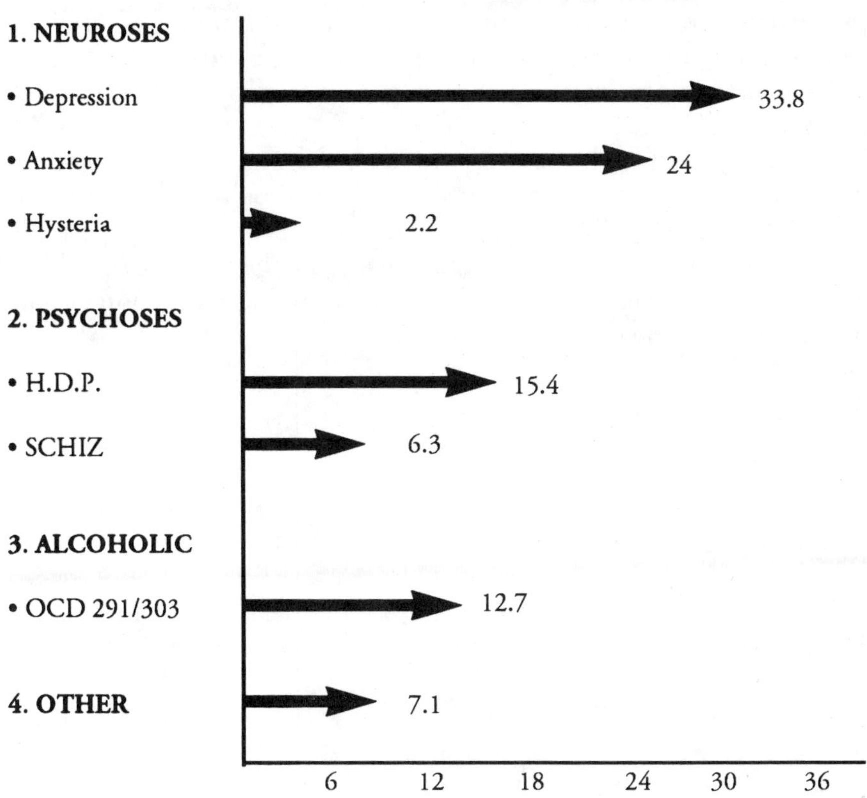

CONCLUSIONS

In light of these findings, it appears possible for the primary health care worker to use the differentiating queries to identify psychiatric cases. In the author's view, the primary health care worker can also manage these patients in the rural clinic setting or at the primary health care level, nearer patients' homes. Involvement of a social

To improve the mental health care delivery system, training primary care workers to detect psychiatric disorders should be considered; attention to the indicators identified above should be included. If possible, this process should be supplemented with psychiatrists' visits to rural clinics and with the training of primary health care workers at the health center or dispensary in the use of Essex and Gosling's charts (1983) as guides to correct diagnosis and management.

Not only could such measures improve the mental health services in rural areas but, in the author's view, they would also reduce the size of the general clinic load by reducing repeat visits by patients with chronic psychiatric disorders. Finally, in the days of shrinking health budgets, these steps would conserve our scarce resources and maximize the value of skilled manpower.

REFERENCES

Essex, B., Gosling, H.: An algorithmic method for management of mental health problems in developing countries. British Journal of Psychiatry 143:451-459, 1983

Goldberg, D. P., Cooper, B., Eastwood, M. R., et al.: A standardized psychiatric interview. British Journal of Preventive and Social Medicine 24:18-23, 1970

Harding, T. W., DeArango, M. V., Baltazar, J., et al.: Mental disorders in primary health care: a study of their frequency and diagnosis in four developing countries. Psychological Medicine 10:231-234, 1980

Mustafa, G.: Mental health and mental disorders, in Health and Disease in Kenya (Edited by Vogel et al.) Nairobi, Kenya, East African Publishing House, 1974

Muya, W., Muhangi, J. M.: Mental health services in Kenya. Presented at an APA workshop in Lusaka, Zambia, 1976

Nie, N. H., Hull, C. H., Jenkins, J. G., et al.: Statistical Package for the Social Sciences (SPSS). New York U.S.A., McGraw-Hill, 1975

World Health Organization: International Classification of Diseases, 8th revision (ICD-8). Geneva, Switzerland, WHO, 1965

Chapter 13

The Role of EEG in Diagnosis and Management of Nuerotic Disorders in Nairobi

by

S. G. GATERE, MD,
Department of Psychiatry,
Faculty of Medicine,
University of Nairobi,
Nairobi, Kenya

ABSTRACT

EEGs were performed on 119 neurotic patients in Nairobi, Kenya. The percentage of patients 17 or older who had theta waves was comparable to the proportion among patients 12 to 16 years old, indicating questionable physiological maturity. The four cases described improved after treatment with anticonvulsants alone or in combination. These findings, although preliminary, should sensitize psychiatrists to the possibility of biophysiological factors in the etiology of neurotic disorders.

INTRODUCTION

This paper originated from my observation that a considerable number of patients referred to psychiatrists by general practitioners in Nairobi were diagnosed with what we categorize as "neurosis." The patients had been thoroughly examined and had been treated for these ailments for long periods without much success.

My interest arose from the clinical observation of the failure-to-cope syndrome, which was characteristic of patients with different neurotic disorders. A similar situation was seen in form II and III schools, among children aged 14 to 16 who had previously been brilliant. Many of these children declined academically. Many were diagnosed as hysterical, as delinquent, or as having behavior disorders. These children also developed failure-to-cope syndrome as they reached adolescence and perhaps went to boarding school. The condition was also seen in students at the O, A, and university levels. Previously brilliant students seemed unable to cope well, especially at examination time.

RESEARCH

Encephalograms (EEGs) were performed on 119 neurotic patients. In this paper I present preliminary results. The age and sex distribution of 115 patients is shown in Table I. The EEG wave patterns changed at 12 to 15 years of age. Theta waves dominated until this maturational point (4-7 Hz; 5-7 Hz). The emotional capacity to handle problems seemed impaired in those who had more theta waves than expected for their age. I wondered whether the EEG patterns of the older patients would relate to those of the patients 12 to 16 years old. Among the patients who were 17 or older, 67% had EEGs with theta waves. At these ages, only 10% of the general population have theta waves. The percentage among these older patients was compared to that found in the patients 12 to 16 years old, indicating questionable physiological maturity. This could, then, be part of the explanation of their emotional immaturity, which is associated with a lower stress threshold. It may have resulted in failure to cope and been manifested as various neurotic disorders.

Table I

AGE AND SEX DISTRIBUTION OF 115 NEUROTIC PATIENTS IN NAIROBI

AGE RANGE (years)	MALE	FEMALE	TOTAL NUMBER	PERCENT
12-16	20	19	39	33.9
17-30	26	13	39	33.9
31-40	6	14	20	17.4
41-50	2	4	6	5.2
51-60	7	4	11	9.6
Total	61	54	115	100.0

The conditions observed among these patients included obsessive neurosis, phobia, hysteria, depression, and hypochondriasis. The relationship between theta waves and specific signs and symptoms is shown in Table II.

The acute form of the failure-to-cope syndrome has been called brain fag syndrome, which occurs in students and is characterized by reductions in sleep, concentration, memory, temper threshold (i.e., increased irritability), energy, interest in general, appetite for food and sex, positive mood, and work output. This results in academic decline. In other cases, maladaptive traits develop to enable the individual to survive and cope with the psychologically perceived stress. These are the cases we refer to as neuroses, in the psychological realm, or psychosomatic disorders, in the physical realm.

Table II

RELATIONSHIP BETWEEN EEG THETA WAVES AND THE SIGNS AND SYMPTOMS OF 119 NEUROTIC PATIENTS IN NAIROBI

SIGN/ SYMPTOM	THETHA 6 - 7	THETHA 5 - 7	THETHA 4 - 7	TOTAL	(%)
HEADACHE	5	8	3	25	21.0%
DEPRESSION	5	7	7	19	15.9%
SEIZURES	4	2	12	18	15.6%
REDUCED CONCENTRATION	2	4	5	11	8.8%
PSYCHOTIC SYMPTOMS	1	2	7	10	8.4%
DIZZYNESS	3	2	3	8	6.7%
INSOMNIA	3	1	3	7	5.8%
MENTAL PROBLEMS	1	3	1	5	4.2%
BRAIN INJURY	–	2	1	3	2.5%
INFECTION	1	2	–	3	2.5%
PANIC ATTACK	–	1	1	2	1.6%
DYSANNESIA	–	2	–	2	1.6%
NAUSEA	–	1	–	1	0.8%

CASE STUDIES

The following four case studies are discussed in relation to the manifestation of specific neurotic symptoms.

Case 1: Hysteria.

A. N., a 16-year-old girl in form III, had hysterical periods during which she would hyperventilate and have palpitations and hot flashes. Sometimes she felt pain in her chest and would have extreme dyspnea with a sense of choking in her throat. She could not concentrate and declined academically

During hyperventilation, A. N.'s EEG showed a burst of slow and sharp waves through all regions. They were bilaterally synchronous and symmetrical, with occasional slow waves showing markedly on the left side. Nine weeks later there was marked excess of diffuse slow activity, occasionally appearing with central and postcentral emphasis. Six months later the EEG showed a marked excess of widespread activity, and ventilation activated bursts and discharges of slow and sharp waves through all regions. The waves were bilaterally synchronous and symmetrical.

A. N. was treated with anticonvulsants, especially carbamazepine, for 12 months. She was excused from strenuous physical activities and is now well, having passed her level exams.

Case 2: Phobic Neurosis.

S. G. M., a 26-year-old university graduate, presented with phobic neurosis (social phobia), which made it impossible for him to teach at the college where he was employed. Students had to look at him, which made him shake and tremble with uncontrollable fear and, thus, abandon the lesson.

An EEG showed occasional bursts and discharges of slow and symmetrical wave activity through all areas. He was treated with carbamazepine (800 mg/day) and trifluoperazine (10 mg/day) for 12 months and is now well.

Case 3: Behavior Disorder.

C. K. was 15 years old and presented with behavior disorder. She was aggressive and picked fights. Her only complaint was an intractable headache, and she was found to be irritable and to have poor concentration.

The initial EEG showed no sharp or spike wave activity. However, a marked excess of slow waves was noted. After 3 months, a slight excess of diffuse slow frequencies was noted, but no discharges were observed.

Treated with anticonvulsants, including carbamazepine and phenytoin, C. K. improved. Her behavior was better, and she had no complaints.

Case 4: Narcolepsy.

J. N. was a 20-year-old young woman who slept excessively and would fall asleep while people were talking to her. She had a very poor academic record and experienced severe headaches. Diagnoses of hypothalamic lesion and Kleine-Levin syndrome were considered.

An EEG showed low- to moderate-voltage slow wave activity at 3-7 Hz through all areas, which was attenuated by visual stimuli. J. N. was treated with carbamazepine (600 mg/day) and is now well and back to work.

CONCLUSION

Although this paper has not provided the in-depth information necessary in a work with major implications for the management of some of the most common psychiatric disorders—namely the neuroses—it has attempted to sensitize psychiatric professionals to the importance of considering biophysiology, especially neurophysiology, in determining the etiology of neurotic disorders. Further, since anticonvulsants, such as carbamazepine, influence the stability of slow brain waves, they should be considered as an important component in the chemotherapy of psychiatric disease, especially the neuroses.

Chapter 14

Major Mental Illness in Two Kenyan Outposts

by

Lawrence E. Banta, MD
Department of Psychiatry,
School of Medicine,
Creighton University,
Omaha, Nebraska,
U.S.A.

ABSTRACT

The author served as a general practice physician in two rural districts in Kenya. The Pokot tribe had experienced many cultural disruptions and severe drought. They had lost the ability to grieve effectively, and psychosomatic illnesses were common. The Samburu District had undergone much cultural change but fewer major disasters; both major mental illness and psychosomatic illness were less common than in the West Pokot District. Psychosocial interventions with these populations included designing ways to solve specific social problems caused by cultural transition, e.g., helping the Pokot redevelop effective mourning practices.

INTRODUCTION

Over a 20-month period from mid-1982 to early 1984, I served as a general practice physician in two clinics in rural Kenya. One clinic was in the West Pokot District and the other in the Samburu District. The clinics were both primary health clinics, set up to care for basic health needs and not specifically for mental health. Each was run by a clinic doctor, a nurse, and paramedical staff. I reviewed the records for the approximately 17,000 patient visits registered while I worked in these clinics to determine a rough prevalence of mental disorder and to assess the need for mental health facilities or local mental health programs.

These areas are representative in many ways of the typical disruptions prevalent in many of the tribal societies, especially in Africa. I will first present an overview of each area and then look at the rough incidence of mental disorder in these areas.

WEST POKOT DISTRICT

West Pokot is in the northwest portion of Kenya on the border with Uganda. Many of the Pokot tribal people freely cross the border into Uganda and do not seem to recognize that they are subjects of the Kenyan government.

This area is relatively isolated. At the time of my work there, the majority of the population was living more than 100 miles from the nearest government health center. This has changed recently with the opening of several government clinics in the territory.

The Pokot are a tribe that has experienced a number of social and cultural disruptions over the past several decades. Because of overgrazing and sporadic rainfall, the soil has become very dry and much less productive than it formerly was. From 1979 through 1981, the severe drought resulted in a major famine. This affected nearly every family, and most families experienced the death of at least one member. The Pokot are also frequently at war with neighboring tribes.

The basic economic system of the Pokot tribe uses cattle rather than money. It has been traditional for the tribes in that area to raid other tribes to steal cattle and bring them to their own territories. Over the past 10 years, sophisticated weapons have been obtained by many of the tribes in the area, including grenades and machine guns. This has greatly increased the morbidity and mortality associated with cattle raids and has also increased the already tremendous fear that is prevalent whenever it becomes known a raid is imminent.

During a raid some years ago, an enemy tribe attacked the Pokot just after all the young men had been circumcised. The tribe suffered a great defeat and there was a tremendous loss of lives. Because of this, much of the rite of passage for young males was discontinued. At the present time, the government is attempting to curtail the rite of passage for young women, which also includes circumcision and has been outlawed by the Kenyan government.

During the one year I lived in this area there were episodic increases in certain types of illness. One such type, praan mut, was only the complaint of a headache. At first I felt this might represent a subclinical form of malaria, which was quite prevalent in this area, or be simply a headache. It became obvious that these headaches occurred when the society was under a great deal of stress, either from threatened raids or from late or ineffective rains. As I began to learn some of the language, I found that it was very deficient in several areas related to emotional expression. There was no way to adequately describe anxiety, depression, or various moods or feelings. As in many tribal areas, these moods and feeling were described more in a somatic sense than in terms of emotion. For example, headaches might mean anxiety, feelings I can't express, depression, etc. Also, pain in the liver or stomach could represent these types of feelings. I did not find any tendency to relate specific organs to specific feelings, other than an association between the heart and extreme sadness.

This society, owing to famines and subsequent disasters, had also lost the ability to grieve effectively for those who died. When I first arrived in the area, it was common practice, after a time of wailing, to simply throw the deceased into the nearest ditch and leave. No further mention was made, especially if it were an infant. Adults and the elderly were generally left in the huts where they died, and the entire village would simply relocate. In the past, the fathers had usually had no part in the grief or in the care of small children. When asked about this, many of them told me that they did not want to become too attached to something they might lose.

Marital and family relationships have also been affected somewhat by the famine. Wives have always been considered property and are purchased for a price of 15 to 50 cattle. The loss of a wife is often regarded as the loss of a prized possession rather than that of a beloved partner. Many husbands and fathers possess many wives and remain aloof from all of them, visiting occasionally as needs arose. The women traditionally have been responsible for planting, cultivating, and providing food. The men were hunters in the past; now they still occasionally wage war against other tribes to increase the number of their cattle.

The famine has disrupted their cultural pattern. It has been necessary for the men to find work, to be involved in planting fields, and to provide for the family. As a result of this change in roles, many men have become somewhat invested in their families, and it was not uncommon for a man to bring his desperately ill child to the clinic. It was then necessary for a man to recognize the loss when a child or spouse died. This was not easily accomplished, however.

The people in this area have extremely poor health and nutrition. They seem to be highly susceptible to malaria and other parasitic diseases because of their poor living conditions and lack of clean water. However, many of the patients seen had psychosomatic types of illness wherein no specific organic causes could be found after thorough investigations were performed.

The major problems encountered were a wide variety of anxiety disorders, a few cases of chronic anxiety and phobic anxiety, and a large number of psychosomatic cases, which represented 25% or more of the cases seen in the clinic. There was one episode of mass hysteria in a local primary school. There were occasional identifiable depressive episodes. In each village area there seemed to be at least one person with chronic schizophrenia. The prevalence of schizophrenia, based on the estimated population of the area, was probably less than 0.5%. There were at least two known episodes of attempted suicide. No completed suicides were reported during my one year of residence in the area. Intrafamilial violence was extremely common, perhaps an indication of the underlying rage from poorly resolved grief and the difficulty these people had in maintaining their society and culture under the prevailing conditions.

SAMBURU DISTRICT

The Samburu District is in north-central Kenya. It is situated mostly on a high plateau, but some areas are completely deserted. The area on the high plateau is relatively healthy; the absence of malaria is due to the altitude and lack of mosquitoes. There is, however, a high prevalence of pneumonia and parasitic disease.

This society is undergoing changes basically due to the encroachment of Western practices and values. The economy is in a transitional state; both money and cattle are used. A high percentage of men are absent from home, working in cities 200 to 300 miles from home. This leaves the entire responsibility of raising the children to the wives. For 11 months out of the year there is no contact between spouses, as most of them are illiterate. Many wives do not know whether their husbands are living or dead but expect them to come back during a certain time of the year. The rites of passage remain for those who follow tradition. After circumcision, the males become warriors, Lmurran, but there are no wars to fight. This leaves them idle and often in trouble. They often commit violent acts, including rape and murder. Other traditions remain fairly intact, and the traditional grieving practices are still followed.

The area has been relatively free of major disasters. Cattle raids are infrequent, and the government army has been successful in giving protection. Anxiety in this society seems to be primarily due to the uncertainties caused by westernization, changes in family structure, the need for economic security, and uncertain rainfall.

In general, this area had less major mental illness than psychosomatic illness. There were several cases of panic disorder, major depression, bipolar disorder, and schizophrenia. The prevalence of schizophrenia seemed to be roughly the same as in the Pokot area, although it would be difficult to quantify it.The town of Maralal is in the center of the Samburu District. It has many amenities, including electricity, occasional running water, more use of cash in the economy, and less tribal tradition. This area had many cases of peptic ulcer disease, coronary artery disease, alcoholism, and addiction to a local plant called Miraa. There was also an incident, not far from town, in which a 7-year-old child murdered his father, who was in the act of beating his wife.

Intrafamilial violence occurred sporadically in the district, but generally was not brought to the attention of health care providers. At least 10 cases of rape were reported during my 8 months in the Samburu District. These were committed primarily by teenagers, still in the dubious role of warrior.

SUMMARY

Of the patients seen in both districts, approximately 25% to 30% could have benefited from purely psychosocial intervention. Of these 25%, perhaps 20% (5% of the clinic population) were suffering from probable mental illness. Of those who came to the clinics, primarily because of mental illness, psychoses were diagnosed in only 4%-5%, which is less than 1% of the clinic population. This, however, would not represent the actual prevalence since in both areas mental illness is often regarded as a spiritual disease and many people come to the clinic only when physical problems occur. During our visits to villages, we saw many untreated mentally ill, but help was not accepted. Actual incidence and prevalence in these areas would be impossible to estimate at present.

We provided psychosocial intervention to help reduce morbidity in several areas. We helped the Pokot redevelop an effective way to mourn the loss of a loved one. A burial service was designed through the local church. This was accepted by people over a large area and appeared to reduce the psychosomatic and violent reactions that followed many deaths. In the Samburu area, a project was designed to help occupy the time of the idle warriors. Work is still under way, and its impact is not yet known.

It would be of great benefit to identify other aspects of the evolving culture that contribute to mental illness and design ways of promoting healthy behavior without disrupting the cultural identity.

CONCLUSIONS

These experiences in two African cultures were seen through the eyes of a general practice physician. After returning to the United States to train in psychiatry, I realized that psychiatric intervention at the level of primary health care could be very beneficial and even perhaps reduce morbidity and mortality in some areas.

There is obviously a need for more study, but the real need is for program development. We know mental illness is present. We must now continue to find the best ways to meet those special needs.

Chapter 15

Case Study of James Peter, An Example.of Transitional Group Psychotherapy in Malawi[1]

by

Karl Peltzer, Ph.D.
Institute of African Studies,
University of Zambia,
Lusaka, Zambia

INTRODUCTION

In the following case study, I wish to combine the view of the anthropologist and the requirements of a coherent clinical approach. I talked to James Peter from 1983 until 1986, in about 65 sessions. Each session was held in privacy and lasted more or less one hour. The guideline of the conversation with him was to associate one episode with another, one dream with another, without bothering about sequence or chronology. When he ran out of material, I would intervene and ask him to be more explicit about specific data. Therefore, the organization of The Story of James Peter is not chronological. Each episode is like a punctuated high point in which

James reinscribes his past. In a series of discrete scenes and acts that refer to coded messages, the unconscious positioning of the narrator will become evident.

At first, I shall deal with his narrative or his autobiography which is structured in three major periods:

1. James' interaction in his environment without illness and spirits.
2. How the spirits and witchcraft made him sick.
3. How the spirits have taken over a healing function.

Finally, I analyze his narrative using the three-dimensional model as frame of interpretation. Occasionally, I offered him money, which he used for school fees and shared with relatives. Before the final version of this paper was written, it was discussed, word by word, with James Peter. (Compare Boroffka, 1980; Obeyesekere, 1977; Parin, et al., 1971; Peltzer, 1981/82; Zempleni, 1977.)

SESSIONS WITH JAMES PETER

I was born in 1959 (in Blantyre). We used to stay in a well-to-do area, and we had a totally comfortable life. We were at least amongst those Africans who were thought to be important at that time, especially because my father worked hand-in-hand with white people. We used to live in a very big house with servants' quarters. It was a fine life.

I am the eldest in the family. The second is a boy. The third also a boy, and fourth are twins. It was two years after these twins were born that my mother died. After her death, my father decided to take another wife. When he took another wife, what happened was quite an experience. There have always been conflicts between the stepmother and us the stepsons.

When I was young, I never liked participating in any games. My favorite game was going to the heap of saw dust which was close to our house and play the cowboy games we saw every Sunday at the show grounds.

Discipline or obedience started sometime early. My father was a strict man and a whip was always next to him. He used to whip us like mad—i.e., my younger brother, the one who comes after me, and my distant cousin, who was staying with us. The two would leave and go to the film show even during times we were not supposed to go out. After I had helped them sneak into the house, they would start discussing what they had seen and they put on superior airs. This made my company awkward, so much so that there were times when fights would start in the house. My younger brother used to whip me. I was such a fool that, whenever I got whipped, I would go out and tell my mother and my mother would whip me again... Then, one day I whipped my brother to the extent that he lost one of his teeth... When my father came back, instead of whipping me, he whipped my brother again. This annoyed me very much. My brother was punished by being locked in the room and given no food for the whole day. I gave him his food through the window. I was very sad, and I remember tears running down my cheeks. That was the last fight I had with my brother and from then on he started respecting me.

My brothers and I were sent to the same school. At first, it was the junior primary school from Standard 1 to Standard 2; then to the primary school... Then, there was something there I didn't like, maybe I was a person who liked being alone... I was always waiting for my father to come and when he came, I was always with him. I never enjoyed mixing with friends... I told my father that I want to change school... The new school was very beautiful. It had good bricks and everything about it was fine and superb, whereas the other one was very old and colonial-looking. I enjoyed the new school and it was there that I met my first friend, Oliver Phiri... There was a conflict between the old and the new school whenever I came home. All my brothers would say a lot of things, including that I would be sent to the Coventry, and that I didn't want to mix with them because I came from the new school, and that I was stubborn and proud of the new school... but I was not very proud...

In the earliest stages before the death of my mother, I was very brilliant. In school I used to be number one, number one, number one, number two, number two, and number two until Standard 5 when the intelligence died with the death of my mother... It is here that I remember that my mother was very important to my life and then she made it a point that I become intelligent. I remember writing a well-phrased letter to my aunt on Likoma Island from

Blantyre during my Standard 2. After the death of my mother things started changing. All of us became careless boys, our clothes were not as clean as they used to be... The mother who came never cared for us. She was only interested in her own kids and the welfare of her own relations.

In Standard 6, I managed to become number four. I remember I ran home feeling very happy, and saw my father and told him I was number four, and my father was very glad and became proud of me. My father always encouraged me to read, and I used to read a lot. On every birthday, my father used to buy a set for me, and then I would read all those books... And when I was at the new school, I met these boys who used to read in the library. I read all the series of "Tin-Tin" that were there and all sorts of literature by Standard 7. I enjoyed Tin-Tin very much because, perhaps I liked to see comic things in people. When it came to films I enjoyed very much those of Charles Chaplin. Usually, when I attended such films, my voice would go because of laughing.

I enjoyed the company of Oliver. One important thing was that I usually found myself helping Oliver. I used to buy shoes for him. If his father did not buy shoes for Oliver, I would take my own pair and give it to Oliver. When I told my father that I didn't have shoes, he would shout at me and do all sorts of things.

I remember one day I answered my father rudely for being so unwise and unreasonable and attacking me.

We were taught to sing the National Anthem in English and to say the Lord's prayer in English. My friends at the old school never knew anything about it. Almost all the neighborhood kids used to attend the old school. I was the only exception.

I remember a certain boy, he was called Robert. I don't remember the name of his father. He was the son of some white man's houseboy... I never liked girls, I never liked any form of company. I never liked violence and I was quiet.

One day I mixed with a group... We would go to Kamuzu Stadium, mix and do all sorts of things, like the Rallys... This was the time when I developed pride for my country and I was very proud of everything, especially whenever the Malawi Army Band was coming at the gate and I was inside. I really liked it, not only the Army Band but the Police Band and the Pioneer Band as well. It was this time that I thought I would become a drum major in the Army Band after school. I also liked to watch soccer. The sight of our own President, as he was coming into the Stadium, made me happy.

But, there was a group of boys my uncle hated. I liked these boys, they were good company. But, all the same, these boys used to smoke cannabis. We had bought a packet of Rothmans cigarettes. Then, the other boy said, why have you brought this boy here, I told you to leave him behind, he doesn't know the game. They started shouting at me and bullying me... Anyway, they still liked me, perhaps because I had a lot of money.

Later I did my standard 8 and failed the exams, and so was not selected for secondary school. I was very annoyed because I did not expect this. Then my father had a car accident. That was in 1969. This was the most important point in my life because it marked the end of stay in a yard in a three bedroom house, the modern type of life. My father was forced to retire. I went to Likoma Island where I did my standard 8. The first term I failed totally, but in the second and third semesters I was really fine... I was always regarded as a hero. I don't know why, maybe it was because I used to make a lot of noise during break, cracking jokes of all sorts of things. I was a good talker. During this time, I was not interested in girls. One day, I came out only to find these milky things coming out of my manhood and, when I saw this, I thought I was sick. I wanted to tell my father but my friends told me to do so, and said, "You are grown up, you should start looking for girls now." Then I said, "oh, my good Lord," and that was the end of everything.

My grandfather, whom I loved so much, gave all kinds of advice. One day, my father sent me K5 and I gave it to my grandfather to keep it for me in his grocery. It stayed one year, the whole of that year, until I finished writing the examinations.

When I went to secondary school, the first thing that happened was teasing. I was teased from Nkhata Bay Boma right up to the school. This affected me very much. I hated school, but I had to go anyway... To my surprise, I was one of the best mathematicians in class.

I loved ladies through letters. I had several ladies through letters. We used to write one another, but we never exchanged sex. The only thing I used to do was drink beer.

One important thing, which I was proud of, is that I was the school platoon leader for Malawi Young Pioneers' activities. I enjoyed drill. I must admit, I have got the mentality of a soldier. This could not have started mainly because of that Army Band. There are fast and energetic strides, which meant to me courage and bravery, and the beautiful colors of the marchers gave me courage all the time.

There is yet one point I would like to make; all my English, the English I have so far got, is a result of Brother Ronald of Santa Barbara in the United States of America. I have read several literature books at the secondary school under his guidance. These books are guiding spirits to me.

One day in Form III, I had a headache. I felt something hard, as if a stone was moving right behind my neck, and I was failing to read. That was the beginning of the problem... It was around 1975... I had a dream about my girl friend. She was mad and I was at Nkhata Bay. Then I said, "why are you mad?" and later it was me who got mad. There I was very mad; I got sick.

Like my father, I did not believe in any form of traditional medicine. I was told by my grandfather that it was actually my father who snapped the string which was tied around my neck. That string had medicine meant to make me strong as an African child... The beginning of my sickness was at the point when this string was snapped from me.

I went first of all to the hospital in 1975. I was given medicine at the hospital. The treatment was composed of four chloroquine and two aspirin tablets. Soon after this, I started getting sick... I got confused, I felt like jumping into the forest, or going into the mountains. My heart would beat hard, then slowly, my body would burn like fire. I felt something moving in the head. I thought the thing in my neck was now moving right into my head, as if a stone, a red hot stone was moving in the head. When it came to the center of the head, I felt like crying. There were times when I would cry, cry, and cry.

The cook in my school advised me to visit a witchdoctor. He told me that I had been bewitched by a man who lived in a house near my house. I could not believe all this and I threw his medicine in a river on my way back to school. I told my friend that I can't be mad. That man is crazy. There is nothing like witchcraft... Then the same things started happening again... I was no longer attending class. I spent most of my time in my room, and then slowly the sickness worsened. And, then, somebody said I should try a famous witchdoctor. Here I was immediately shaven and I found myself in the process of bloodletting from my head. I had to buy the heart of a cow which was very bitter to eat because of the herbs... It was only after I tried to write the second paper that I got sick again and I was asked to leave school, tears rolling all over my eyes.

In 1981, my uncle took me back to Likoma where I was taken to a famous healer. The trouble began when the healer wanted to see all my parents. My father and everybody else were unwilling to help me stay at the healer's place because they feared his powers. My father wanted me to be sent to the mental hospital. He thought I was a cannabis smoker and heavy drinker and that was why I was sick.

I was taken to the mental hospital in Lomba where I was given doriden and valium. These two drugs from that time on started ruling my life. I used to visit the mental hospital almost every time to collect these drugs. But still, I combined my efforts with African traditional medicine. I stayed with a certain healer who said that I had been fitted with a child's penis to soften and destroy me. This man gave me much confidence... I stayed with him for two months. He said that what he saw was that there was a conflict between the mother's and the father's side about us children. I asked my parents if this was true... My uncle and my grandfather on my father's side said it was true and that I was bewitched. I used to bathe with medicine at the pit where wastes were dumped... Then, I went home and my parents were now getting organized. My father's side and my mother's side were all ready. My distant uncle from my mother's relation, the cousin of my mother, and my relatives took me to the healer. The healer told my relatives that I should stay with him for the treatment. I was asked to bring a sheep for chilopa... That was the beginning of another life. My stay at the healer's place was educational on its own. I had never liked mixing but now I found myself mixing with other people. I ate together with them. The first day I tried to eat with them, but because I was used to eating alone I was left behind. I learned that there were people who suffered more than I did. These were people who cared much for the one tambala they had. I started chatting with my friends, started telling them stories that I once was very intelligent.

They listened to my stories and I also got to hear their stories. We would join together working, got to bathe together, drink, and close our eyes when drinking our medicine. The doctor was almost a father to me. He gave me wisdom when he was explaining things—he was so good. He explained very interesting things about culture proverbs, and he taught us good manners. There were cases where quarrels erupted, and the doctor would call us all, joining patients from different parts. Some came from Mozambique, others came from Likoma, others from Nkhota-Kota, and even from Karonga. The kind of life we Africans lead consists of helping one another, so we shared many things. Somebody would have a packet of sugar and somebody would have a packet of salt... I stayed there until exams time came.

I went to school where I met my friend Roger Gondwe, who kept on helping me right until the day of exams. He kept on encouraging me till I wrote my exams all right... When I was taking medicines from the healer, I felt encouraged. After every paper I would apply medicine on my upper eyelids and upper eyebrows. The problem was eyes tearing; but, at last, I managed to write, and I said maybe it was this encouragement that I lacked the first time I was writing. I had about four or five friends. I also had a girl friend. This girl friend took my picture and gave it to her boy friend. I must admit I was a bit frustrated, but the frustration was disguised by the sickness. The girl went to college and the boy went to Chancellor College when I was still sick. I was not selected for college. So I started working in the bank. I applied to go to college; then, in the name of the Lord, I was sitting in the bank, I saw this telegram coming to me, that James should report to Chancellor College on 1st October 1978.

I stayed at college. I was not very good in the first year and in the second year... Mind you, all this time, I was still taking valium. Whenever I felt a bit of pain in my head, I took valium straight away. I would go to the mental hospital and get valium. Then I reached a point where I used to mix drugs with beer, especially doriden. When I had three packets of Chibuku with doriden, I was very drunk. I enjoyed these drugs.

All sorts of things happened. I was very free with my tongue at Chancellor College. I would join any company; any group. The boys I loved most at Chancellor College were George and this boy Robert. I liked the way they spoke English. They became my idols... But, then, these boys did not come back, and I felt that the departure of these boys was the beginning of the end of authentic students at Chancellor College. From that point on, I started hating Chancellor

College. I had this fear, and my life was full of misery...

On holiday, while I was staying at the healer's place, I saw my lady. She became mine and I hers. This means a lot to the building up of my character.

The second phase of my life is very delicate and important. It had to be handled carefully. It involves certain things that I do not want to expose to anybody or any form of technology.

My stay at the mental hospital was bad. I didn't like it and I do not intend to go there again. The mental hospital simply destroys the mind.

The second part of my life is the experience I have had ever since I was initiated into the field of healing... The most important thing was dancing vimbuza, which is not a joke. It is a dance which the youth consider traditional and primitive. Secondly, to dance vimbuza, means everybody thinks and believes you are mentally ill... To begin with, it was in April 1981, I think, when I got sick and then, after that, I was given another chilopa. This time it was more painful than the first time... The training was that anybody could abuse me. They would say: "Look, he thinks he is the best person on earth." "You are nothing; you stink." I would stay for the whole day without food and nobody cared for me. Then, when I was angry, immediately what followed was that all of them said, "No food for you. " Then I would say "Ah!" I was going to kill myself... I remember that I dreamt that I was tied behind and there were soldiers trying to kill me. That was the most painful moment in my life. The doctor was preparing me to face the world, the art of healing needs brave men... I felt that I was in the world of fear.

When I came to school, I realized that the whole treatment I had undergone was much more painful than what I met here. There were people who were mocking me. I said, this is nothing; what I have experienced was much more painful. Then, I started challenging them to the extent that I lost fear.

At first, I did not respect anybody. I thought I could do anything because of the mere fact that I am at the University. I thought I could do anything and shout at anybody. I could go in the corridors and say, "Even though you are in authority I don't care. " When I went to a beer place, I fought easily... I also thought that you (the author) and the doctor had conspired that I should be killed.

When I came to college this time, I wasn't sure of myself. You remember, we met in the library... I thought I was followed by authorities wherever I went. I did not become angry any more, and slowly I started getting all right. Now, I am very strong and brave. I fear nothing.

My spirits seem to be directing me towards healing and witch-catching. But, I am not interested in all of these because I know, at one point, they will destroy my feeling concerning my education.

As I said, I wanted to sleep; now these things (spirits) are coming into me and they are very powerful. They tell me to go to my mother's grave and hunt for something that is in a wastebin—a broken clay pot; and I will try to call the spirits and, then,put the medicine on me .

I could become angry and I was going to shout. But I was silent. So, I think, my spirits, the spirits, the mungoma, that is why they came to the doctor and said, this boy should not go to school; we don't want him to die so early. This is my speculation in search for answers to some of the problems I was facing.

I mean, I am answered through spirits, and the spirits help me; when I want anything, they help. They guide me, they protect me. You see, these spirits are somewhere in the mountains. Especially in the morning hours, they spread to different individuals they protect.

I went with my friend to the market. When I entered the market, I felt vyanusi come in. I sensed that the spirit was coming in. I felt then, like electricity, they entered into my head as I was entering the gate of the market. When such things happen, it means that they are just protecting me from something else. If somebody thinks that he can destroy me at the market because I like going there, he fails.

The mungoma spirits want me to be at the hospital (healing centre), and the spirits of my mother and my grandfather would like me to go to school. But I don't want to work in the hospital; I would prefer to die because my father has done much efforts to send me to school.

In the eyes of the elders, my truth and my being knowledgeable is either bound to irritate them or their dignity is threatened. They will be frustrated and there will be shame in their eyes. So, it is this that I don't want to see happening. So, if an elderly person who is illiterate would say, I know this thing, my only comment would be, you are very wise.

Right now the spirits want me to sleep. We have been discussing for quite a long time and all of a sudden I feel sleepy. That means that the mungoma spirits have got something to tell me... (you can sleep)... It will come, maybe I'll sleep.

It is now that I have discovered that it is these spirits that tell me to read African leaders, for example Steve Biko.

ANALYSIS

In the following, the three-dimensional model is being applied to the nosology, etiology, and therapy of James Peter.

Authority Dimension

1. Nosology and Etiology

Father: He is very strict and he was associated with the upper class. He had a severe accident and his remarried wife divorced him. He praised James for academic achievement, but he refused to visit him at the healer's place. He also snapped a string with specific power, which James was wearing around his neck when he was small against the will of the elders. He shouted at him when he was holding his girl friend in public.

Mother: She was strict. She died when James was eight years old. The mother's spirit felt unhappy since she had been neglected.

Grandfather: He was important to James. However, he died when James was 15 years old. The grandfather's spirit felt unhappy since he had been neglected.

Authorities or big people, as James called them: James was either very quiet or rude towards authorities. He did not always accept their power, based on ascribed status, which contradicted his belief in achieved status. He, for instance, corrected the English of some authorities, which was considered rude. The more his illness proceeded, the more he projected his problems onto the mother-spirit and the grandfathers spirit (participative projection).

2. Therapy

At first James tried Western medicine; but, as time went on, he shifted more and more to traditional healing. He got psychosocial care in the healing setting which he did not receive in the Western setting. However, it is not so clear here as to how he could completely take over traditional religious concepts since he grew up in an urban and Western milieu. Only later in our conversation did we discover that he was exposed to tradition when he played with his relatives—i.e., singing malpenga in the servant's quarters, being told stories about village life, etc. However, following a Western socialization, he kept these experiences out of his consciousness. Moreover, he realized that, after he went to the village, town life was not everything.

He said that, at first, he missed the comfort of town life, but later he discovered and experienced the positive aspects of traditional life in his village. He also started learning and loving his grandfather. The healer gave him confidence, parental love, wisdom, courage, and taught him manners. James felt proud of him, although he disliked the restrictions of his freedom.

The (directly) related spirits which possess James are:

The mother spirit: For her, the chilopa and mboni ceremony has been performed, and the afflicting aspect of the mother spirit has been transformed into a healing aspect.

The grandfather spirit: For him, the chilopa ceremony has been held. Part of the chilopa was that James was given a necklace to wear. When he was alive, the grandfather was annoyed when his son snapped that string from his grandson. The breaking of the string was seen as a causative factor to James' illness. Now, at this discharge ceremony of the chilopa, he was reinitiated from disease to health (life) by being given a new life string.

The grandfather's brother spirit: guides James mainly on African literature.

The great-grandfather spirit. For him James made an offering at his grave.

These related spirits mainly helped in the process of his own recovery. As James became initiated into a trainee to become a healer, he also got possessed by other nonrelated spirits. This enabled him to articulate his conflict between traditional and Western education after he reconciled with his own relatives on a community or societal level and not just the familial level. Gradually, more and more nonrelated spirits came into him and formed an alliance with his related spirits. At first, he projected his hopelessness, despair, and suffering onto ancestral spirits, which formed a replication of his parent-child relationship. Later, he became more concerned with his community and its problem and developed a nonrelated spirits' relationship which reflected his clan-child experiences. This goes beyond his family and involved other patients. Thereby, the focus of attention, which often disturbs autonomous processes of healing and problem-solving, is directed to positive thinking and other objectives; anxiety disappears and is replaced by self-confidence and self-esteem (Figge forthcoming). In the following chief spirits, it becomes evident that those spirits, which have formed an alliance with his ancestral spirits, signify a projection which is both a mechanism of defence and a system of security (compare Obeyesekere, 1976, p. 235). The major spirits which possess James are:

Mungoma, which is the name of a Ngoni spirit. James patrilineal ancestors are Ngoni. Mungoma is against James' formal education, but he protects James from evil influences and from becoming uncontrollably aggressive.

Vyanusi is his trainer's (healer's) mother spirit, who is the guiding spirit of the healing centre, especially for those who have been initiated there. The incorporation of a spirit of his healer and trainer reflects his strong participative projection with them.

There are more ally spirits like mungomi, which also protect and get him involved in dancing. These allies or signifiers may refer to other signifiers, which have already come at random, but not yet in a pronounced form. It is this assertion that propels him from the position of a sick or simple possessed person to that of a healer. He is no longer imprisoned in the web of his old imaginary identifications with near ancestral relations, but is on the way to a symbolic identification with cultural heritage in the form of the alliance between ancestral and unrelated spirits (compare Collomb and de Prenant, 1982). The latter provide him with the philosophy to live peacefully, try to do good, live in good company, have a good conversation, etc. In addition, he should live in conformity with the desires and prescriptions of one's personal protecting spirit, which reflect the rules of the group.

Group Dimension

1. Nosology and Etiology.

Brothers: James is the first born, but had to fight in order to gain respect from his younger brothers. Due to his delayed education and his illness, he was unable to take responsibility for his younger siblings, which made him feel like a failure, especially after his father became an invalid. The expectations of first-born sons very often lead to emotional disturbances (Ebigbo and Ihezue, 1983).

Classmates: James' classmates used to tease him a lot. Since he was good in class his classmates were jealous of him, which the healer interpreted as witchcraft. He had enemies in college.

Peer group: The peer group did not accept him. James easily got into a fight when he was drunk.

Close friends: Two of James' close friends did not come back and, as a result, he did not develop confidence in new friends. One of his friends keeps running away from him, because there are times he comes and James does not talk.

Girls: James was not interested in girls, they frustrated him.

People: James feels that people would abuse him, and that he is being followed by people who want to take personal things away from him and who want to destroy him. James' relationship with the group was characterized by persecutory ideas (projective identification).

2. Therapy

As an inpatient with the healer, James experienced real community life with the other patients. He started having real friends with whom he could share his painful experiences. During that time, he got to know his girl friend with whom he developed an intimate relationship. He found a real friend who helped him a lot to pass his exams. When the people were still troubling him, he underwent an initiation ceremony to face life. His real friends from the healing centre, with whom he developed confidence in the world around him, gave him behaviour therapy. They confronted him in a drastic way with the negative aspects of the world and yet they accepted him. They pointed out his weak points and, by going through this dramatic experience which was marked by nightmares and fear of death, James was better able to face negative experiences. He was made to feel strong and to lose fear of his school environment. After all, he had experienced something much more painful. After he had mastered such a dreadful experience, in return, he gained the confidence to face and accept people who were against him. He no longer felt being followed by people, and no longer became aggressive if someone were against him. In addition to the group psychotherapy he went through as an inpatient with a healer, he was provided with protection incisions, and other measures, which gave him more confidence and security in the group dimension.

Body-Mind-Environment Dimension:

1. Nosology and Etiology

Body: Recurring headaches, stone hitting his neck, heart beating, something moving in the head, eye tearing, snap in heart, becomes thin, gets paralyzed on one side, and experiences pains of pins in the abdomen. James was never interested in sports.

Mind: James was brilliant in primary school. He failed Standard 8 exams, but later was very good in mathematics and English literature in secondary school. Then, he got confused. He could read and listen to what the teacher was saying, but he could not grasp the meaning. He heard people talking in school who were trying to be against him.

Environment: At first, James stayed in a very big house in an upper-class area. At first, he went to an old school, but then he became very proud that he had changed to a new school out of bricks and everything. From there, he was forced to stay in a village on Likoma Island. As an inpatient in the mental hospital, he felt totally uneasy. He worked in a bank for a short period until he went to Chancellor College.

2. Therapy

Body-Mind-Environment: At first James received pharmaceutical drugs—e.g., aspirin, valium, doriden. Then he shifted to herbal remedies, danced malipenga, vimbuza, and mungoma. Moreover, he received massage. Through African philosophies, like muzimuism-i.e., the attitude towards life based on the belief of mizimu—songs, etc., to which he was exposed in conversations with the healer and fellow inpatients, he gained insight into how his own biography is connected with his authority and group dimension, as well as with the society at large, especially the conflict between traditional and Western culture, as well as environment—town versus village; new and old school; modern and traditional hospital (compare 6.1. Milieu therapy).

NOTES:

1. Names have been changed.

REFERENCES:

Boroffka, A. (1980) Benedict Nto Tanka's commentary and dramatised ideas on disease and wicthcraft in our society, Frankfurt, M. P.O. Lang

Figge, H.H. (forthcoming), Controlled Spirit possession as a form of group psychotherapy in Brazil. In: Peltzer, K. and Ebigbo, P.O. (eds.).

Katz, R. (1982b) Boiling energy: Community healing among the Kalahari Kung., Cambridge, Massachusetts: Harvard University Press

Obeyesekere, B. (1977), Psychocultural exegesis of a case of spirit possession in Sri Lanka. In: Crapanzano, V. and Garrison, V. (eds.), pp. 235-94

Parin, P., Morgenthaler, F. and Pari-Matthey, G. (1971) Fuerchte deinen naechsten wie dich Seibst: Psychoanalyse and Gesellschaft am Model der Agni in West Africa. Frankfurt, M. Suhrkamp

Peltzer, K. (1981/82) The work of Nana Afua Saa, an Okomfo (healer) from Kumasi . Ethnomedice 7:47-89

Zempleni, A . ,(1977), From symptom to sacrifice : The story of Khady Fall . In: Crapanzano , V . and Carrison, V. (eds.). pp. 87-139

Chapter 16

Forensic Psychiatry in Africa Today

by

Tolani Asuni, MD, Professor
Department of Psychiatry,
College of Medicine,
University of Lagos,
Lagos, Nigeria

ABSTRACT

In some African countries, revision of the legal systems and mental health laws inherited from colonial powers has been slowed by economic problems, lack of manpower and education, and the need to address survival problems. Where the economic situation is poor and psychiatrists are rare, obviously psychotic persons accused of crimes are still sent to asylums. In many countries, however, psychiatrists are involved throughout criminal cases. A psychiatrist determines the competence of the accused to stand trial, testifies as to the relationship between the accused person's mental state at the time of the offense and the crime itself, and is involved in the treatment of convicted mentally ill persons. Opinion is divided on the subject of separate hospitals for mentally ill offenders; Kenya treats mentally ill offenders in a special unit within its major psychiatric hospital.

INTRODUCTION

One can put forensic psychiatry in Africa in its true perspective only against the background of its colonial heritage, social, economic, and cultural factors, the development of psychiatry in general, the legal systems operating in the different countries, and the availability of trained personnel. It is not possible, therefore, to talk about forensic psychiatry without running the risk of overgeneralizing and, consequently, making mistakes. What can safely be done is to talk about trends emanating from the aforementioned factors and, if possible, to give examples.

COLONIAL HERITAGE

The practice of psychiatry, no doubt, existed before the colonial era, but it consisted mainly of treating psychosis when a psychotic individual's behavior disturbed the smooth running of the community. This does not mean that neuroses and personality disorders did not exist. They either were contained or were regarded mainly as problems of living for which there were social, cultural, or religious remedies. The role of the traditional healers includes social engineering, religious leadership, counseling, etc., in addition to the specific role of healing. This type of healing is holistic, approaching not only the individual, but also the community and the relationship between the two. It also takes into account the spirit world, which includes ancestors.

The colonial powers, in line with the practice of psychiatry in their countries, introduced the concept of asylums and the practice of keeping disturbed psychotic persons in these asylums and in some prisons that were designated as asylums. An obviously psychotic person who committed a criminal offense was regarded primarily as a patient and not a criminal. The less obviously psychotic person was treated as a criminal. A psychotic offender was sent to an asylum or to a prison, usually one that had been designated an asylum. This designation was sometimes simply bureaucratic; a number of prisons not so designated also housed psychotic offenders.

Since alienists, the old term for psychiatrists, were rare, any physician could declare a person mentally ill. As there were also very few physicians, an administrative officer, usually an European expatriate, could also declare a person mentally ill where there was no physician.

In terms of therapy, there was not much difference between asylum and prison, as there was little or no active therapy in either. This was a reflection of the state of knowledge in psychiatry at the time. The situation, unfortunately, remains almost the same in some parts of Africa where the economic situation is poor and psychiatrists are still rare.

This situation has to be seen against a background of extreme poverty, malnutrition, undernutrition, endemic diseases, and killing diseases. It is no wonder that psychiatry is still given low priority. In spite of this, some countries, such as Kenya and Nigeria, are developing psychiatric services for psychotic offenders on the basis of available funds.

To accomplish this in Kenya, additional buildings were planned for Mathari Hospital, the major psychiatric facility in the country.

POST COLONIAL ERA

Some African countries, even after independence, continue to operate under the inherited legal system and the existing mental health legislation. It is gratifying, however, that efforts have been made, and are still in progress, to revise legal systems and mental health legislation in a number of African countries. There is no doubt that the will is there, but the constraints are overwhelming; they include economic problems, lack of manpower and education, and problems of general survival. Furthermore, the teaching of criminology, which can embrace the elements of psychiatry related to offenders, is not well established in most African countries. Even our law schools, which students must attend before they can be registered to practice law, are still not very strong in the relevant subjects. The academic departments of psychiatry, whose clinical bases are teaching hospitals, are not equipped with adequate security to enable them to handle accused psychotic persons. The best they can do in such situations is to interview and examine accused subjects in out patient clinics or carry out such exercises in prison. Training in forensic psychiatry for both medical students and residents is therefore bound to be deficient. A number of academic departments of psychiatry have close links with service hospitals that are equipped, in terms of security, to accommodate the accused or convicted mentally ill. With such collaboration, which includes the appointments of service psychiatrists as associate lecturers in the academic departments, the teaching of psychiatry becomes stronger and exposes medical students to some forensic psychiatry.

In view of the shortage of psychiatrists in Africa, it has not been possible to develop subspecialties in the academic and service areas. This does not mean that the subspecialties are not recognized. Indeed, in practice, many general psychiatrists focus attention on the subspecialties of their interest or subspecialties in which they are, by the nature of their duties, called on to perform. For instance, most psychiatrists working in psychiatric hospitals have to handle forensic psychiatric cases in the course of their duties. In due course, they develop considerable expertise in the forensic subspecialty, for which they are eventually recognized. This development is built on what they learned during training and, sometimes, what they learned during specialized exposure after training.

PRACTICE OF FORENSIC PSYCHIATRY

The practice of forensic psychiatry in Africa, as in other countries, can be divided into three stages— pretrial, trial, and posttrial.

Pretrial Stage

The pretrial stage is mainly to ascertain the competence of the accused person, in terms of his mental state, to participate effectively in the trial process. It is not necessary to explain the ingredients of this competence, as they are universal. It is appreciated, however, that it is risky to depend only on the interview and examination of the accused, as he can readily fake mental illness. This is why it is vital to get information about the accused from other relevant sources. With the information from these other sources, it has been possible to issue a report on the competence of the accused after examination on an outpatient basis. Unfortunately, this is not possible in most cases, as there are usually no other identifiable sources of information and the accused persons have to be hospitalized for observation. This observation is sometimes done in prison with the collaboration of the prison officers. The officers are requested to record the behavior of the accused person and his relationships and interaction with other inmates and prison staff. Often the pretrial observation is performed in a psychiatric hospital, where there is a dearth of clinical psychologists to participate in this exercise.

Some psychiatrists do not restrict themselves to observation only. If they find that the accused is incompetent by virtue of his mental state (usually psychosis), they proceed to give him treatment. The reason for this is that the accused is mentally ill and in need of treatment. Why delay treatment until the court gives the order, since it will be given eventually in any case? If the accused had malaria fever or meningitis, should the physician in charge wait for the court order to administer treatment? Court orders usually take days, if not longer, to process. I am not aware that such professional action has been challenged in any court in Africa.

One problem with this system is that accused persons sent for pretrial reports on competence are sometimes forgotten (for want of a more appropriate word) and are left in the hospital indefinitely. This requires an aggressive move by the psychiatrist in charge to call the court's attention to the situation so the accused person can be removed from the hospital. If the court is not ready to hear the case, the accused person is kept in a prison. Some accused persons who have regained competence after treatment and have been transferred to prisons have relapsed because their maintenance medication has not been administered. It is embarrassing when the actual condition of the accused cannot be reconciled with the certificate of competence issued by the psychiatrist. If the psychiatrist is present in court, he can easily explain that the accused was removed from his care and was not kept on his maintenance medication.

Trial Stage

The role of the psychiatrist in the trial stage is to establish the relationship between the mental state of the accused at the time of the offense and the occurrence of the offense. One of the major problems encountered by psychiatrists in Africa, and perhaps in some other countries, is the time between the offense and the psychiatric examination, which may be months. In addition, the information usually available to the psychiatrist is so sketchy as to be useless. The information gathered by the police is geared toward making a viable charge and no more. The cadre of officers, like probation officers, is not readily available for collecting information that may assist the psychiatrist in formulating a profile of the accused and reconstructing the event of the offense. The level of confidence with which the psychiatrist makes his report and gives evidence to the court is, therefore, determined by the quality and quantity of relevant information available to him.

It is not enough to say that the accused is suffering from a particular diagnosis, as not all people suffering from that entity commit such offenses. It is more meaningful to state which symptoms associated with the diagnosis led to, contributed to, or were related to the behavior. The genesis of the illness is not relevant to the needs of the court in making its primary decision of guilty or not guilty. This approach does not leave much room for contention, which often does great damage to the image of psychiatry, especially when psychiatrists are on opposing sides and are interpreting the same sets of facts, not symptoms, in different ways.

Since there is a shortage of psychiatrists in Africa, the practice of having psychiatrists on both sides of a case is very rare. This puts a great deal of responsibility on the only psychiatrist in the case to be as objective and scientific as possible and to assist the course of justice. He must not be compelled to take one side against the other in the case, economic incentive notwithstanding. The court's practice of maintaining a panel of psychiatrists, as in some states of the United States, is commendable. This panel is responsible for giving expert psychiatric evidence to the court.

Another area in which African psychiatrists can make a healthy departure from practices elsewhere is the legal issue of responsibility and diminished responsibility. This concept is not a psychiatric concept, and it is not fair to ask psychiatrists to make a pronouncement on an issue that does not belong exclusively to the area of their competence.

Psychiatrists in Africa are still held in high esteem, especially by the courts. This situation can be used, and is being used, by psychiatrists to educate the courts in matters relating to the mental health of offenders, especially when the psychiatrist is humble and the patient does not pontificate. From time to time, one comes across some aggressive advocates who are very irritating because they are armed with only partial knowledge. One can bring them down by demonstrating superior knowledge in a nonpedantic manner.

In interacting with an accused person for the purpose of assessing mental state, one needs to establish considerable rapport to win his confidence.

Would it not be a betrayal of this confidence to give a report that is likely to go against the accused person, especially if the psychiatrist as a citizen believes that the consequent penalty is too severe or unacceptable? This area demands the detachment of the psychiatrist's personal orientation from his professional findings if we are to keep the profession as clean and scientific as possible and if we are to make our evidence in courts reliable. The practice of having a panel of psychiatrists maintained by the court tends to water down the personal idiosyncrasies of the panel members and lend greater credibility to their reports.

Post Trial Stage

The involvement of psychiatry in the post trial stage centers around treatment as a condition of the sentence or mandatory treatment. The old laws inherited from the colonial era specify that those who have been found guilty but insane or not guilty by reason of insanity must be kept in custody, but they are silent on the issue of treatment. This might have been appropriate in the days of asylums. However, today a hospital is, by definition, a place of treatment, so anyone committed by the courts to a hospital has to be treated. The issue of refusal to receive treatment in a psychiatric hospital generally does not arise in Africa.

If anyone who has been found by a professional to be mentally ill, especially if he is psychotic, refuses treatment, then he should not be kept in a hospital. If he has been committed to the hospital by the court, the logical implication is that he should be treated. The hospital is obliged to carry out the treatment, as that is the purpose for which it has been established. This is the case in Africa where treatment resources are available in the hospital. However, for reasons of economics and other pressing needs, not all psychiatric hospitals have adequate treatment resources and facilities, be it for civil cases or criminal cases.

If a psychotic offender has been committed to a hospital and improves enough to become articulate and refuse treatment when continued treatment is considered necessary, he should be transferred to a prison. A hospital is not a place of incarceration. If a person has to be incarcerated in the hospital, it is only for treatment; otherwise, he should be kept in prison.

This raises the issue of separate hospitals for mentally ill offenders. Opinions appear to be divided among psychiatrists in Africa. Some hold the view that such institutions are needed. Others hold that such institutions are not needed and that secure units should be created in general psychiatric hospitals to accommodate those committed by the courts. The argument in support of the latter position is persuasive because of economic considerations and, perhaps more important, because the patients are more likely to identify the secure custody, which will have to be built into the institution, with the caregivers. A secure unit within a hospital setting will be perceived as part of the hospital and not a prison. There is no special orthopedic hospital for prisoners needing orthopedic treatment, to name only one specialty, and I know of no special hospitals for mentally ill offenders in Africa. In Kenya, as was stated earlier, a unit for mentally ill offenders or convicts has been built within Mathari Hospital. This is in keeping with the position of those who argue against the establishment of a special hospital.

CONCLUSION

African psychiatrists need to develop their practice of forensic psychiatry to meet their needs, taking into account social, economic, and cultural factors. We do not have to copy practices in other countries exactly. Rather, we should learn from the problems and mistakes created by those practices. We should not allow the rights of the individual to override the rights of his family and community and the protection of the professional in the execution of his caring duties. At the same time, we should make use of the sociocultural support of the individual where it still exists, remembering that no man is an island unto himself, especially in Africa.

Chapter 17

Crime and Mental Illness in Africa: A Restrospective Study of Court Referrals to A Provincial Psychiatric Clinic in Kenya

by

F. G. Matete, MD, MBChB, MRCPsych
Consultant Psychiatrist
Nyanza Provincial General Hospital
Kisumu, Kenya

ABSTRACT

The relationship between crime and mental illness is complex, and in Kenya there is still a dearth of data on the subject. This retrospective study was designed to determine the level of psychiatric morbidity among the 51 subjects referred by Kenyan courts to a provincial forensic psychiatric clinic during 1984. The cohort had a mean age of 28.8 years, the ratio of males to females was 9:1, and 86.3% of the subjects were found to be mentally ill. Of the mentally ill, 70% had been ill for over 1 year, 20% had previously been admitted to psychiatric facilities, and 15% had been convicted of crimes in the past.

INTRODUCTION

The statistical relationship between crime and mental illness is a complex one because the two concepts are largely unrelated. On the one hand, criminals can be expected to have mental illness just like anyone else. On the other, mentally ill people may also commit crimes (Gunn, 1977; Trick and Tennent, 1981). Furthermore, crime statistics have a number of shortcomings; not all crime is reported or detected, and criminals with less obvious mental health problems may be missed by the referring magistrates (Muluka and Acuda, 1978).

With these pitfalls in mind, I set out to study the case records of all criminals referred to the forensic psychiatric clinic of the Nyanza Provincial General Hospital in Kenya during 1984. The aim was, first, to determine the level of psychiatric morbidity in that cohort and, second, to delineate the pattern of crime in the study sample.

METHODS

A retrospective review was made of the case files of all 51 persons held by criminal remand who were referred to the forensic psychiatric clinic at Nyanza Provincial General Hospital during 1984. All referrals had come from law courts in Nyanza Province. I examined each subject in an assessment interview lasting an average of 45 minutes. The mental state examination was modeled on the Maudsley format (Institute of Psychiatry, 1978).

Clinical diagnosis was mainly based on presenting signs and symptoms, mental status examination, course of illness, and premorbid personality. Schizophrenia was diagnosed on the basis of Research Diagnostic Criteria (Feighner et al., 1972), while the diagnosis of dementia was based on criteria set by the Royal College of Physicians (1982). Mental handicap was viewed as a result of incomplete development of the mind—a condition that may have existed before the age of 18 years. Stress was laid on educability and social competence rather than intelligence (Hill et al., 1979).

The data were analyzed by age and sex and by diagnostic category and crime.

RESULTS

There were 46 males and five females, a male-to-female ratio of 9:1. The mean age of the cohort was 28.8 years (range, 15-61). Of the 51 subjects, 44 (86.3%) were found to be mentally ill, and of these 44, 70.5% had had symptoms for over 1 year, 20.5% had previously been admitted to psychiatric hospitals because of symptoms, and 15.9% had previous convictions. No patient had been undergoing treatment at the time of the crime.

Table I shows the crimes committed by the cohort. Crimes against individuals accounted for 70.5% of all the crimes committed by the cohort; they included assault, homicide, creating a disturbance, and abandoning an infant. Crimes against property amounted to only 29.4% of all crimes, and they included arson, trespassing, criminal damage, and theft. It is important to note that all the cases of arson involved economically significant targets—e.g., a house and a sugar cane plantation.

Table I

TYPES AND NUMBER OF CRIMES COMMITTED BY 51 OFFENDERS REFERRED TO A FORENSIC PSYCHIATRIC CLINIC IN KENYA

CRIME	NUMBER OF CASES	PERCENT OF TOTAL
Assault	15	29.4
Homicide	14	27.5
Arson	7	13.7
Creating a disturbance	6	11.8
Trespass	5	9.8
Criminal damage	2	3.9
Theft	1	2.0
Abandoning an infant	1	2.0

Table II indicates the relationship between diagnostic category and type of crime.

Table II
RELATIONSHIP BETWEEN DIAGNOSTIC CATEGORY AND TYPE OF CRIME AMONG 51 OFFENDERS REFERRED TO A FORENSIC PSYCHIATRIC CLINIC IN KENYA

CRIME	NUMBER OF CASES	PERCENT OF TOTAL
Assault	15	29.4
Homicide	14	27.5
Arson	7	13.7
Creating Disturbance	6	11.8
Trespass	5	9.8
Criminal Damage	2	3.9
Theft	1	1.9
Abandoning Infant	1	1.9
TOTAL	51	99.9

RESULTS

Of the 14 subjects in this cohort who had committed homicides, all but two were found to be mentally ill. The only female murderer was a widow with pathological grief who was forced into traditional remarriage and later hacked her second husband to death. The homicide victims were 12 adults and two children; 10 were male and four were female. All the homicide victims were well known to their murderers. One was a traditional healer who was drowned by his client during a dawn cleansing ceremony in a river. Thirteen of the 14 homicide victims died instantly, indicating the vicious nature of the attacks. Two murderers committed double murders, but none was a recidivist. Table III shows the means used by the murderers to commit their crimes; all the weapons were simple and readily available.

Table III

WEAPONS USED BY 14 MURDERERS REFERRED TO A FORENSIC PSYCHIATRIC CLINIC IN KENYA

WEAPON	NUMBER OF CASES	PERCENT OF TOTAL
Blunt instrument, e.g., fist, stick	8	57.1
Nonexplosive missile, e.g., stone	4.3	21.0
Carbon monoxide	1	7.1
Sharp instrument, e.g., knife	1	7.1
Drowning	1	7.1
Unknown	1	7.1

DISCUSSION

This kind of study has a number of pitfalls, as already outlined. The prevalence of mental illness among this cohort (86.3%), however, is quite close to that found by Mustafa and Muya, as reported by Muluka and Acuda (1978). The male-to-female ratio of 9:1 is similar to findings in Europe and to the earlier local finding of 7:1 (Muluka and Acuda, 1978). Age 17 has been reported elsewhere as the peak age for criminal behavior, but the mean age of 28.8 years in this study cohort also supports the observation that crime is most commonly committed by the young. For example, one of the subjects in this cohort was a 15-year-old girl in a boarding school who managed to conceal her pregnancy. She delivered the baby secretly within the school compound and threw the infant across the school fence. This incident and the numerous other reports of adolescent pregnancies call for study to determine the exact incidence of adolescent pregnancy in our country with a view toward developing a course of national action to cope with the problem.

None of the 44 mentally ill subjects had been receiving treatment at the time of their crimes. Twenty-three (51.3%) were schizophrenic. Because schizophrenia has an incidence of 15-20 new cases per 100,000 population (Kendell et al., 1983) per year and is a chronic disease, it is important that we devise and institute comprehensive community-based psychiatric services, lest what has happened in the United Kingdom, described so poetically by Rollin (1969) and Gunn (1974) also happens here.

Three subjects (two schizophrenic and one demented) had been vagrants at the time of their arrests, reminding us of the sociological concepts of migration and social mobility, particularly the drift hypothesis, and again pointing to the need for community psychiatric services for the chronically mentally ill. Such a community-based system would also provide avenues for research into local psychosocial factors that, when combined, precipitate vagrancy in the mentally ill (Caplan, 1974; Freeman, 1985; Lamb, 1984). In Kenya, as in other developing countries, dementia is already becoming apparent. This reminds us of the World Health Organization's observation that dementing disorders of later life have become recognized as a major public health problem in our society (WHO, 1981).

REFERENCES

Caplan, G.: Social Support and Community Mental Health. New York, Behavioral Publishing, 1974

Feighner, J. P., Robins, E., Guze, S. B., et al.: Diagnostic criteria for use in psychiatric research. Archives of General Psychiatry 26:57-63, 1972

Freeman, H. L.: Mental Health and the Environment. London, England, Churchill Livingstone, 1985

Gunn, J.: Prisons, shelters, and homeless men. Psychiatric Quarterly 48:505-512, 1974

Gunn, J.: Criminal behavior and mental disorder. British Journal of Psychiatry 130:317-329, 1977

Hill, P., Murray, R., Thorley, A.: Essentials of Postgraduate Psychiatry. New York, U.S.A., Academic Press, 1979, pp. 141-153

Institute of Psychiatry: Notes on Eliciting and Recording Clinical Information. Oxford, England, Oxford University Press, 1978

Kendell, R. E., et al.: Companion to Psychiatric Studies, 3rd ed. London, England, Churchill Livingstone, 1983, pp 283-284

Lamb, H. R. (ed.): The Homeless Mentally Ill: A Task Force Report of the American Psychiatric Association. Washington, D.C., U.S.A., APA, 1984

Muluka, E. A. P., Acuda, S. W.: Crime and mental illness: a study of a group of criminal patients in Mathari mental hospital. East African Medical Journal 55:360, 1978

Rollin, H. R.: The Mentally Abnormal Offenders and the Law. London, England, Pergamon Press, 1969

Royal College of Physicians: Organic Mental Impairment in the Elderly: Implications for Research, Education and the Provision of Services. London, England, Royal College of Physicians, Committee on Geriatrics, 1982

Trick, K. L. K., Tennent, T. G. G.: Forensic Psychiatry, An Introductory Text. London, England, Pitman, 1981, pp 23-30

World Health Organization: Dementia in Later Life: Research and Action: technical report series no. 730. Geneva, Switzerland, WHO, 1981

Chapter 18

Psychosomatic Structuring Among Africans

by

Sobbie A. Z. Mulindi, PhD,
Lecturer,
Department of Psychiatry,
Faculty of Medicine,
University of Nairobi,
Nairobi, Kenya

ABSTRACT

The term alexithymia has been used for a group of functional psychological disturbances often found in patients with psychosomatic diseases: poor fantasy life, poor dream recall, inability to express feelings with words, and thinking that is concerned only with conscious psychic processes. The author discusses studies on the relationship of alexithymia to early development and the association between individual adjustment and social factors. To assess the effect of rapid cultural change on African individuals, the author determined the prevalence of alexithymia among patients in a psychiatric consultation-liaison clinic in a teaching hospital in Kenya. Alexithymia was more common among single, separated, or divorced subjects, students with difficulties at school, those who had experienced sudden changes of environment, and members of the Kikuyu tribe. The patients tended to have multiple vague symptoms, to lack psychological insight into their problems, and to engage in doctor shopping. Africans experiencing rapid cultural changes have not had the social support necessary for successful adaptation, and this failure to cope has resulted in a high prevalence of psychosomatic disorders. The Kikuyu, for instance, experienced the Mau-Mau rebellion during the fight for independence and live close to an urban area which is associated with multiple stresses.

INTRODUCTION

This paper is an outgrowth of extensive research in doctor-patient communication and psychosomatic disorders. This presentation is part of my research project for the doctor of science degree at the University of Rene' Descartes V, The Sorbonne, Paris. Its title is Sociocultural Mutations and Psychosomatic Structuring, African Study.

As far as I know, no research has been done in this area on the African continent, especially in the Anglophone countries. Much of the systematic research on African psychosomatic patients has been in French West Africa and can be found in Psychopathologie Africaine. Scientists associated with this type of research are Collomb, Zemple'ni-Rabin, Avbin, and M. C. and E. Ortigues.

THEORETICAL FRAMEWORK

Psychosomatic medicine studies the influence of psychosocial factors on physical health. It has undergone marked conceptual shifts in the past two decades.

First, theorists today believe that there are no psychosomatic diseases per se and that all physical diseases have psychosocial components. These components may predispose to illness, initiate it, or maintain it. Second, previous studies in psychosomatic medicine were oriented toward symptoms and disease rather than toward the relationships and mental functioning of the here-and-now patient

(Mulindi, 1983). The concept of alexithymia arose as a result of this shift toward thinking in terms of the communication patterns of psychosomatic patients.

DEFINITION OF ALEXITHYMIA

The concept of alexithymia has medical, cultural, and social implications. Briefly, it refers to persons whose bodies speak for them in times of stress. Such patients have been observed to experience little intrapsychic conflict and to lack psychological insight.

Marty et al. (1963, 1976a, 1976b) identified a style of thought and expression elicited in psychodynamic interviews from patients with classic psychosomatic illnesses—e.g., asthma, rheumatoid arthritis, ulcer— that they called la pensee operatoire, or operational thinking, an extension of Piaget's conceptualization of intelligence development.

According to this conceptualization, patients with psychosomatic illness manifest a certain concrete, inert quality in that thought is not linked to fantasy, thinking simply replicates past actions but does not enlarge upon it, and there is little dream recollection and little ability to fantasize.

In the United States, Shands (1958, 1975), in working with psychosomatic patients, found similarities to pensee operatoire in material from interviews with these patients but not with other psychoneurotic patients. Sifneos (1973, 1977) observed similar characteristics in a psychiatric clinic at the Massachusetts General Hospital during the years 1954 to 1967. Deriving from the Greek, a for lack, lexis for word, and thymos for emotion, he coined the term alexithymia, or absence of words for feelings, for the patients he observed. Alexithymia has, therefore, been used to describe certain psychological characteristics that have been observed in patients suffering from a variety of psychosomatic diseases, as well as the mental state of some individuals who are not necessarily ill.

The invention of the term alexithymia does not signify discovery of a new object or structure but, rather, recognition of certain functional psychological disturbances, which are worth studying in detail to determine their nature, origin, and significance in individual patients and normal people. Furthermore, the degrees and type of alexithymic characteristics vary between individuals and may vary at different times in the same person's life.

Therefore, the term psychosomatic disorders is not restricted to a small group of specific disorders with structural lesions, but encompasses equally functional disturbances related to stress, behavior disturbances, and conversion hysteria.

DEVELOPMENTAL AND PSYCHODYNAMIC ASPECTS OF ALEXITHYMIA

As noted earlier, the characteristic features of alexithymic patients are impoverished fantasy life, poor dream recall, inability to express feelings with words, and a mode of thinking concerned with conscious psychic processes that have no appreciable relation to unconscious fantasies. Stephanos (1975), the Paris group (e.g., de M'Uzan, 1974), Wolff (1977), and McDougall (1974) have attempted to trace the genesis of alexithymic characteristics to faults in the earliest object relationships of the infant.

Likewise, Mitscherlich (1977) and Gaddini (1977) have emphasized the significance of the early infant- mother relationship and the way children handle transitional objects, in the sense described by Winnicott (1958, 1966, 1982), whereas Nemiah (1973) has elucidated the neurophysiological rather than the psychological explanations. Kernberg (1972) has tried to bridge the two. These contributions enable us to understand how physical, psychological, and social factors contribute to the development of a particular condition, symptom, or behavioral abnormality in a particular person and at a particular time. Of prime importance are the structure of the psychic apparatus and the nature of defense mechanisms employed for adaptive purposes in an individual in a given environment.

THE SOCIOCULTURAL POSITIONS

Winnicott (1982) pointed out the importance of cultural heritage in assuring individual continuity. According to him, cultural heritage is a potential link between the individual and the environment. It is through culture that the personal psychic and social codes are articulated. The personal psychic code comprises structure of identifications, personal fantasy, object relations, defense system, etc. The social code is a system of values, social rapports, etc. If civilization is a system of enlightened institutions for maintaining security, when these break down the cultural heritage is unable to assure the continuity of existence. In other words, when there are rapid sociocultural changes, the relationship of the individual to the group is menaced and his security is threatened. The breakdown of a culture has disorganizing effects on the individual's socially organized psychic defenses.

A person can only adapt to change if the initial mother-group-cadre was good enough. Recent years have witnessed a revival of interest in the question of why and under what circumstances those with certain physical risk factors are more likely than others to develop the symptoms of physical illnesses. My concern in this paper is to consider this issue and, in particular, to consider the main theoretical standpoints from which explanations of research findings have been advanced.

A single major theme that has emerged from recent research on stressful life events, personality, and illness has been the significance of social factors in the onset and course of a wide range of physical and psychiatric disorders. It has been well established that life events which threaten health do so primarily because of their social meaning to the individual (Engel, 1971; Rahe, 1972; Struening and Rabkin, 1976; Dohrenwend, 1974; Brown, 1976; Cassel, 1976; Brown and Harris, 1978; Totman, 1979a & 1979b).

Some studies have shown high rates of illness after bereavement and other forms of loss (Rowland, 1977; Totman, 1979a & 1979b). Other circumstances have been linked to enhanced susceptibility to illness or poor adjustment to a new job or role (Parens et al., 1966; Jacobs et al., 1970; Hinkle, 1974). They include social mobility (Marks, 1967; Jenkins, 1976), exposure to different social status environments (Syme et al, 1965; Cohen, 1974), frequent residential moves (Syme et al., 1965 Rowland, 1977), and poor adaptation to an unfamiliar culture after leaving a primitive social order (Cassel, 1976; Kaes, 1979).

The overall conclusion from what is now a very large body of findings is that, especially in the Western world, social traumas of various kinds have adverse effects on health independent of the effects of diet, exercise, smoking, and other proven physical risk factors. The greatest danger seems to come from changes that somehow disrupt or threaten the social continuity in a person's life, particularly social deprivation, such as the loss of a relationship or social role that had previously given direction and purpose to a person's efforts (Brown and Harris, 1978; Kaes, 1979).

The likelihood that an individual will adjust to these kinds of social upheaval, which constitute a risk to health, is moderated by the presence of social support (Cobb, 1976), the availability of compensating social involvement (Totman, 1979a & 1979b), and the enduring characteristics of the person himself. The latter, presumably, determine his resistance in critical situations as a result of early learning and experience (Lazarus, 1966; Kaes, 1976).

Psychological defenses generally act in favor of consistency; they also act in favor of low susceptibility. This confirms the hypothesis that an individual's general defense competence will be positively associated with low susceptibility to disease. A large number of studies have linked unsuccessful psychological defenses to rapid progression of cancer and auto-immune conditions. Strong psychological defenses have been associated with good prognosis for survival with renal dialysis, whereas, poor psychological defenses have been associated with somatization—i.e., the substitution of somatic preoccupation for dysphoric affect in the form of complaints of physical symptoms and even illness (Kleinman, 1980).

Particularly intriguing are descriptions of a pattern of alternation between physical and psychiatric symptoms in patients such that the onset of physical symptoms coincides with remission of psychiatric symptoms and vice versa (Dubin, 1977). These findings point to the irregularity of the mental functioning in many patients with psychosomatic disorders. They elucidate, furthermore, the relationship between physical, mainly neurophysical, aspects and psychosocial aspects. Relating human experience and brain function remains difficult. However, Kohut (1971), focusing on the disorder of a self-experience, has added a new dimension to our understanding of the complexities of mental mechanisms.

THE AFRICAN CONTEXT

PREVALENCE OF ALEXITHYMIA

Using the theoretical framework just outlined, I assessed the prevalence of alexithymia among patients seen through a psychiatric consultation- liaison clinic in a teaching hospital, the Kenyatta National Hospital. More than 200 patients were seen between 1984 and 1986. About 75% were aged 15 to 35 years and the majority were female. The education level of the patients ranged from the functional illiteracy of older patients, about 25% of the sample, to university level. The prevalence of alexithymia was high among single, separated, or divorced subjects, those with difficulties at school, and those who had experienced sudden changes of environment. The prevalence of ulcers was high among adolescents.

In the majority of the patients, however, the presentation was characterized by vagueness, multiple symptoms, frequent changes, and lack of sharp boundaries between ideas and experience. Most of the patients lived in towns and cities, rather than rural areas. There was no evidence of a high prevalence of alexithymic characteristics among the lower socioeconomic group. However, there was a high prevalence among the Kikuyu tribe.

DESCRIPTION OF PATIENTS

The patients tended to do a great deal of doctor shopping before they landed in a psychiatric consultation- liaison clinic. They had limited self-exposure and self-reflection and lacked psychological insight into their problems. They had difficulty describing their feelings and tended to give detailed accounts of events without any form of association. During interviews these patients used fewer affect-laden words than did psychoneurotic patients.

In psychotherapy, these patients were silent for longer periods and the therapist tended to be more active. They dreamed infrequently and lacked interest in the content and meaning of their dreams. They appeared to require a great deal of supportive psychotherapy, rather than traditional insight- oriented psychotherapy. The most effective supportive psychotherapy was the holding type described by Winnicott. Patients who were not treated with this approach decompensated and developed severe psychiatric disturbances.

EFFECTS OF CULTURE

Africa is undergoing more rapid sociocultural changes than anywhere else in the world. It is experiencing the equivalent of the West's Middle Ages, Industrial Revolution, and twentieth century all at the same time. Rapid technological advancement has had a serious impact on the lives of many people. Children and adults are able to watch Maradona play football 10,00 kilometers away or the launching of the space shuttle from Cape Canaveral, Florida, U.S.A., while at the same time adhering to magicotraditional beliefs and values. There has been a rapid shift from traditional values and customs to new values without sufficient anchoring to assure individual psychic security.

The monetary economy encourages migrations from the communal climate of intense interpersonal exchange and security to an insecure and anonymous urban setting. The individual in crisis has no framework of support. New situations arise to which the lonely individual cannot adapt. All these changes disrupt the individual's continuity of existence and sense of security, which previously had been assured by the group psychosocial apparatus (Kaes, 1976). The inability to cope with numerous life events and stresses is manifested in the high prevalence of various types of psychosomatic disorders encountered in clinics.

If the ultimate objective of psychosomatic research and behavioral medicine is to provide a scheme for preventive and remedial measures, then a principal objective must be a causal theory about the psychosocial determinants of illness, which this study has attempted to provide. Moreover, the more general, more encompassing the causal model, the greater will be the range of derivative programs for intervention and prevention.

We now have findings from a large number of studies of life events, personality, and illness that, taken together, point to some definite themes and patterns. Several contemporary authors have remarked that a causal theory about the psychosocial determinants of illness must make sense out of these patterns as they apply to a particular environment or sociocultural setting. The higher prevalence of alexithymic characteristics among the Kikuyu tribe than among the other ethnic groups can be accounted for by the following factors.

The Kikuyu society seems to have undergone drastic sociocultural changes due, first, to the Mau-Mau rebellion during the fight for independence and, second, to its proximity to an urban area, with its associated life stresses. The result of these sociocultural disruptions is a high frequency of psychological, behavioral, and psychosomatic disorders within this tribe. This fact is validated by my observation of the range of age groups affected.

The other reason, which seems to be culturally biased, is the fact that among the Kikuyu tribe the public expression of feelings, especially of anger or sadness, is not encouraged. Furthermore, like many African languages, the vocabulary lacks words to express mental states. For example, the word feeling is equated with hearing if literally interpreted. Thus, if a doctor asks a patient, "How are you feeling?" in Kikuyu, "Uraigua atia?", it literally means, "How are you hearing?" This has important semantic implications for the patient's explanatory model (Helman, 1984).

Further research is necessary to determine the etymological significance of language use in this context. Some authors have tried to attribute the high frequency of somatization in Africans to rearing patterns, especially the prolonged weaning period (from 6 to 18 months) and intense body contact in infancy. As an etiological explanation, it remains to be demonstrated how neural mechanisms and human interactions account for the transformation of physiological experiences into psychological representations. They result in a capacity for symbolization and, eventually, acquisition of a language for expressing emotions. In this context, psychophysiological studies of alexithymic patients may help to clarify some of the relationships among bodily sensations, perception, cognition, imagination, and verbal behavior. It would appear that alexithymic patients lead an automatistic, mechanistic life and experience a psychosomatic regression to a primitive system of defense and to the earliest stages of somatic development. The irregularity of mental functioning in these patients accounts for the characteristics so far observed, especially from the psychodynamic and behavioral perspectives.

CONCLUSION

This pilot study allows few conclusions. Clinical observations confirmed the high prevalence of alexithymic characteristics in patients with somatoform disorders, psychogenic pain disorders, substance use disorders, and other stress-related symptoms of depression. These findings are similar to characteristics observed in other cultures and thus confirm the existence of psychosomatic phenomena, pensee operatoire, or alexithymia. They support the hypothesis that these characteristics are products of sociocultural change.

The concept of alexithymia has immense clinical value in both medical and psychiatric settings. The consultation-liaison psychiatrist should seek to identify alexithymic characteristics in medically ill patients in order to avoid misdiagnosis and inappropriate treatment. Further, to avoid unnecessary doctor shopping and iatrogenic diseases, the techniques and skills involved in the doctor-patient relationship should be modified so that the doctor can understand patients' communicative styles and provide effective consultation.

REFERENCES

Brown, G. W.: Social causes of disease, in An Introduction to Medical Sociology. Edited by Tucker, D. London, England, Tavistock, 1976, pp. 291-333

Brown, G. W., Harris, T.: Social Origins of Depression. London, England, Tavistock, 1978

Cassel, J.: The contribution of the social environment to host resistance: the Fourth WadeHampton Frost Lecture. American Journal of Epidemiology 104:107-123, 1976

Cobb, S.: Social support as a moderator of stress. Psychosomatic Medicine 38:300-314, 1976

Cohen, J. B.: Socio-cultural change and behavior patterns in disease etiology. PhD dissertation, University of California at Berkeley, Berkeley, Calif., U.S.A., 1974 de M'uzan, M.: Psychodynamic mechanisms in psychosomatic symptom formation. Psychotherapy and Psychosomatics 23:103-110, 1974

Dohrenwent, B. S.: Stressful Life Events: Their Nature and Effects. New York, U.S.A., John Wiley & Sons, 1984

Dubin, W. R.: A study of the relationship between psychological defenses and endocrine function in a patient with cardiovascular disease. Transactions and Studies of the College of Physicians of Philadelphia 45:65-73, 19797

Eiser, J. R.: Sudden and rapid death during psychological stress: folklore or folk wisdom? Annals of Internal Medicine 74:771-782 (1971)

Gaddini, R.: The pathology of the self as a basis of psychosomatic disorders. Psychotherapy and Psychosomatics 28:260-271 , 1977

Helman, C.: Culture, Health and Illness. Bristol, England, John Wright & Son, 1984

Hinkle, L. E.: The effect of exposure to cultural change, social change and changes in interpersonal relationships on health, in Stressful Life Events: Their Nature and Effects. Edited by Dohrenwent, B.S. New York, U.S.A., John Wiley & Sons, 1974

Jacobs, M.D., Spilken, A. Z., Norman, M. M., et al.: Life stress and respiratory illness. Psychosomatic Medicine 32:223-242, 1970

Jenkins, C. D.: Recent evidence supporting psychologic and social risk factors for coronary disease. New England Journal of Medicine 294:987-994, 1033-1039, 1976

Kaes, R.: In L'appareil psychique groupal: constraction du groupe. Paris, France, Dunod, 1976

Kaes, R.: Crise, rupture et depassement. Paris, France, Dunod, 1979

Kernberg, O.: Early ego integration and object relationships. Annals of the New York Academy of Science 193:233-247, 1972

Kleinman, A. M.: Patients and Healers in the Context of Culture. Berkeley, Calif., U.S.A., University of California Press, 1980

Kohut, H.: The Analysis of the Self. New York, U.S.A., International Universities Press, 1971

Lazarus, R. S.: Psychological Stress and the Coping Process. New York, U.S.A., McGraw-Hill, 1966

Marks, R. U.: Social stress and cardiovascular disease—factors involving social and demographic characteristics: a review of empirical findings.
Milbank Memorial Fund Quarterly 45 (supp): 51-108, 1967

Marty, P.: In L'appareil psychique groupal: Construction du groupe. Paris, France, Dunod 1976

Marty, P.: Les mouvements individuals de vie et de mort. Paris, France, Payot 1976

Marty, P., de M'uzan, M., David, C.: L'investigation psychosomatique. Paris France, Presse Universitaire, 1963

McDougall, J.: The psychosoma and the psychoanalytic process. International review of Psychoanalysis 1:437-459, 1974

Mitscherlich, M.: The significance of the transitional object for psychosomatic thinking. Psychotherapy and Psychosomatics 28:272-277, 1977

Mulindi, S. A. Z.: The importance of the relationship value in the genesis, maintenance and healing of psychosomatic patients: study of mental functioning of regressive nature. PhD dissertation, Universite' Lyon II, Lyon, France, 1983

Nemiah, J. C.: Psychology and psychosomatic illness: reflections on theory and research methodology. Psychotherapy and Psychosomatics 22:106-111, 1973

Parens, H., McConville, B. J., Kaplan, S. M.: The prediction of frequency of illness from the response to separation: a preliminary study and replication attempt. Psychosomatic Medicine 28:162-171b, 1966

Rahe, R. H.: Subjects' recent life changes and their near-future illness reports. Annals of Clinical Research 4:250-265, 1972

Rowland, K. F.: Environmental events predicting death for elderly. Psychological Bulletin 82:349-384, 1977

Shands, H. C.: An approach to the measurements of suitability for psychotherapy. Psychiatric Quarterly 32:500 (1958)

Shands, H. C.: How are "psychosomatic" patients different from "psychoneurotic" patients? Psychotherapy and Psychosomatics 26:270-285, 1975

Sifneos, P. E.: The prevalence of "alexithymic" characteristics in psychosomatic patients. Psychotherapy and Psychosomatics 22:255-262, 1973

Sifneos, P. E., Apfel-Savitz, R., Frankel, F. H.: The phenomenon of "alexithymia": observations in neurotic and psychosomatic patients. Psychotherapy and Psychosomatics 28:47-57, 1977

Stephanos, S.: The object relations of the psychosomatic patient. British Journal of Medical Psychology 48:257-266, 1975

Struening, E. L., Rabkins, J. G.: Life events, stress and illness. Science 149: 1013-1020, 1976

Syme, S. L., Hyman, M. M., Enterline, P. E.: Cultural mobility and the occurrence of coronary heart disease. Journal of Health and Human Behavior 6:178-189, 1965

Totman, R.: What makes "life events" stressful? a retrospective study of patients who have suffered a first myocardial infarction. Journal of Psychosomatic Research 23:193-201, 1979a

Totman, R. G.: Social Causes of Illness. London, England, Souvenier Press, 1979b

Winnicott, D. W.: Through Pediatrics to Psychoanalysis, London, England, Tavistock, 1958

Winnicott, D. W.: Psychosomatic illness in its positive and negative aspects. International Journal of Psychoanalysis 47:510-516, 1966

Winnicott, D. W.: Playing and Reality (1971). New York, U.S.A., Methven, 1982

Wolff, H. H.: The contribution of the interview situation to the restriction of fantasy life and emotional experience in psychosomatic patients. Psychotherapy and Psychosomatics 28:58-67, 1977

Chapter 19

The Relationship of Psyche and Soma as Viewed by American Psychiatrists

by

David R. Hawkins, MD,
Director, Consultation-Liaison Service &
Professor of Psychiatry,
Department of Psychiatry,
Michael Reese Hospital and Medical Center
and
Professor of Psychiatry,
Pritzker School of Medicine,
University of Chicago,
Chicago, Illinois,
U.S.A.

ABSTRACT

The author traces the history of psychosomatic medicine from the first use of the word psychosomatic by the German psychiatrist Heinroth in 1818 through the ascendancy of psychoanalysis to the recent emphasis on organic causes of behavior. Systems theory holds that biological events can be viewed at multiple levels, and different scientific disciplines provide knowledge and generate hypotheses for each other.

The neurosciences in particular have begun to yield findings linking psyche and soma. Important examples are studies relating neurochemistry, REM sleep, and brain lateralization to information processing.

Scientists working at different levels of organization can now see the relevance of findings in other disciplines to their own work, and medicine will be better able to understand human biology if it addresses psychological and social issues as well as physical and chemical facts.

HISTORY OF PSYCHOSOMATIC PSYCHIATRY

The question of the relationship of psyche to soma and vice versa has intrigued and plagued man at least since the time of classical Greece. There has been an ongoing debate as to whether they should be viewed as separate entities or as different aspects of an indivisible whole. Since the development of science, many reductionists have taken the position that ultimately behavior and mental illness will be understood in terms of the biochemistry of the brain.

The term psychosomatic has been used to focus attention on the importance of both psyche and soma in medicine and to emphasize that the organism is a single entity. Unfortunately, the term itself emphasizes a division and is often used to imply psychogenesis of illnesses with somatic signs and symptoms, a concept more appropriately termed psychophysiological illness.

The term psychosomatic was first used in 1818 by the German psychiatrist Heinroth, who considered insomnia a psychosomatic disorder because both physical and psychological events could cause it. The term, however, did not come into common usage until the 1920s and 1930s. Several lines of study and theories of mental function, which began at the end of the last century and the beginning of this one, drew significant attention to psychosomatic medicine.

Freud, through his study of patients with conversion hysteria, had demonstrated how unconscious psychological conflicts could lead to illness that apparently involved the body. In this model, the unconscious psychic conflicts could be resolved through expression of bodily symptoms that symbolized the unconscious conflict. Pavlov had demonstrated the role of the conditioned reflex in behavior and showed how manipulation of the conditioned reflex in conflict situations could lead to the development of severe neurotic responses, which included profound physiological changes. Walter Cannon, the most distinguished American physiologist of the early half of the twentieth century, had demonstrated the physiological concomitants of pain, fear, rage, and other emotional states.

In 1937, the National Research Council sponsored a conference that brought together investigators from those and other relevant backgrounds (Liddell, 1962).

That meeting demonstrated to many scientists that others, with different points of view and from different backgrounds, were approaching many of the same problems and that it would be worthwhile to establish relationships which would foster further interdisciplinary communication and research. After this meeting, representatives of the Josiah Macy, Jr. Foundation were instrumental in helping establish the journal, Psychosomatic Medicine, in 1939, and in 1942, the American Psychosomatic Society and its journal, Psychosomatic Medicine, were established.

From the mid-1930s until the late 1950s, meetings concerned with psychosomatic medicine attracted scientists from a variety of disciplines and clinicians from a variety of specialties. During this same period psychoanalysis flourished and psychodynamic psychiatry was in the ascendancy. Most of us now think there was an overemphasis on psychoanalysis, which led to an excessive reaction in the organic direction.

After an exciting period in which psychological events were correlated with the onset or exacerbation of a variety of illnesses, it became increasingly apparent to those investigating psychosomatic relationships that research needed to focus on end-organ pathophysiology and on brain mechanisms.

Many became disillusioned with the psychosomatic point of view. At the same time, the discovery of the usefulness of neuroleptics in treatment of mental illness led to an enormous increase in psychopharmacological research and neuroscience in general.

Unfortunately, the enormous advances in so-called biological psychiatry were accompanied by disparagement of psychological aspects of medicine.

In the ongoing irrational bipolar struggle between psyche and soma, the somaticists were again in the ascendancy. After World War

II and until the late 1960s, most academic psychiatry departments were chaired by psychiatrists who had been trained in psychoanalysis. Nowadays, most medical schools are looking only for biological psychiatrists.

BIOLOGY'S RESTORATION OF THE PSYCHE TO PSYCHOSOMATIC

The discovery of neuroleptics for treatment of mental illness and the subsequent development of other psychotropic drugs have led to an enormous amount of first-rate neuroscientific research. The present period in psychiatry is spoken of as the era of biological psychiatry. The majority of the best young research psychiatrists are specializing in neuropsychopharmacology rather than psychosocial studies. This tendency to make major swings in areas of interest is typical in the United States. It would seem to represent our capacity for great enthusiasm, which does not always make for proper balance. Nevertheless, the recent major strides in the methodology and technology of neuroscience studies have led to enormous increase in knowledge that is relevant to medicine. Unfortunately, this has strengthened the arguments of those who would understand and treat psychological problems in an overly simplistic and mechanistic fashion. The polarity of psyche versus soma, or the psychological versus the organic, is again being stressed.

The real challenge, of course, is to understand how these different levels of integration relate to each other. General and living systems theories have been of enormous conceptual value in this regard (von Bertalanffy, 1968; Miller and Miller, 1985). Briefly, a system is a set of units with specific and hierarchical relationships to each other. This model allows for an understanding of how progressively more complex hierarchical systems influence each other.

In Wilson's model (1977), every scientific discipline has an antidiscipline, and this view helps clarify the relationships in the hierarchy of ever-increasing complexities. According to this concept, psychology is the antidiscipline for sociology and neuroscience is the antidiscipline for psychology. The antidiscipline typically requires more rigor than the formulations of the related discipline, which in turn is likely to develop concepts or problems that are important for the antidiscipline to investigate.

It is enormously useful that the human mind is constantly trying to understand how things work by reducing them to their simplest terms. Useful as this propensity is, it can be a trap, and in situations that need more complex analysis, reductionism has betrayed many a scientist.

As Mayer (1982) has so clearly demonstrated, many biological events have to be viewed at different levels. He divides biology broadly into functional biology and evolutionary biology. The former explains the fact that a certain species of bird starts its migration at a certain time by showing that a change in the amount of sunshine influences sex hormone levels that, when they reach a certain point, trigger migration. The latter can explain how the mechanism evolved and what function it serves for the preservation of the species. The bird's adaptation has to be related to complex geographic and climatologic characteristics.

THE ROLE OF NEUROBIOLOGY

I believe that some of the recent strides in neurobiology will soon make psychological issues again respectable to most biological scientists and will demonstrate that to understand behavior one has to understand not only the underlying biochemistry but how it relates to information processing. Let me use a few examples to illustrate how better understanding of basic neuroscience issues will enhance acceptance of the psychological level of integration.

Kandel (1983) and his colleagues have been studying learning and development of a primitive form of anxiety in the giant snail, Aplysia. The number of neurons in this organism that are responsible for certain learned protective behaviors is so small that it is possible to demonstrate the neural connections responsible for learning a conditioned aversive response. In other words, it is now possible to demonstrate the actual neural basis for what had heretofore been possible to study only behaviorally. Moreover, the biochemistry of process is being worked out. This means that we are now becoming able to study the physical and chemical basis for information processing in the nervous system. An important aspect of these studies is the demonstration of the plasticity of the mechanism, and the important dimension of the process is the handling of information.

I predict that understanding the underlying mechanism will legitimize the attempt to understand anxiety and avoidance learning at the information-processing or psychological level as well.

One is reminded of the reaction when the existence of enkephalins was first demonstrated. The placebo reaction was now legitimized. However, the fact of the placebo response is still demonstrated only in clinical investigation, and the question of what psychological perception triggers the enkephalin in a placebo response is still as big as ever.

The field of research that has probably shed more light on the connection between psyche and soma than any other is the study of dreams and dreaming. Freud was the first to deal scientifically with dreams, although leading philosophers throughout history have written and speculated about dreaming. Freud's single greatest work was The Interpretation of Dreams, published in 1900. He demonstrated that the dream is a meaningful production of the mental apparatus and is amenable to interpretation and, hence, understanding. In the last chapter of that book, he discussed his view of the process of dreaming and outlined his conception of the human mental apparatus. In the process he laid the framework for all his subsequent psychoanalytic views.

There was little revision of his views of dreaming until almost the middle of the century, when psychoanalysts, such as French (1954) and Erikson(1954), provided evidence that dreaming has a certain type of emotional problem-solving function.

At almost the same time, Kleitman, a distinguished physiologist whose field of investigation was sleep, and junior colleagues demonstrated the existence of periods of rapid conjugate eye movements (REM) during sleep and showed that dreaming occurred during this phase of sleep (Aserinsky and Kleitman, 1953; Dement and Kleitman, 1957). Gradually it was shown that this stage of sleep consists of a unique state of intense neurophysiologic activity in the central nervous system and a temporary paralysis of the general motor system. It has also been shown that the REM phase of sleep developed phylogenetically in the most primitive of mammals and is seen in all the subsequent mammals.

Animal studies, and some suggestive studies of humans, have indicated that REM sleep plays a role in the consolidation of memory. Moreover, the hippocampus, which has been shown to be crucial for consolidation of long-term memory, shows a pattern of constant theta-wave activity during REM sleep when measured by electroencephalography. Theta activity in the hippocampus is seen in the waking state only during certain activities crucial to species preservation and not at all in non-REM sleep.

On the basis of these and other findings and the analogy of the computer, many have hypothesized that a major function of REM sleep is to process information (Hawkins, 1966; Palumbo, 1978). REM sleep clears the circuits involved in the immediate processing of the previous day's activities and sorts and stores new information in appropriate memory banks. In so doing, it may modify the approach to that particular life issue and may permit some creative activity in relation to future life events. The latter represents the problem-solving dimension. An overall statement of this line of theorizing has been best expressed in the book Brain and Psyche: The Biology of the Unconscious by Winson (1985), a neuroscientist at the Rockefeller University, whose own investigations have chiefly focused on the hippocampus. He maintains that REM sleep allows off- line information processing in the mammalian brain. He hypothesizes that the functioning and mechanisms developed as REM sleep are the neurophysiological basis for the unconscious. Moreover, study of the material of dreams gives us some beginning indication of the way the brain processes information. It is increasingly clear that the brain operates far differently from the logical conscious thinking of which we are aware.

The history of the study of sleeping and dreaming illustrates the futility of the either/or psyche versus soma debate and shows how studies in the disciplines and antidisciplines enhance each other. Many of the early studies performed after the discovery of the REM phase of sleep were set up to test hypotheses derived from psychoanalytic dream theory. An early example is the first human REM sleep (dream) deprivation experiment (Dement, 1960). It was postulated that dream deprivation would not permit periodic discharge of the unconscious and would, therefore, lead to psychological difficulties. Although the initial study suggested this was the case, subsequent similar experiments failed to confirm the original finding, but much was learned from the studies. The knowledge gleaned from psychophysiologic studies of sleep require considerable revision of the classic dream theory.

The functional biological sleep studies aimed at understanding mechanisms are amplified by the evolutionary biological studies demonstrating the correspondence of the development of REM sleep to the evolution of the mammalian brain, which ensures such great plasticity of behavior. This and other discoveries from comparative species studies provide major clues to the information sorting, storing, and memory-consolidation functions of REM sleep.

Another line of investigation in the neurosciences not only is providing much information about how the brain (the organ of the mind, or psyche) works, but is also adding convincing evidence of the importance of psychological mechanisms and confirming aspects of psychological theories, including psychoanalysis. This is the remarkable series of studies of split-brain preparations, initially with animals and subsequently with human beings in whom the corpus callosum and anterior commissure were severed. The pioneer in these studies and the mentor of subsequent investigators was Roger Sperry (1968), who received the Nobel Prize for this work.

Among other things, these studies have demonstrated the relative independence of the two cerebral hemispheres when the huge pathway that ordinarily keeps them in constant communication is severed. Both hemispheres can process conflicting information simultaneously and independently. Moreover, there is evidence that there is a difference in the specialized strategy of information processing (Levy et al., 1972)

One investigator (Gazzaniga, 1985) has postulated that information is processed simultaneously in many areas of the brain. He believes that one is not conscious of this because most of the brain areas are nonverbal and cannot internally communicate with the dominant hemisphere's language and cognitive system. He relates this to Freud's concept of unconscious process. These concepts are much too complex for brief explanation, but I use them to illustrate that scientists studying complex brain mechanisms in a variety of disciplines increasingly see processes which parallel complex psychological formulations, including psychoanalytic ones.

Up to this point, I have not dealt directly with medicine, which is the unifying force and provides the motivation for spending money on biomedical research. There are pressures both for and against attention to psychosocial issues by physicians. Engel (1977) has written compellingly, logically, and intellectually of the need for a new medical model. He proposes that the biomedical model be replaced with a biopsychosocial model. He makes it clear that the traditional biomedical model is no longer scientific but, rather, has become the Western world's dominant folk model of disease. In a subsequent paper (1980), he demonstrated, by carefully studying the clinical case of a patient with an acute myocardial infarction, how the systems theory can be of enormous help in understanding multiple events, their impact on the individual and vice versa, from the level of the community to that of the molecule, and how events at different hierarchical levels are related.

Persuasive and illuminating as these and other papers have been, it seems unlikely that the most convincing arguments for the importance of understanding information processing and, hence, psychosocial dimensions of human biology will come from the neuroscientists whose work in explicating fundamental central nervous system processes provides an understanding of the basic mechanisms underlying behavior. Moreover, when a mechanism is understood, we can see that it serves rather than causes information processing.

CONCLUSION

Current neurobiological research is leading to enough basic understanding that scientists working at different levels of integration can begin to respect each other's fields and understand the relevance of these other findings to their own work. As we learn more about the function and mode of operation of the primitive nervous system and the human brain, it becomes more apparent that the crux of operation is information processing in the service of adaptive behavior and that psychological and social issues must be attended to along with physical and chemical ones. Neurobiology may be the means of restoring the psyche to psychosomatic.

REFERENCES

Aserinsky, E., Kleitman, N.: Regularly occurring period of eye motility and concomitant phenomena during sleep. Science 118:273-273, 1953

Dement, W.: The effect of dream deprivation. Science131:1705-1707, 132:1420-22, 1960

Dement, W., Kleitman, N.: The relation of eye movements during sleep to dream activity: an objective method for the study of dreaming. Journal of Experimental Psychology 53:339-346, 1957

Engel, G. L.: The need for a new medical model: a challenge for biomedicine. Science 196:129-136, 1977

Engel, G. L.: The clinical application of the biopsychosocial model. American Journal of Psychiatry 137:535-544, 1980

Erikson, E. H.: The dream specimen of psychoanalysis. Journal of the American Psychoanalytic Association 2:5-56, 1954

French, T.: The Integration of Behavior, II: The Integrative Process in Dreams. Chicago, U.S.A., University of Chicago Press, 1954

Freud, S.: The Interpretation of Dreams (1900), in Complete Psychological Works, standard edition, vols. 4,5. London, England, Hogarth Press, 1953

Gazzaniga, M. S.: The Social Brain: Discovering the Networks of the Mind. New York, U.S.A., Basic Books, 1985

Hawkins, D. R.: A review of psychoanalytic dream theory in the light of recent psychophysiological studies of sleep and dreaming. British Journal of Medical Psychology 39:85-104, 1966

Heinroth, J. Ch. A.: Lehrbuch der Stoerungen des Seelenlebens. Leipzig, Germany, 1818

Kandel, E. R.: From metapsychology to molecular biology: explorations into the nature of anxiety. American Journal of Psychiatry 140:1277-1293, 1983

Levy, J., Trevarthen, C., Sperry, R. W.: Perception of bilateral chimeric figures following hemispheric deconnection. Brain 95:61-78, 1972

Liddell, H. S.: The origins of Psychosomatic Medicine and the American Psychosomatic Society. Psychosomatic Medicine 24:10-12, 1962

Mayer, E.: The Growth of Biological Thought. Cambridge, Mass., U.S.A., Harvard University Press, 1982

Miller, J. G., Miller, J. L.: General living systems theory, in Comprehensive Textbook of Psychiatry, 4th ed. Edited by Kaplan, H. E., Sadock, B.J., Baltimore, Md., U.S.A., Williams & Wilkins, 1985

Palumbo, S. R.: Dreaming and Memory: A New Information Processing Model. New York, U.S.A., Basic Books, 1978

Sperry, R. W.: Mental unity following surgical disconnection of cerebral hemispheres. Harvey Lectures 62:293-323, 1968

von Bertalanffy, L.: General System Theory. New York, U.S.A., Braziler, 1968

Wilson, E. O.: Biology and the social sciences. Daedalus 2:1270-104, 1977

Winson, J.: Brain and Psyche: The Biology of the Unconscious. Garden City, N.J., U.S.A., Anchor Press/Doubleday, 1985

Chapter 20

Homoracial and Heteroracial Behavior in the United States

by

Chester M. Pierce, MD,
Professor, Education and Psychiatry,
Harvard Medical School
and
Harvard Graduate School of Education,
Cambridge, Massachusetts,
U.S.A.

and

Wesley E. Profit, PhD,
Director, Forensic Services,
Bridgewater State Hospital,
Bridgewater, Massachusetts,
U.S.A.

ABSTRACT

This is one of a series of investigations conceived and administered by blacks for the purpose of experimenting on whites. Such experimental focus is lacking sorely, but it is much needed in behavioral sciences research. There is a crucial clinical need for blacks to learn how whites behave when they are not in the presence of blacks. Without studying whites as well as blacks, we can know little of why blacks defer to whites. The object of the experiment was to document differences in group dynamics between single- race groups and mixed groups. Our conclusions speak to racism in the United States but may be relevant anywhere where blacks and whites interact. Applications of the investigation may best be made by blacks in our never-ending effort to banish racist behavior by means of hypervigilant self-monitoring and elective action.

INTRODUCTION

It has been postulated that whites' behavior toward blacks is different from their behavior toward each other. Further, in almost all instances, blacks permit, if not invite and demand, others to degrade, demean, and minimize them. Also, there seems to be nearly universal confusion among blacks in distinguishing between being accepted by whites and being tolerated by them.

The chief manifestations of racism are incessant, often gratuitous and subtle offenses, or microaggressions against blacks by whites. The delivery of these assaults, largely kinetic and nonverbal, is so predictable in black-white relationships that they can be anticipated and counted with a mathematical exactitude which delights the physicist. This is because the fabric of racism is based on an etiquette in which both races nearly always arrange for the white's use of space, time, energy, and mobility to take precedence over and to be resolved to the disadvantage of the black's use of time, space, energy, and mobility. If this is so, particularly when a corollary theory of body language is establised, pictures of heteroracial and homoracial groups could document the theory.

METHOD

The subjects were 18 to 20 years old, were paid volunteers, did not know each other, had low incomes, and had no college education. Each group was made up of four persons in homoracial or heteroracial units. There were six heteroracial and 12 homoracial units; half were all-male and half were all-female. Thus, there were three groups of black men, three groups of black women, three groups of white women, and three groups of white men. The heteroracial units comprised three groups of two black and two white women each and three groups of two black and two white men each.

At the taping site, the subjects were asked to give away $50 in a legal manner. The $50 bill was shown to them and they were assured that their decision would be implemented. The group process was filmed and the dialogue was transcribed. Before the study, race-specific behavior was predicted in 165 verbal and nonverbal areas—e.g., who talks more, who gives or takes advice, which body parts are exposed or protected.

An interracial team of men and women, technically trained for the tasks, conducted the analysis. The analysis included qualitative assessment of verbal and nonverbal content. Only a small part of the results will be presented.

STATISTICALLY SIGNIFICANT RESULTS

The following significant differences in behavior are accompanied by the relevant p values. The black women showed no difference in the measured areas between their behavior in front of other black women and their behavior in front of white women.

Behavior of Blacks

Compared with their behavior in the presence of white men, black men in the presence of other black men:

- demonstrated more inhibited thinking (e.g., "We can't do this") (.003)
- talked more about drugs (.019), clothes (.038), mothers (.034), families (.009), brown people (.018), race (.027), and illegal possibilities for donating the money (.036)
- used more words (.013)

Compared with their behavior in the presence of whites, blacks in general (male and female) demonstrated the following behaviors in the presence of other blacks:

- made more suggestions (.017)
- talked more about food (.012) and clothes (.028)
- considered more illegal possibilities (.05)

Behavior of Whites

Compared with their behavior in the presence of black men, white men in the presence of other white men:

- used more words (.009)
- made more suggestions (.003)
- were more specific in their suggestions (.016)
- made more suggestions in the negative form (e.g., "Let's not do . . .") (.008)
- made more tentative suggestions (e.g., "We could try .")
- asked for more advice (.020)
- talked more about children (.010), death (.052), violence (.055), and food (.017)
- were more often ignored by their peers (.017)
- discussed more illegal possibilities (.010)

Compared with their behavior in the presence of black women, white women in the presence of other white women:

- talked more about cleanliness (.020), athletics (.017), drugs (.026), and Native Americans (.016)
- made more requests for information (.043)
- made more suggestions in the negative form (.013)

Compared with their behavior in the presence of blacks, whites in general (male and female) demonstrated the following behavior in the presence of other whites:

- used more words (.011)

- talked more about food (.005), starvation (.025), death (.026), cleanliness (.022), drugs (.011), children (.046), and Native Americans (.018)
- made more requests for information (.019)
- asked more questions (.027)
- gave more suggestions (.005)
- made more specific suggestions (e.g., "Let's send the orphans from the Little-Children-of-the-Poor House to the baseball game this Friday") (.011)
- made more suggestions in the negative form (e.g., "I don't suppose. (.0005)
- made more tentative suggestions (.011)

QUALITATIVE RESULTS

The research team perceived no differences in the originality, usefulness, effectiveness, or humanity of the solutions presented by the groups. For instance, one group decided to give the money to the Red Cross, another to give it to CARE.

Homoracial black male groups could be characterized as tolerant of individual deviation from the assigned task. Also, they confessed openly, in front of the camera and strangers, self- incriminating activities. They dwelled on what could not be done.

Homoracial black female groups could be characterized as sociable. They established support with amazing celerity and worked in a relaxed, friendly manner.

Homoracial white male groups could be characterized as confident. Further, they were the most intolerant of individual deviation from the assigned task, even though they thoroughly examined means to procure the $50 for themselves illegally. That is, they considered the most options and did so in an almost leisurely fashion.

Homoracial white female groups could be characterized as inquiring. When away from blacks, they used many more words and had a lively cognitive exchange.

In the heteroracial same-sex situations, the men were more tense and wary than women. The black men were deferential and hesitant and allowed the white men to finalize decisions and use more space. In the female heteroracial interaction, there was the appearance of equality. In both the male and female heteroracial situations, the whites delivered the final decisions and were markedly less likely to express group weakness or self-doubt. The whites were disposed to give commands and not ask blacks for suggestions.

In our efforts to become more certain of our identity and indigenousness, blacks must learn how we differ from whites in what we do or do not do. This study indicates that even when blacks are designated as actual coequals, they may allow whites to determine legitimacy and decide the course of action. All homoracial groups talk more freely and more intimately, but at subtle levels, homoracial white and black groups differ considerably. Firmer knowledge about and awareness of these differences would be especially useful in education of and service to black people.

CONCLUSIONS

The three conclusions presented herein are only a few of the numerous distillates that the full data suggests. For the sake of brevity and the purposes of this presentation, the distillates address practical areas of concern to black clinicians.

Overdisclosure by Blacks

The dynamic of overdisclosure in front of whites has different origins in black men and black women. The men, perhaps because of eroded confidence and despair over the ability to control their destiny, gratuitously revealed unflattering and negative things about themselves. Overdisclosure may result from their habitual talk when they are by themselves about what cannot be accomplished.

Unlike any other group, black women showed no alteration of behavior in front of the other race, perhaps because of their historical forced intimacy with white females. They showed more evidence that, given the opportunity, they could be competitive with their counterparts. It could be argued that increased guile and artfulness by black women, even to the extent demonstrated by other groups in heteroracial circumstances, might favorably influence race relations.

Whatever the true and complete meanings of black overdisclosure, its continuance has weighty implications for future black male-female relationships, as well as black-white relationships.

Role of White Women in Racism

White men were the only group that had no significant discussion of race. White women were the most immersed in racial concerns. Given the role of white women, particularly as wives and mothers of those who exert power, it is important to find out what role they have in shaping and sustaining racism. This view differs from the more common belief that racism is to a large extent related to efforts by white men to protect/control white women. Because of competition and strain between black and white women, the perpetuation of racism may be due to active female behavior more than is usually believed.

Recognizing that racism itself may be one reason white gatekeepers do not allocate funds for blacks to study their children, black psychiatrists may be obliged to design inexpensive studies that can be performed in an indirect or unobtrusive manner. It matters not that blacks may resent that whites have never themselves directly studied black children.

Black Cognitive Styles

Blacks exhibited a style of thinking that could be characterized as defensive. In addition, it was rapid, geared toward end results rather than process, and more impressionistic than precise. The blacks considered fewer options but arrived at a comparable answer 10 times as fast as whites—i.e., it took them 3 minutes to decide to give the money to CARE, whereas whites took 30 minutes to give it to the Red Cross.

Perhaps it is irrelevant whether or not this is a consequence of incessant offensive thinking and behavior by whites. What is less in contest is that such defensive thinking modes must have huge survival value for blacks. However, to dilute the withering effects of racism, it may be important to make a systematic analysis in biological, as well as psychosocial, terms of how we think. The biological aspects would have to include the neurosciences, chemistry, and genetics.

Further, especially for the purpose of education, we should consider the common cognitive styles of whites, such as making more requests for information, asking more questions, being more specific and exact, and, especially, making more suggestions in the negative form. Maybe some of these can and should be modified for common use by blacks. At minimum, we need to be aware of how their use by whites affects black-white interactions. Despite their routine use by whites, they are concealed or modified when blacks are present.

Lastly, we must become more keen in appreciating the difference between positively charged microaggressions and negatively charged microaggressions. A frequent consequence of a microaggression is deferrence to a white's decision. Any assault or insult, whether minor or major, can be delivered with various degrees of cheerfulness. Thus, an insult or assault delivered in an ugly, confrontational manner is much more likely to be resisted than an equally damaging one that deceives by being delivered in a kind but firm and definite manner.

Differentiation of such microaggressions, whether in an experimental, social, or clinical situation, is crucial in negotiating one of the most perplexing aspects of being black. That is, blacks, especially in any direct interaction with whites, must develop ways of knowing when and how to resist victimization versus when and how to accept victimization. At minimum, blacks must be more in control of deciding things for themselves without white guidance, suggestions, or advice. The essence of oppression is permitting others to use and abuse your space, time, energy, and mobility.

SECTION III:

Child Psychiatry

Chapter 21

Child Psychiatry in Kenya

by

F. G. Njenga, MD, MRCPsych,
and
L. Wairimu Ndirangu, MA, MSW
Nairobi Kenya

ABSTRACT

Estimates of the prevalence of psychiatric disturbances in African children and adolescents range from under 10% to 24%. Most studies of childhood psychiatric illness in Kenya, however, have been impressionistic. The social revolution following independence has had a large impact on families and children, and emotional and conduct disorders in children are common. The first psychiatric clinic for children was established in Nairobi in 1981, and the authors used a multi-axial system to assess 71 children referred to the clinic over 7 months. Neurotic disorders were diagnosed in 46%, hyperkinetic disorders in 11%, conduct disorders in 10%, and psychoses in 6%. Primarily, organic disturbances were infrequent. Family interviews were invaluable in obtaining information and stimulating family communications, and the symptoms of 23% of the children could be directly related to abnormal intrafamilial relationships. In the future, emphasis should be placed on educating psychiatric and pediatric care givers and on establishing child guidance clinics in the provinces.

OVERVIEW

Prevalence

The prevalence of psychiatric disturbance in adults in Africa is now estimated to be between 17% and 21% (German, 1972; Ndetei and Muhangi, 1979). Giel and Van Luijk (1969) studied psychiatric morbidity in two Ethiopian villages. They found that 3% to 4% of all children under the age of 10 years and 10% of those 10 years old or older showed psychological abnormalities. In Uganda, Minde (1974) found the prevalence of psychiatric disturbances among primary school children to be 18%—10.5% in rural areas and 24% in urban areas. In Kenya, Sindandi and Acuda (1979) found that 12% of the adolescents in a rural secondary school were mentally ill. Cederbland (1968) studied 1,716 Sudanese children aged 3 to 15 with respect to stuttering, sleepwalking, enuresis, encopresis, and sleep disturbances. There was an 8% prevalence of these symptoms alone.

Difficult as it is to compare these figures with those collected elsewhere, because of methodological differences, it is pertinent to cite figures obtained elsewhere. In their 1-year Isle of Wight study in England, Rutter et al. (1976a and 1976B) found a 10% to 15% prevalence of psychiatric disorders in 10-year-old children. Another group of children reported marked suffering associated with psychiatric symptoms but their problems were not evident to parents and teachers. When these children were included, the prevalence rose to 21%, a figure close to that reported by Minde (1974) in his Uganda study. Leslie (1974) found a prevalence of 21% in boys and 14% in girls in his study at Blackburn, an industrial town in northern England. In Australia, Krupinski et al. (1967) found rates of 10% and 16% for children and adolescents, respectively.

As of 1981, no systematic investigation had yet been done in

Kenya to establish the prevalence of psychiatric illness among children. Most of the work done with children so far has been impressionistic (Izuora, 1970; Asuni, 1970). The information available, however, suggests that children and adolescents in Kenya are just as prone to psychiatric illnesses as those elsewhere. It is believed that the number of children with psychiatric disorders is high and that the diagnostic profile is similar to that in London or Uganda (Minde, 1974).

Historical Perspective

Much of the practice of medicine in Kenya is modeled on the British system for historical reasons. Great Britain was a forerunner of child psychiatry because of the interest shown by Victorians in the welfare of their children.

Kenyatta (1937) was the first to observe human behavior in Kenya. He did not have psychiatric training, but his writings, especially in relation to mother and child, are insightful. He described mothers teaching their children through the medium of lullabies "so that it becomes easy for the children to assimilate early teachings without any strain." He further described how the child was taught to walk and, in later stages, to relate to his peers and elders.

Kenyatta also described the social pressures on parents of children who did not seem to be growing in the proper manner and emphasized the importance of personal relations. He stated, "It is with personal relations that the Kikuyu education system is concerned rather than with natural phenomena." Later he stated: "Europeans assume that, given the right knowledge and ideas, personal relations can be left largely to take care of themselves and this is, perhaps, the most fundamental difference in outlook between Africans and Europeans."

I have quoted Kenyatta generously because the fears expressed in other chapters of his book relating to the breakdown of the social fabric seem to have come true, especially among those living in post-independence Kenya.

Rutter and Mudge (1976) commented on the secular trends in Great Britain and noted that they are similar to those in America (Bronfenbrenner, 1975). Families are becoming smaller, people are marrying later, the rate of illegitimate births is increasing, and divorce, family breakdown, and single-parent families are more common.

Kenya, especially urban Kenya, is also experiencing rapid social change, and, as in Western societies, the implications for children and adolescents are unknown, but the conditions are likely to make normal development more difficult. The children of people born in the forties and fifties seem to be suffering the brunt of this post-independence social revolution.

Emotional and conduct disorders are prevalent but are not yet well understood by parents and physicians. The current absence of facilities for addressing the emotional needs of the 50% of the population under age 15 is indicative of the general neglect of this age group.

In time these services will develop. I believe, however, that these resources must first be developed within the available services in a way that lends itself to evaluation. There is a particular need for trained social workers, psychologists, and paramedics, if a meaningful program is to be developed.

PATIENTS IN A CHILD PSCHIATRIC CLINIC

The first child psychiatric clinic in Kenya was set up in 1981 by the Department of Psychiatry of the University of Nairobi. This clinic was necessary because, prior to that time, children under the age of 15 were seen in a busy psychiatric outpatient clinic primarily designed for adults.

In the new clinic, children were seen, examined, and managed by a psychiatrist, a psychiatric social worker, a psychologist, and senior house officers undergoing training for higher degrees. Formulations were based on a multiaxial system that required the coding of the following axes: axis I—clinical psychiatric syndrome, axis II—developmental disorders that are present or apparent from the history, axis III—intellectual level, axis IV—medical or physical conditions, and axis V—psychological factors or situations in the patient's environment.

From studying 71 children over 7 months, it was possible to conclude that multiaxial classification of child psychiatric disorders can be applied routinely in Kenya. A number of problems, however, continue to cry out for solution; one is the lack of a method of measuring the IQ of children in the Kenyan setting. The most obvious limitations of the available measures are language difficulties, but the diverse social experiences of Kenya children are also a barrier to standardized measurement.

During the study, it was found that 60% of the children referred to this clinic were 11 to 15 years old, and no children below the age of 5 were referred.

An interesting and rather surprising finding was the relative infrequency of primarily organic disturbances in referred patients. Neurotic disorders were diagnosed in 46%, hyperkinetic disorders in 11%, and disorders of conduct in about 10%. Six percent of the children were psychotic when first examined. The relative infrequency of psychosis may be related to the fact that this service did not have a backup emergency service, so acutely ill children with psychoses or extreme disturbances of behavior were seen elsewhere.

Thirteen children with epilepsy were seen and managed during this period. Their referral was precipitated by secondary disturbances of behavior, most often during or after seizures.

The Family

An inescapable conclusion was the fact that, laborious as it may be, a family interview is an integral part of the diagnosis and management of childhood psychological disorder. A family interview may be the first time members of a family talk to each other about their common problem(s). Various family alignments or alliances may become apparent to the interviewer.

Seeing the family as a whole may also reveal the frequent but often missed situation in which a desperate family brings a relatively normal and mentally healthy child to the hospital or to a doctor when their main problem and source of anxiety is actually another child who is mentally retarded, physically handicapped, or even mentally ill. For example, they profess that the child they have brought has a severe conduct disorder in the hope that somehow they may be able to get help for their real problem. The other child may not be mentioned at all in the history, and routine questions like "Are the other children alive and well?" more often than not are answered by a quick but anxious "Yes, doctor." Only a family interview (or a home visit) is likely to clarify the otherwise incomprehensible actions of parents who return a normal child to the hospital, where the child may finally be labeled as neurotic or as having supratentorial syndrome as a way of saying that no diagnosis has been reached.

Even more common are parents who are themselves ill (e.g., depressed) and project their symptoms onto a child. Nine percent of the children in this study had such parents. As mentioned earlier, a family interview may be the first time all members of the family talk about their common problems openly. This serves the double purpose of eliciting information for the interviewer and providing therapy. The family interview also offers a good opportunity for the team looking after the child to explain the situation to the family and to impress on them their role and importance in cooperating in the subsequent management of the child.

Twenty-three percent of the children seen came from homes with overt evidence of abnormal intrafamilial relationships. The presenting symptoms could be related directly to that situation.

In the practice of child psychiatry in Kenya, one comes across a number of complexities peculiar, in some respects, to this society. A recent case illustrates this point.

A 5-year-old girl was referred for the management of what appeared to be grand mal epilepsy but was, on closer observation, a functional condition representing anxiety. For 2 months, this girl's home had been bombarded by rocks and other missiles ostensibly thrown onto the roof by ghosts. This matter was reported extensively in the local media and had reached alarming proportions in the locality. The key to the mystery was the presence of some degree of marital difficulties in the family. As long as the child remained ill, the family remained together, as the parents continued their country wide search for a solution to the ghost attacks. The family moved from traditional healers to their local hospital, back and forth, and yet no solution could be found in either place. Even the grandmother's prayers did not seem to resolve the rift between the child's parents.

THE FUTURE

The Department of Psychiatry at the University of Nairobi is in the process of setting up a child and family therapy unit. This unit is expected to not only provide much needed services in Nairobi, but also enable doctors, social workers, and medical students to acquire skills relevant to the practice of child and family psychiatry. Postgraduate students in pediatrics should also be exposed to the practice of child psychiatry so that they can use these skills in their practice as pediatricians.

The wider problem seems more difficult to tackle. The number of children at risk is great, but the number of trained personnel is small. Child guidance clinics are needed in the provinces. These could be manned by social workers and psychologists, who could work in conjunction with local psychiatrists.

REFERENCES

Asuni, T.: Problems of child guidance of the Nigerian school child. West African Journal of Education 14:49-55, 1970

Bronfenbrenner, U.: In Child Psychiatry: Modern Approaches. Edited by Rutter, M., Hersov, L. London, England, Blackwell Scientific Publications, 1975, p. 416

Cederbland, M.: A child psychiatric study on Sudanese Arab children. Acta Psychiatrica Scandinavica Supplement 200:1-23, 1968

German, G. A.: Aspects of clinical psychiatry in sub- Saharan Africa. British Journal of Psychiatry 121:461-479, 1972

Giel, R., Van Juijk, J. N.: Psychiatric morbidity in a small Ethiopian town. British Journal of Psychiatry 115:149-162, 1969

Izuora, G. E. A.: Mental health problems of children in developing countries, in Proceedings of the 2nd Pan Africa Psychiatric Workshop. Mauritius, 1970, pp. 36-65

Kenyatta, J.: Facing Mount Kenya (1937). New York, U.S.A., Random House, 1962

Krupinski, J., Baikie, A. G., Stoller, A., et al.: A community health survey of Heyfield, Victoria. Medical Journal of Australia 1:1204-1211, 1967

Leslie, A.: Psychiatric disorders in the young adolescents of an industrial town. British Journal of Psychiatry 125:113-124, 1974

Minde, K.: The first 100 cases of a child psychiatric clinic in Uganda: a follow-up investigation. East African Journal of Medical Research 1:95-108, 1974

Rutter, M., Graham, P., Chadwick, O. F., et al.: Adolescent turmoil - fact or fiction? Journal of Child Psychology and Psychiatry 17:33-56, 1976a

Rutter, M., Madge, N.: Cycles of Disadvantage — A Review of Research. London, England, Heinemann Educational Books, 1976B

Sindandi, P. O., Acuda, S. W.: Psychiatric morbidity among secondary school students in rural Kenya. Nairobi Journal of Medicine 10: 36-39, 1979

Chapter 22

Black Children in Psychiatric Outpatient Treatment in the United States

by

Harry H. Wright, MD, MBA, Associate Professor
and
Elisabeth A. Cole, BS, Biostatistician
Department of Nueropsychiatry,
William S. Hall Psychiatric Institute,
School of Medicine, University of South Carolina,
Columbia, South Carolina,
U.S.A.

ABSTRACT

The authors discuss general issues involved in the diagnosis and treatment of black children in the United States and review the demographic and clinical variables of preadolescent black children in South Carolina who attended clinics at the 17 community mental health centers and at a research and teaching hospital. The percentage of black children treated at the hospital's child outpatient clinic increased from 7% to 25% during the 15 years studied. The authors discuss factors related to the underrepresentation of black children in the treatment programs and make suggestions for improving access to and utilization of services by black children and their families.

INTRODUCTION

Children growing up in stressful environments are at a greater risk of developing emotional, behavioral, developmental, and social problems than those in average environments (Garmezy, 1974; Brenner, 1979). The poor and politically powerless are particularly affected and black children are disproportionately represented in both of those groups. For example, one out of every two black children in the United States lives in poverty (Children's Defense Fund, 1983). In addition, the percentage of black children living with both parents dropped from 58% to 41% over the last 15 years. Racial prejudice directed against blacks and social policies that have denied a disproportionate number of black families the opportunity to obtain resources needed for adequate family functioning are two of the major factors that increase the stress on many black families. It is not surprising, then, that many black children present at mental health settings with learning, social, emotional, and/or behavioral problems. In fact, some authors state that black children have been relatively worse off in the 1980s than they were in the 1960s (Gibbs, 1984), implying a gradual deterioration in the environments in which black families raise their children.

Social policies have also had an impact on the understanding of the nature of the presenting problems of black children and have resulted in a lack of early identification, errors in diagnosis, and inadequate and/or inappropriate treatment for many black children and their families. Even when poverty is not a major issue, as with black children from families in the middle and upper social classes, racism still has a devastating impact on their development and their risk of emotional and behavioral problems.

Despite racial prejudice and an array of other adverse conditions, most black children and families make healthy social and psychological adjustments to the environments in which they live (Billingsley, 1968) and cope with racism to the best of their abilities. Many children and families, however, do require therapeutic intervention from outside their families and are referred for treatment.

When a child is referred, the first task of those in the treatment setting is to assess whether or not the child has a disorder that needs treatment. The fact that the child has been referred indicates that someone has a concern. The reason for concern may turn out to be a normal stage of development, a minor problem that does not require treatment, a problem that requires minimal therapeutic intervention, or a major individual or family problem that requires significant therapeutic interventions over a period of months to years.

A comprehensive assessment requires a basic understanding of the social-cultural context from which the child comes, as well as the individual assets and liabilities of the child. For the black child, this is often difficult because of the numerous stereotypes that exist about black children and families (Bender, 1939; Wilkinson and Spurlock, 1986; Ten Houten, 1970; Bennett, 1986; Bradshaw, 1978). Many of these stereotypes continue to drive the therapeutic interventions recommended for black children and their families long after they have been refuted and extensively discussed. In addition to the individual psychopathology of black children and their families, there is a complex relationship between the mental health of black children and the economic, political, and social policies of the community and society. Race and socioeconomic status have been reported to have a significant impact on the psychiatric treatment of black children and their families (Jackson et al., 1974; Stehno, 1982).

Several reports have indicated that the type of therapeutic intervention recommended by providers is associated with race (Lewis et al., 1980; Griffith, 1977). Black patients are more likely to be seen for diagnosis only (Jackson, 1974) and are judged to be less suitable for insight therapy (Flaherty and Meaghen, 1980). Black adolescents are more likely to be referred to nonmental health services (Lewis et al., 1980; Stehno,1982). Additionally, studies indicate that blacks are more likely to drop out of treatment at predominantly white settings (Warren, 1972), and if they continue in treatment, many issues must be addressed by the therapist if a positive outcome is to result (Ridley, 1984; Gardner, 1971; Griffith, 1977; Jones and Gray, 1983). Most often, these issues are not addressed during treatment (Brantley, 1983).

Misdiagnosis of black patients of all ages has been well documented (Jones and Gray, 1986; Lawson, 1986; Mukherjee et al., 1983; Adebimpe, 1981). Misdiagnosis is a particular problem when black children are involved since the type of intervention, or lack of it, has more, long-term consequences for these very malleable young patients. In addition, the biases, myths, and misconceptions about black children have lasted for decades and continue to guide interventions, long after they have been pointed out and refuted (Wilkinson and Spurlock, 1986). One of the major myths about black children is that certain diagnoses, such as conduct disorder and psychosis, occur more frequently than in whites. In fact, the prevalences of most psychiatric disorders in blacks do not differ from those in whites when standardized diagnostic protocols are used (Abramson and Wright, 1981; Adebimpe, 1981; Lawson, 1986).

It is important that the therapist understand that race and ethnicity may play a major role in determining how a patient seeks help, what he defines as a problem, and what he views as a useful intervention. Unless race and ethnic variables are taken into account, therapeutic interventions are sure to fail (Sue, 1981; Acosta et al., 1982). A patient's feelings, ideas, beliefs, values, gestures, intonations, perceptions, and evaluations can only be understood in the context of the patient's sociocultural environment (Parson, 1985).

TREATMENT

Although the data in this paper focus on preadolescent black children in outpatient psychiatric care in the public mental health system in South Carolina, the circumstances in other states are similar. There are 17 community mental health centers that provide public outpatient psychiatric services for children and their families in South Carolina. Over the last 15 years, there has been an increase in the number and percentage of black preadolescent children seen in the outpatient clinics of many of the mental health centers. In 1985, a total of 1,097 black children 12 years of age and under were seen in the mental health centers across the state. This was 21.7% of the total number of children seen in mental health centers in that year—less than the 30% black population in South Carolina. The range for the centers, in terms of percentage of black preadolescent children seen, was 3.8% to 37.2%.

More extensive data are available for a state- supported teaching and research hospital with a child psychiatry outpatient clinic. Table 1 summarizes the data on the number of black preadolescent children seen in the years between 1970 and 1980.

Table 1
BLACK CHILDREN IN OUTPATIENT TREATMENT AT A TEACHING HOSPITAL IN SOUTH CAROLINA, U.S.A., 1970-1985

Year	Number of Black Children Seen	Percent of all Children Seen
1970	4	7
1975	18	15
1980	20	14
1985	27	25

Between 1980 and 1985, a total of 146 black preadolescent children were seen for the first time. Although the percentage for the teaching hospital is slightly above average for the mental health centers, the changes there reflect the trends in most of the mental health centers over the 15 years. The referral sources are listed in Table II.

The self-referral rate was nearly twice that of the entire population of children seen in the clinics. Almost 35% of the black children had had previous mental health treatment, and 10% had been patients in psychiatric hospitals. Nearly 11% had been treated with psychotropic medication before referral to the clinic. Eighteen percent had been hospitalized for medical problems in the past. A profile of the parents' marital status is shown in Figure 1. The proportion of single, never-married mothers is twice that for the overall population of children seen in the clinic.

Table II
REFERRAL SOURCES OF BLACK CHILDREN SEEN AT A TEACHING HOSPITAL IN SOUTH CAROLINA, U.S.A.

Referral Source	Percent of Children
Physician	36
Self	24
School	23
State department of social services	20
Mental health center	12
Speech and hearing clinic	6

Figure I
MARITAL STATUS OF PARENTS OF BLACK CHILDREN SEEN AT A TEACHING HOSPITAL IN SOUTH CAROLINA, U.S.A.

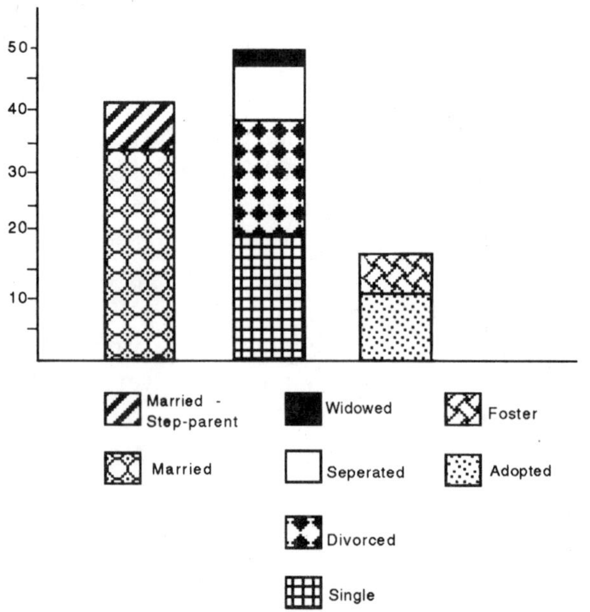

For the children seen in mental health centers, the most frequent diagnoses were adjustment disorder, V codes, no diagnosis, and conduct disorder (Table III).

Table III

PSYCHIATRIC DIAGNOSES OF 1,097 BLACK PREADOLESCENT CHILDREN SEEN IN MENTAL HEALTH CENTERS IN SOUTH CAROLINA, U.S.A.

Diagnosis	Number	Percent of Total
Ajustment disorder	338	30.8
V codes	169	15.4
No mental disorder	137	12.5
Conduct disorder	125	11.4
Attention deficit disorder	76	6.9
Other disorders	70	6.4
Anxiety disorders	69	6.3
Schizophrenia	22	2.0
Mental retardation	15	1.4
Pervasive developmental disorders	12	1.1
Affective disorders	10	0.9

Two mental health centers had significantly higher than average percentages of conduct disorder, and two other centers had significantly higher than average percentages of black children with diagnoses of anxiety disorder (Table IV).

Table IV
MENTAL HEALTH CENTERS WITH HIGHER THAN AVERAGE PERCENTAGES OF BLACK CHILDREN WITH CONDUCT DISORDER AND ANXIETY DISORDERS IN SOUTH CAROLINA, U.S.A.

Mental Health Centers	Percent of Black Seen at Center	Percent of Black Children with Conduct Disoder Diagnosis
A	12.7	25.6
B	20.9	22.2
All Centers	21.7	11.4
C	35.1	17.7
D	27.8	13.5
All Centers	21.7	6.3

DISCUSSION

Although the trend in South Carolina and in the United States in general has been toward increased access and utilization of public mental health services for black preadolescent children, there remain significant barriers to full utilization of mental health services by black families for their children.

Social policy issues have been described by other authors (Comer, 1985; Gibbs, 1984; Comer and Hill, 1985) and will not be repeated here. The referral source has an impact on utilization of service by black families. Both the self- and school-referral rates for black preadolescent children were twice those of the general clinic rates for these sources. At least for self-referrals, this should have significant implications for the mental health center. Black families must feel welcome and comfortable in the facility if they are expected to come back and refer other families. Although many factors are involved in establishing this type of environment, the most critical is the composition, attitude, and behavior of the staff. Following are two examples of interactions between mental health center staff and black children, with discussions of relevant data.

Example A

A mental health center with a catchment area population that was 38% black saw very few black preadolescent children. The center had three clinicians who worked at least part-time with children and adolescents. None of the clinicians had formal training in child mental health care. None of the professional or clerical staff members was black. Black patients who came to the clinic rarely returned for more than one or two visits.

In many public mental health outpatient clinics for children, the staff involved in evaluating and training children does not have formal training in child mental health care. This becomes a major problem for black preadolescent children. When the staff does not have general knowledge and skills in mental health intervention with children, it is certainly unlikely to have the knowledge and skill to deal with the more complex issues of black children. Staff members must be trained to 1) assess and treat young children in general and 2) gain experience in assessment and treatment of black children—i.e., learn something about variation in child development and black family functioning.

In this clinic there are no black staff members despite the large population of blacks in the community. It is unlikely that the average black patient will feel comfortable in this environment. If a black family happens to make it into this center, they will probably not tell anyone else to go there, regardless of the type of service they received. Remember the high percentage of self-referrals among black patients. The center should make an effort to recruit and hire black staff members. Few blacks seek help for serious personal problems in the mental health clinic. Both the stigma and the ineffectiveness of the "help" have contributed to this lack of utilization. Involvement of black staff would enhance services for at least some black families, although hiring black staff members should not be viewed as the answer to this problem.

The therapist (black or white) should make every effort to know and understand the sociocultural environment and value system of the black preadolescent patient, and he should also examine his own attitudes, beliefs, and feelings as he works with the patient psychotherapeutically (Wilkinson and Spurlock, 1986).

Several reports have focused on psychotherapy and black patients (Carter, 1979; Gray, 1987; Jones and Gray, 1983), and a few have focused on psychotherapeutic interventions with black children (Spurlock, 1985; Hencock, 1980). Most of the reports on therapeutic intervention with black children have focused on children from poor families (Hallowitz, 1975). Very little has been written about therapeutic interventions with black children from middle-class families (Bagarozzi, 1980; Scanzoni, 1971; Frazier, 1966). The therapists in the public mental health clinic, if they are to be effective, must be aware of the common as well as the different issues brought to treatment by the family of poor and middle-class black preadolescent children.

Example B

A white therapist in a child psychiatry clinic in a public mental health center was seeing a number of black children and their families but could not connect with them. There were misunderstandings on both sides of the potential therapeutic relationship. For example, the therapist felt a child's mother was overprotective of her 9-year-old child because he was unaware of the real danger in the neighborhood in which the family lived. He made many assumptions without asking questions about the situation.

Careful collection and interpretation of clinical data is essential in making appropriate decisions about assessment and treatment of black preadolescent children. The therapist must know what questions to ask. Accurate, honest communication is the basis for establishing trust with the child, and an interest in and some understanding of the issues is essential in building an alliance with the families of black children.

Misdiagnosis of the problem has been discussed by many authors in the literature (Wright et al., 1984). To decrease the frequency of misdiagnosis of black preadolescent children, the use of appropriately validated rating scales and behavior checklists has been suggested. Review of the statistical data on diagnosis of black patients over a 2- or 3-year period may help a treatment facility to identify problems in treating black patients. It is also important to remember that studies of treatment rates are inadequate for estimating the distribution of psychiatric disorders in the population of preadolescent black children.

Misconceptions about black families lead to inappropriate treatment interventions. The black family in the United States has a strong sense of survival. In fact, several authors have written of black families' amazing ability to grow and advance after confronting years of discrimination and demoralization (Wilson, 1970). For many years, reports on black families have focused on the so-called dysfunction structure and behavior within the family (Ten Houen, 1970; Moynihan, 1965; Rainwater, 1966). Today most authors acknowledge that black families are not so different from other ethnic families in structure and function (Gutman, 1970; Pinderhughes, 1982; Hall, 1982). Like other families, black families struggle to provide for the needs of their members.

SUMMARY

While this report has examined only the public mental health services utilized by families of black preadolescent children in South Carolina, the findings are applicable to other states and treatment settings. The underrepresentation of black children in treatment programs is not a puzzle to be solved but represents a natural consequence of past and current social policies, as well as a lack of adequate knowledge and skill in the use of therapeutic interventions with black children.

A review of the facilities' data on past treatment of black children can help guide the development of a plan to improve access and utilization of treatment resources by black families for their children. Most of the time, this leads to organizing specific educational and training programs for the staff, but attitudes may be the most important consideration.

While some gains in variety of treatments and appropriateness of treatment settings for black preadolescent children have been made, there remains a considerable amount of work to be accomplished in this area if black families are expected to utilize fully the services offered.

REFERENCES

Abramson, R. K., Wright, H. H.: Diagnosis of black patients (letter). American Journal of Psychiatry 138:1515, 1981

Acosta, F. X., Yamamato, J., Evans, L.: Effective Psychotherapy with Low Income and Minority Patients. New York, U.S.A., Plenum, 1982

Adebimpe, V. R.: Overview: white norms and psychiatric diagnosis of black patients. American Journal of Psychiatry 138:279-285, 1981

Bender, L.: Behavioral problems in Negro children. Psychiatry 2:213-228, 1986

Bennett, L.: The 10 biggest myths about the black family. Ebony 41(10):123-133, 1986

Billingsley, A.: Black Families in White America. Englewood Cliffs, N.J., U.S.A., Prentice-Hall, 1968

Bradshaw, W. H.: Training psychiatrists for working with blacks in basic residency programs. American Journal of Psychiatry 135:1520-1524, 1983

Brantley, T.: Racism and its impact on psychotherapy. American Journal of Psychiatry 140:1605-1608, 1983

Brenner, M. H.: Influence of the social environment on psychopathology: the historical perspective, in Stress and Mental Disorder. Edited by Barrett, J. E., New York, U.S.A., Raven Press, 1979

Children's Defense Fund: A Children's Budget: An Analysis of the President's FY 84 Budget and Children. Washington, D.C., U.S.A., Children's Defense Fund, 1983

Comer, J. P.: Black children and child psychiatry. Journal of American Academy of Child Psychiatry 24:129-133, 1985

Comer, J. P., Hill, H.: Social policies and the mental health of black children. Journal of the American Academy of Child Psychiatry 24:175-181, 1985

Flaherty, J., Meaghen, R.: Measuring racial bias in inpatient treatment. American Journal of Psychiatry 137:679-682, 1980

Gardner, L. H.: The therapeutic relationship under varying conditions of race. Psychotherapy: Theory, Research and Practice 8:78-87, 1971

Garmezy, N.: Children at risk: the search for the antecedents of schizophrenia, part 1: conceptual models and research methods. Schizophrenia Bulletin 8:14-90, 1974

Gibbs, J. T.: Black adolescents and youth: an endangered species. American Journal of Orthopsychiatry 54:6-21, 1984

Griffith, M. S.: The influence of race on the psychotherapeutic relationship. Psychiatry 40:27-39, 1977

Jones, B. E., Gray, B. A.: Black males and psychotherapy: theoretical issues. American Journal of Psychotherapy 37:77-85, 1983

Jones, B. E., Gray, B. A.: Problems in diagnosing schizophrenic and affective disorder among blacks. Hospital & Community Psychiatry 37:61-65, 1986

Lawson, W. B.: Racial and ethnic factors in psychiatric research. Hospital & Community Psychiatry 37:50-54, 1986

Lewis, D. O., Shanok, S. S., Cohen, R. J., et al.: Race bias in the diagnosis and disposition of violent adolescents. American Journal of Psychiatry 137:1211-1216, 1980

Mukherjee, S., Shukla, S. S., Woodle, K., et al.: Misdiagnosis of schizophrenia in bipolar patients: amulti-ethnic comparison. American Journal of Psychiatry 140:1571-1574, 1983

Parson, E. R.: Ethnicity and traumatic stress, in the study and treatment of post traumatic stress disorder. Edited by Figly, C. New York, U.S.A., Brunner/Mazel, l1985

Ridley, C. R.: Clinical treatment of the non-disclosing black client. The American Psychologist 39:1234-1244, 1984

Stehno, S.M.: Differential Treatment of Minority Children in Service Systems Social Work :39-45, 1982

Sue, D.W.: Counseling the Culturally Different. New York, Wiley, 1981

Ten Houten, W.D.: The Black Family Myth and Reality. Psychiatry 33:145-173, 1970

Warren, R.: Different Attitudes of Black and White Patients Toward Psychiatric Treatment in a Child Guidance Clinic Amer J Ortho Psychiat 42:301-302, 1972

Wilkerson, C.B., Spurlock, J.: The Mental Health of Black Americans. In Wilkerson (ed): Ethnic Psychiatry. New York: Plenum, 1968

Wright, H. H., Scott, H. R., Pierre-Paul, R., Gore, T.A.: Psychiatric Diagnosis and the Black Patient. Psychiat Forum 1:65-71, 1984

Chapter 23

Innovations in Mental Health Care for Children and Adolescents in the United States and Britain

by

Felton Earls, MD
Professor of Child Psychiatry
School of Medicine,
Washington University,
St. Louis, Missouri,
U.S.A.

INTRODUCTION

While my primary purpose is to describe some of the innovations in child mental health services that are currently taking place in the United States and Great Britain, I do so anticipating that this discussion will have relevance to the growth of child psychiatry in Africa. It should not be necessary for African psychiatrists to follow the same course as that adopted in the West, for the history of child psychiatry in the West is spotted. Over the past 80 years, child psychiatry has struggled to find a place for itself as a science and as a medical service. During this period, innovations and promises have come all too readily and none have been greater than the mental hygiene and child guidance movements that gave this field its foundation.

Over 30 years ago, in an address to the American Psychiatric Association, David Levy (1952) pronounced these innovations a failure. One important reason for this, he noted, was that the preventive and early intervention approaches had been practiced in geographically and intellectually isolated child guidance centers. This isolation had encouraged an uncritical evaluation of psychiatric services for children and an unbalanced orientation toward therapeutic work that favored psychodynamic interpretations over others.

From the time of Levy's pronouncement until now, evidence has continued to accumulate that the promise of inoculating children against mental disorder has not been fulfilled. In fact, there is evidence that rates of psychiatric disorder in children have increased (Rutter, 1980) and that disorders not formerly recognized, such as prepubertal depression (Puig-Antich, 1980) have emerged. At the same time there is evidence, albeit still meager, that our treatments have either modest or no effects at all. So, while there is a need for innovations—one might say even a desperate need— this pause to view our horizons is sobering.

But a look at the history of child psychiatry is not a cause for pessimism. Just in the past decade, research productivity has increased sharply, and the design and methods employed in these investigations have become more sophisticated. Methods to improve the diagnostic precision of specified childhood disorders have become available (Herjanic, 1984), the familial aggregation of both adult and child disorders has been demonstrated for the most frequent disorders in the population, psychopharmacological approaches have been expanded (Greenhill, 1984), and the search for biological and developmental markers in children for adult-onset disorders, such as schizophrenia, has advanced (Neuchterlein, 1986). It is against this background of current progress that innovations in concepts and the organization of mental health services for children must be considered.

One other point should be made before a discussion of new directions in the care and treatment of children. This pertains to the relationship of child psychiatry to pediatrics and to general psychiatry. This is a complicated affair. In an effort to embrace the medical model and to help child psychiatry become a more legitimate subspecialty of psychiatry, the American Academy of Child Psychiatry has recently recommended that child psychiatry become more hospital-based and, at the same time, more strongly aligned with general psychiatry. This stance implies that child psychiatry must strive for two possibly contradictory objectives. Becoming increasingly hospital-based, or tertiary, in its orientation means a stronger alliance with pediatrics and the care of physically ill children. More direct alignment with academic departments of psychiatry means that child psychiatry will participate in scientific efforts to unravel developmental links between genetics, brain mechanisms, childhood experiences, and disorders in adults. Of course, they may both be taken as challenges to contemporary child psychiatry, but it is unlikely that any one program will be equally well developed in both. As is the case in all medical disciplines, individual centers may develop particular expertise in one aspect or another of child psychiatry, while the field as a whole develops on several fronts (Earls, 1982).

In this paper, three separate innovative projects will be described. Each relates to a different developmental phase of childhood and adolescence and, conceivably, to different types of biological or social processes involved in the etiology and maintenance of psychiatric disorders. Together they represent frontiers on which child psychiatry as a medical discipline is advancing.

For the first of these projects, the delivery of comprehensive health care to adolescents evaluation is currently under way. For the second project, the use of school-based interventions for disturbed children, the data have already been published. The third project, which deals with the prevention of conduct disorder in high-risk infants, is presented as a research prospectus of considerable interest in the field. In each case, the innovation has been designed as a research project rather than as a demonstration. This connection between new approaches to design of services and research is essential if the field is to continue to evolve as a medical science.

CONSOLIDATED HEALTH CARE FOR ADOLESCENTS

Just over the past decade the notion has emerged that adolescence is a phase of the life cycle which warrants a special approach to health care.

Adolescence is a distinctive developmental period that has become particularly salient in American culture. Much of the rationale for this view is the observation that the health needs and complaints of teenagers are different from those of children and adults. The major causes of mortality and morbidity in this age group seem to be related to life-style, behavior, and social factors rather than to organ deterioration (Perkins et al., 1982).

The major initiative in defining this new field of medical care has come from pediatricians, with the assistance of obstetrician-gynecologists, internists, psychiatrists, psychologists, and social workers. Training programs in departments of pediatrics have been established, and residents are being prepared for the practice of adolescent medicine. Because the new morbidity that inspired this development is so clearly linked to mental health, the relationship between adolescent medicine and mental health is inevitably addressed. Health care for this age group involves the treatment of medical problems, psychiatric conditions, impaired relationships with parents and peers, and problems resulting from failure at school. This objective of providing comprehensive health care for adolescents encouraged the Robert Wood Johnson Foundation to establish a large fund to foster development in this new area.

In 1981 the Foundation awarded grants to 20 medical schools for development of consolidated approaches to adolescent health care. No one approach was advised. Rather, proposals were chosen on the basis of creativity and the strength of administrative ties between medical school departments and between these departments and important community health and social agencies providing care to youths. In each case, a medical school had to demonstrate that the academic-community network of health care resources would serve a population of adolescents who were at higher than average risk for the major health conditions and types of death for this age group.

Seven conditions were listed: homicide, suicide, depression, alcohol abuse, substance abuse, early pregnancy, and sexually transmitted diseases. It was also recognized that adolescents with chronic diseases and a variety of other conditions, ranging from multiple injuries to legal problems, might also be at high risk for one of these seven targeted problems. The location of most American medical schools in inner-city areas meant that many were already serving high-risk populations, at least insofar as this connotation is demographically defined. In all but one case, departments of pediatrics served as the grant holders and coordinators of the consolidated programs. Each program, while strengthening health services for adolescents, also assumed responsibility for a training program in adolescent medicine.

The 20 programs varied in a number of ways. Some were principally situated in neighborhood health care settings, others were hospital-based, and in a few instances they were based in schools. The approach to consolidation always involved a multidisciplinary effort, usually with a pediatrician as the pivotal team member. The other professionals involved included internists, nurses, social workers, psychologists, and psychiatrists, although the actual composition of the teams varied. In most cases, an existing clinic program was augmented by special sessions for adolescent patients that were organized and conducted by the multidisciplinary team. In a few instances, totally new programs were established. In previously established programs it took time to evolve a truly comprehensive approach, since a number of administrative and clinical barriers had to be overcome.

Within 3 years of initiation, interest in these consolidated programs shifted to an evaluation of their effectiveness. To obtain an answer to the question Did consolidated services make a difference?, a research design was needed that met several requirements.

1. An appropriate comparison for the consolidated programs had to be found. This necessitated close attention to variations among the consolidated programs, for they differed in many ways, including the degree to which they succeeded in meeting the goal of consolidation.
2. The most accurate means of assessing the impact of health care would be to interview the adolescents directly. This required sampling an adequate number

of youths from a variety of consolidated and nonconsolidated programs. It also required that the youths be reassessed some months after receiving the health care they had sought to judge how effective it had been.

3. The assessment of the youths had to be as broad and comprehensive as the medical care they ideally were to receive.
4. The evaluation had to be conducted independently of the programs to minimize bias in the evaluators.

These requirements were incorporated into a research design, and the evaluation began in 1984 under the direction of Dr. Lee Robins and myself. The design called for a comparison of several of the consolidated programs and a number of traditional programs. Because of the variation in the consolidated programs, it was decided that seven of the 20 were required to reflect adequately the different approaches taken. Three traditional programs were selected on the grounds that they did not provide specialized care to adolescents, they were not associated with training programs in adolescent medicine, and they were located in cities other than those where the consolidated programs were. This latter criterion eliminated the possibility that an adolescent might receive care from a consolidated and a nonconsolidated program within the same time interval.

The sampling strategy involved selecting youth between the ages of 13 and 18 who attended each of the services during a 6-month period. The aim was to interview between 300 and 400 youths in each of the programs. In most cases this objective was reached, but in four of the programs it was not, because fewer than the expected number of youths in the designated age range used the service. However, the final sample size of 2,791 was judged adequate to detect differences in outcome between youths presenting with most, if not all, of the seven health conditions targeted by the Foundation.

The interview designed for the study consisted of 10 sections and covered the following areas:

- Health service utilization over the past year
- Medical problems such as injuries, chronic diseases, and common minor abnormalities

- Lifetime and current symptoms of psychiatric disorders from which DSM-III diagnoses, such as major depression, conduct disorder, somatization disorder, alcohol abuse and dependence, and substance abuse and dependence could be derived
- Family history of physical and mental disorders
- Family and peer relationships and current stressors
- School adjustment; social, religious, and recreational activities

The interview required about an hour to complete and was given at two times: at or near the time of the youth's request for help and 10 to 12 months after this initial interview. At follow-up, the interview was augmented with more detailed questions on treatment, compliance with recommendations received from medical personnel, and the outcome of targeted conditions. In addition, the medical records of the youth were systematically reviewed. Of the 2,791 youths interviewed initially, 87%, or 2,417, were reinterviewed. Table I below (next page) gives the number of completed interviews at the two times for each of the 10 participating programs.

In the remaining part of this section, I will present demographic data on the types of youths using the services, the frequency of their presenting problems, and the prevalence of various risk factors for major forms of morbidity and mortality in this age group. A specific hypothesis will be tested that has direct implications for the assumption that mental health is a fundamental concern for the successful care and treatment of the great majority of adolescent health problems. The hypothesis is that depressive symptoms, assumed by some to be a developmental correlate of adolescence, are generally related to help-seeking. Thus, it is predicted that depressive symptoms and depressive disorders will be uniformly correlated with the variety of reasons adolescents come for help. If the hypothesis is confirmed, it would suggest that successful health care for adolescents must be directed toward treating their depression in addition to whatever complaints they might have.

Table I

NUMBER OF YOUTHS INTERVIEWED IN CLINICS PARTICIPATING IN THE EVALUATION OF THE ROBERT WOOD JOHNSON FOUNDATION'S PROGRAM TO CONSOLIDATE HEALTH SERVICES FOR HIGH-RISK YOUNG PEOPLE

CONSOLIDATED CLINICS	NUMBER OF YOUTH INTERVIEWED	
	Wave I	Wave II
Boston Youth Program, Boston City Hospital	132	111
Los Angeles High Risk Youth Project, Children's Hospital of Los Angeles	175	121
Project for Teen Health, Cook County Hospital	356	307
Indianapolis Program to Consolidate Health Services for High Risk Young People, Indianapolis University Hospitals	342	287
Dallas High Risk Youth Project, Parkland Memorial Hospitals	362	302
Jackson-Hinds Project, University of Mississippi Medical Center	374	355
Adolescents Services Project, Yale-New Haven Hospital	193	167
NON-CONSOLIDATED CLINICS		
Public Health Clinics of the City of St. Louis	373	345
Charity Hospital, New Orleans	279	240
Family Practice Center, Deaconess Hospital, Buffalo, New York	200	182

Table II
DEMOGRAPHIC CHARACTERISTICS ASSOCIATED WITH TYPE OF PRESENTING PROBLEM

	SEX		AGE			RACE		
PRESENTING PROBLEM	M.	F.	13-14	15-16	17-18	W.	B.	H.
Well Care (886)	52.28	25.71*	33.49	33.64	29.61	20.51	36.23	22.17*
Acute Illness (691)	34.07	22.04*	35.89	24.55	21.34	21.69	25.53	44.34*
Chronic Illness (80)	4.08	2.51	3.11	3.36	2.36	2.54	2.78	4.52
Pregnancy (1069)	---	38.34	20.81	35.73	46.38*	53.22	35.68	22.17*
Mental Health (134)	7.54	4.00*	6.46	5.93	3.39*	5.93	4.20	7.24*
Total (2860)	22.85	77.15	14.99	39.45	45.55	21.17	70.90	7.93

Notes:

* p<.001; Sex: M=Male; F=Female; Race: W=White; B=Black; H=Hispanic

As shown in Table II, the sample was primarily female and black. Utilization increased with age. The major classes of presenting problems for each sex, age group, and race are given in the table. Well care was defined as routine health examinations (not related to pregnancy) or provision of information about health concerns. The acute illnesses were upper respiratory illnesses, other infections, and injuries. The most frequent chronic illnesses were asthma, hypertension, and anemia. The great majority of the females coming for reasons associated with pregnancy were receiving prenatal care. The mental health problems included depression, suicide, stress reactions, and, in a small proportion of cases, problems primarily related to alcohol or substance abuse. Inspection of the table shows that for every type of concern other than pregnancy, the proportion of males exceeded the proportion of females. This unexpectedly high rate of utilization by males may have been due to the school clinics, which attracted larger numbers of males than those located in hospital or neighborhood settings. It also appears that medical and mental health complaints decreased with age while, as expected, pregnancy increases. The whites and Hispanics exceeded blacks for all medical and mental health problems, while blacks exceeded the others in seeking well care.

Table III

DEPRESSIVE SYMPTOMS AND MAJOR DEPRESSIVE DISORDER AS ASSOCIATED WITH TYPE OF PRESENTING PROBLEM

PRESENTING PROBLEM	4+ DEPRESSIVE SYMPTOMS	MAJOR DEPRESSIVE DISORDER (DSM-III)
Well care (886)	23.02*	3.72*
Acute Illness (691)	36.32*	7.67
Chronic Illness (80)	33.75	5.00
Pregnancy (1069)	37.04	6.64
Mental Health (134)	57.46	21.64
Total (2860)	32.03	6.13

Note: * P<.001

Data on the relationship between depression and help-seeking are shown in Table III. Depression was assessed in two ways. A simple count of symptoms that had persisted for at least two weeks was made. The presence or absence of a DSM-III diagnosis of major depression was also determined. The two approaches were used to compare a formal approach to defining depression in adolescents with a less restrictive one. The decision to set the cutoff on the symptom count at four was to ensure that the number of symptoms present was similar to the number required when making a DSM-III diagnosis (although, of course, the rules regarding coexistence of symptoms were not followed). The results, shown in Table III, demonstrate that the hypothesis regarding the pervasiveness of depression was not supported. A higher than expected rate of major depression was only present when, as one would expect, the presenting problem was of a psychiatric nature. In all other conditions, the rates of major depression were similar to the rates for the sample as a whole or, as in the case of those attending clinics for physical check-ups and medical information (well care), significantly less.

It was recognized that presenting problems reflect only part of an adolescent's risk profile, however. For example, a 15-year-old male requesting a physical examination for clearance to try out for the football team might be discovered to abuse alcohol and carry a weapon. These are important health and life-style issues, and successful intervention during the medical management of this youth should reduce his risk for alcoholism, homicide, and violent accidents. Our interview was designed to assess such risk conditions. It was also important to know to what extent the various risk factors were correlated with each other. Again, the popular notion that depression is generally related to risk of major dysfunction or premature death in teenagers was investigated. Many of the consolidated clinics, in fact, regularly screened all their patients for depression. Demographic data on high-risk conditions assessed in the interviews are shown in Table IV, and their relationship to depressive symptoms and major depression is shown in Table V.

As shown in Table IV, pregnancy, carrying a weapon, and multiple injuries were common. Pregnancy was by far the most common problem in females, while conduct disorder, carrying a weapon, and multiple injuries were the most common problems in males. Females had higher rates of dropping out of school, suicide attempts, hopelessness, and running away from home than males, but there were no significant sex differences for having been jailed, alcohol abuse, substance abuse, and sexually transmitted disease.

Also, similar proportions of males and females reported having three or more of these high-risk conditions. These youths with multiple risk factors are the most important ones to involve in treatment, since they may be at the highest risk of life failure and death.

Table IV
DEMOGRAPHIC CHARACTERISTICS ASSOCIATED WITH HIGH-RISK PROBLEMS DETECTED ON INTERVIEW

Problems Detected on Interview	Sex		Age			Race		
	Male (637)	Female (2150)	13-14 (418)	15-16 (1101)	17-18 (1268)	White	Black	Other
Conduct Disorder (861)	38.8	28.5*	23.9	33.1	31.1	50.8	24.2	20.4
Carries Weapon (773)	38.7	24.6*	23.7	29.3	27.9	31.2	26.5	30.8
Jailed (156)	7.3	24.6*	4.3	5.8	5.8	13.4	3.1	7.7
Runaway (496)	12.4	19.4*	11.5	18.9	18.9	37.1	11.9	19.0
School Drop-out (552)	8.3	21.8*	3.1	10.7	30.8*	44.6	10.9	19.5
Suicide attempt (231)	4.5	9.4*	6.2	8.9	8.4	15.4	5.7	12.2*
Hopelessness (436)	10.4	17.3*	11.6	16.2	16.7	26.4	11.8	22.7*
Alcohol abuse (112)	5.8	3.5	1.7	4.3	4.6	12.7	1.2	6.3*
Substance abuse (137)	5.6	4.7	3.1	4.7	5.7	11.5	2.3	9.95*
Multiple Injuries (582)	33.1	17.3	24.2	20.9	19.8	27.3	19.0	20.4*
SexuallyTransmitted Disease (188)	7.0	6.8	1.2	4.9	10.2*	6.8	6.8	7.2
Pregnant (874)	--	41.0	13.5	33.2	56.4*	45.4	41.3	25.3*
3+ problems (810)	25.4	30.1	15.3	26.5	35.7*	52.9	21.6	32.9*

Note: * $p<.001$

Table V
DEPRESSIVE SYMPTOMS AND MAJOR DEPRESSIVE DISORDER ASSOCIATED WITH HIGH-RISK PROBLEMS DETECTED ON INTERVIEW

PROBLEM DETECTED ON INTERVIEW	PERCENT WITH 4+ DEPRESSIVE SYMPTOMS	PERCENT WITH MAJOR DEPRESSIVE DISORDER
Conduct Disorder (861)	51.1	12.5
Carries weapon (773)	48.4	9.4
Jailed (156)	55.8	14.7
Runaway (496)	61.9	15.7
School drop-out (552)	44.4	8.2
Suicide attempt (231)	87.9	26.4
Hopelessness (436)	94.0	29.4
Alcohol abuse (112)	73.2	22.3
Substance abuse (137)	88.2	21.9
Multiple Injuries (582)	40.6	8.1
Sexually transmitted disease (188)	60.7	9.0
Pregnant (874)	35.6*	5.3
3+ problems (810)	60.7	14.8

Note: *N.S.

Only three of the specific high-risk conditions increased with age: dropping out of school, pregnancy, and sexually transmitted diseases. With few exceptions, blacks had lower rates of these problems than the other two racial ethnic groups. The sampling of youths from inner-city areas selected a more representative sample of black than white youths. In fact, the two projects with the highest proportions of whites, the Los Angeles Free Clinic and the public health clinics in Indianapolis, had the highest proportions of youths with multiple risk conditions. We wondered what factors contributed to the selection of high-risk white youths, and one factor emerged. More white than black youths came from middle-class families. By and large, they had become alienated from their families, and their use of public health facilities, rather than private doctors, reflected this situation. The fact that their running away from home, rates of dropping out of school, and substance abuse were higher than the rates for black and Hispanic youths verifies their downward drift in social status.

Table V illustrates how frequently depressive symptoms and major depression coexist with all high- risk conditions except pregnancy. The prevalence of depressive symptoms among youths with behavioral problems (as reflected in the first five conditions listed in Table V) was 1.5 to 2 times as high as in the sample as a whole. Much higher prevalences occurred in youths with alcohol and substance abuse.

It is reassuring that pregnancy, chronic illness, acute illness, and well care are not associated with higher than expected rates of depression (Table III). The data support the conclusion that youth with these problems who seek health services are not at particularly high risk for conditions associated with premature death and major dysfunction.

The main thrust of this analysis is to demonstrate that it is not difficult to target youths at the highest risk for major forms of morbidity and premature death in primary care settings. Proportionally, they are more likely to come to health services with mental health complaints than with other presenting problems. However, another way to look at these data is in terms of the absolute numbers with high-risk profiles. In other words, even though the youths requesting well care had a low rate of depressive disorder, in absolute terms they represented a larger group with this disorder than those presenting with mental health complaints. Also, the number of females seeking help for reasons related to pregnancy who had depressive disorders was more than two and one-half times the number with major depression among those who presented with mental health problems. While it is not difficult to show that the small group of youths presenting with mental health complaints is indeed at high risk, the larger job of screening all adolescents for high- risk profiles is necessary if the treatment provided for them is going to be effective.

Determining how well the staffing patterns and time allotments reflected the needs of these patients was an objective of our evaluation. All of the consolidated programs had either psychologists or social workers directly involved in the diagnosis and treatment of youth, but very few had psychiatrists. While it appears that this lack of direct involvement by psychiatrists is cost-effective for many and perhaps most of the mental health problems presented by youth, it probably does not guarantee the most intensive intervention.

The point of this presentation is to introduce the idea of using adolescent medical services as a general context in which to deliver mental health care to youth who need it. Because it reduces stigma and is convenient and attractive to teenagers, it represents an ideal environment for the delivery of mental health services. The desire to segment care into medical and mental health compartments is particularly unwarranted for this age group, according to our data and the prevailing wisdom of those in adolescent medicine. Developing the skills to satisfactory comprehensive care is quite another matter. It represents a frontier in medical training and in the design of specialized health services.

A SCHOOL-BASED INTERVENTION—THE NEWCASTLE EXPERIENCE

Two other innovative approaches to mental health care of children will be briefly described. These research projects have been selected to provide perspective on the range of new approaches in child psychiatry. The choice of these two is based on the fact that they satisfy basic aspects of research design and evaluation, in addition to being innovation and potentially far-reaching.

One project was a randomized treatment trial for behavioral and emotional disorders carried out by Kolvin and colleagues in Newcastle, England (1981). The program involved a comparison of three different treatment approaches designed for children at two grade levels in the Newcastle public schools. A sample of children entering infant school (aged 7 years) and another sample entering junior high school (aged 11 years) were screened for the presence of psychiatric disorders. Those judged to have such disorders were then randomly assigned to one of four groups: one group received 3 months of group therapy; the second group received behavioral modification, which was administered by the child's classroom teacher; the parents of children in the third group received training in behavioral control techniques for several months; and the fourth group served as a no-treatment control group. The assignment was made without regard for the types of disorders the children had. Almost all had either emotional or conduct disorders. The four groups were blindly evaluated at several intervals up to 3 years after the end of the treatment program. The results of this experiment demonstrated that the group therapy and behavioral modification approaches had dramatic and lasting benefits in terms of symptom reduction, whereas no difference was seen in the control group or in the children whose parents were involved in the parent training.

Three aspects of these results underscore their importance as an innovation.

1. Both the group therapy and the behavioral modification were conducted within the school. Kolvin et al. speculated that this environment provided a naturalistic context, which rendered the treatments more powerful than they would have been in the more traditional context of a clinic.

2. Since the results of the group therapy and behavioral modification were comparable, a strong argument can be made for choosing the group therapy approach. It is less expensive and less time- consuming than other treatment approaches.

3. The treatments that worked must have nonspecific therapeutic properties since they appeared equally effective for children with different types of problems. The results of this large-scale study are presented in detail in the book Help Starts Here (Kolvin et al., 1981).

It is one of the best documented treatment studies on child psychiatry ever published, and the research methods appear sound. The results were surprising, yet understandable in that interventions which take place in schools may reduce the stigma associated with treatment and provide a direct means to translate what is learned in therapy to real-life situations. Yet the work of the Newcastle group has received relatively little attention. To my knowledge, replication has not been attempted in either the United States or the United Kingdom. This is a curious omission given the traditional role of school consultation in child mental health services. The results of the Newcastle experience warrant much closer attention than they have received. In most other fields a result of this magnitude and importance would be immediately tested by others.

A PREVENTION TRIAL TO DECREASE THE INCIDENCE OF CONDUCT DISORDER

For the past few years, Dr. Lee Robins and I have been interested in the feasibility of a project to prevent conduct disorder. The rationale for this idea comes from realization that conduct disorder tends to persist over many years and has a clear developmental link to adult psychopathology (Robins, 1978). In childhood, the disorder is closely related to hyperactivity (Stewart et al., 1981) and in adolescence and adulthood it is related to antisocial personality disorder, criminality, alcoholism, substance abuse, homicide, and suicide (Robins, 1974; Weiss et al., 1985; Gittelman et al., 1985). These relationships have been best documented in samples of males, but results with female samples indicate that depression and somatization disorder should also be kept within the spectrum of outcomes (Robins).

Because childhood conduct disorder and its adult sequelae are all common psychiatric conditions and because they are costly in terms of human life, property destruction, and institutional placements, it is important to develop means of prevention, early detection, and treatment. Nevertheless, the many decades of efforts to treat conduct disorder and juvenile delinquency have met with either overt failure or short-term benefits (Shamsie, 1981). No one particular treatment approach seems promising at the moment, although behavioral modification appears to exert the most sizeable gains over the short run. Recognition of the size of the problem and the dismal record of treatment efforts inspired our interest in the possibility of primary prevention. To this end, we put together the known facts about conduct disorder and proposed a randomized control trial to test its efficacy (Robins and Earls, 1986).

Because conduct disorder is known to develop early, a preventive trial would have to begin in the first years of life. A group at high risk are infants born to women with antisocial personality disorder. One could expect that about half the infants reared by such women will begin to manifest evidence of conduct disorder by the time they enter elementary school. Because women with this disorder are likely to mate with men who have the same disorder, choosing a group of children on the basis of the presence of the disorder in their mothers places them at even higher risk because of assortative mating.

The crucial problem is the content of the intervention. On the basis of the success of the Perry Preschool Program, one of the most thoroughly evaluated of the Head Start projects in terms of improving academic performance and social adjustment (Berrueta-Clement et al., 1984), we have examined and are now testing the feasibility of using an experimental day care curriculum as the intervention. The program would begin as soon after birth as possible and offer a developmentally graded curriculum to offset the known risk factors associated with conduct disorder. Physical and language skills would be enhanced, and the capacity for patience, warmth, and tolerance would be fostered. Parents would be systematically involved in the program so that they could acquire greater sensitivity for the individual temperaments and developmental competencies of their children. Involvement in the program would continue uninterrupted until the child reached school age If promising results were shown by this age, the program could be extended into middle childhood through the addition of an after school program. Ultimate success would depend on being able to demonstrate a lower rate of conduct disorder by age 10 in those exposed to the curriculum than in the control group. There is convincing evidence that childhood antisocial behavior at this age leads to adult antisocial behavior (Robins, 1978). Thus, prevention of conduct disorder by age 10 is tantamount to prevention of antisocial personality disorder, since it almost never appears in adults who did not have childhood conduct disorder.

The negative effects of early group care of infants and young children include exposure to contagious diseases, disruption of maternal attachment at critical ages, and the possibility of aggressive and hard-to-control behavior.

The significance of this agenda rests in the use of infant and preschool day care as a context for the prevention of childhood psychiatric disorder. This project tests how far decreased exposure to chaotic family life and poor parenting and efforts to increase the social and intellectual competence of children can go in offsetting the risk of a specific type of psychiatric disorder. It should also contribute to our understanding of how the familial clustering of certain types of adult and child disorders occurs and, by so doing, clarify the mechanisms involved in familial transmission. For example, the research design leaves open the question of the extent to which antisocial behavior is biologically or socially generated. The intervention should be designed broadly and flexibly enough to permit both factors to operate and either to predominate.

The effort to influence the early environment of a population at high risk for the development of conduct disorder through the use of a day care program is also a promising development for efforts to prevent other types of psychiatric disorder, particularly depressive disorders. On a much broader scale, day care has become a necessary consideration for over half the American mothers with infants (Brazelton, 1986). As a more general benefit to society, the use of day care programs as experimental environments may lead to impairments in their design for normal children as well. The potential for early developmental programs that incorporate preventive health practices and environmental enrichment to become an important health care resource in developing countries should also be carefully examined.

SUMMARY AND CONCLUSIONS

Three innovative approaches to the mental health care of children and adolescents have been discussed. The integration of mental health care into primary health care for adolescents was examined in the most detail because this has been a highly desired objective for many decades in the United States. I believe the demand for adequate health care for this age group necessitates that mental health care become an integral component of total health care. Psychiatry should become as critical to the organization of primary care as pediatrics already is.

Two other approaches were briefly described: school-based services to detect and treat psychiatric disorders in elementary and junior high school students and the use of a day care program as a context for the primary prevention of psychiatric disorders that originate early in development. Each is a strategy for integrating mental health care for children of different ages into existing community institutions. They all reply to Levy's criticism three decades ago that child psychiatry was isolating itself from the rest of medicine while championing a nonscientific orientation toward therapeutic work and the design of services.

In the West, we are now at a critical stage in the evolution of child psychiatry as a medical discipline, and rational-empirical approaches are laying the foundation for what will be a productive future. The three approaches I have described here are worth the consideration of those charged with the responsibility for designing mental health services for children and adolescents in Africa. They represent strategies that would help Africa avoid the isolation that contributed to a period of stagnancy in the development of child psychiatry in the United States.

REFERENCES

Berrueta-Clement, J. R., Schweinhart, L. J., Barnett, W. S., et al.: Changed Lives: The Effects of the Perry Preschool Program on Youths through Age 19. Ypsilanti, Mich., U.S.A., High Scope Press, 1984

Brazelton, T. B.: Issues for working parents. American Journal of Orthopsychiatry 56:14-25, 1986

Earls, F.: The future of child psychiatry as a medical discipline. American Journal of Psychiatry 139:1158-1161, 1982

Gittelman, R., Mannuzza, S., Shenker, R., et al.: Hyperactive boys almost grown up, 1: psychiatric status. Archives of General Psychiatry 42:937-947, 1985

Greenhill, L.: Pediatric psychopharmacology, in The Clinical Guide to Child Psychiatry. Edited by Shaffer, D., Ehrhardt, A., Greenhill, L. New York, U.S.A., Free Press, 1984, pp. 493-518

Herjanic, B.: Systematic diagnostic interviewing of children: present state and future possibilities. Psychiatric Developments 2:115-130, 1984

Kolvin, I., Garside, R. F., Nicol, A. R., et al.: Help Starts Here: The Maladjusted Child in the Ordinary School. London, England, Travistock, 1981

Levy, D. M.: Critical evaluation of the present state of child psychiatry. American Journal of Psychiatry 108:481-490, 1952

Neuchterlein, K.: Childhood precursors of adult schizophrenia. Journal of Child Psychology and Psychiatry 27:133-144, 1986

Perkins, M. A., Valentine, J., Lamb, G. A.: Targeting health services: an approach to identify excess risks in the inner city. Massachusetts Journal of Community Health 8-13, 1982

Puig-Antich, J.: Affective disorder in childhood: a review and perspective. Psychiatric Clinics of North America 3:403-424, 1980

Robins, L.: Changes in conduct disorder over time, in Risk in Intellectual and Psychosocial Development. Edited by Farran, D. C., McKinney, J. D. New York,U.S.A., Academic Press, 00. 227-259

Robins, L. N.: Deviant Children Grown-Up: A Sociological and Psychiatric Study of Sociopathic Personality, Huntington, N.Y., U.S.A., Robert E. Krieger, 1974

Robins, L. N.: Sturdy childhood predictors of adult antisocial behavior: replications from longitudinal studies. Psychological Medicine 8:611-622, 1978

Robins, L. N., Earls, F.: A program for preventing antisocial behavior for high risk infants and preschoolers: a research prospectus, in Psychiatric Epidemiology and Primary Prevention: The Possibilities, Edited by Hough, R., Gongla, P., Brown, V., et al. Los Angeles, U.S.A., Neuropsychiatric Institute Institute, University of California, 1986, pp. 73-85

Rutter, M.: Changing Youth in a Changing Society. Cambridge, Mass., U.S.A., Harvard University Press, 1980

Shamsie, S. J.: Antisocial adolescents: our treatments do not work—where do we go from here? Canadian Journal of Psychiatry 26:357-364, 1981

Stewart, M., Cummings, C., Singer, S., et al.: The overlap between hyperactive and unsocialized aggressive children. Journal of Child Psychology and Psychiatry 22:35-45, 1982

Weiss, G., Hechtman, L., Milroy, T., et al: Psychiatric status of hyperactives as adults: a controlled prospective 15-year follow-up of 63 hyperactive children. Journal of the American Academy of Child Psychiatry 24:211-220, 1985

Chapter 24

Suicidal Adolescents in the USA: A Sociocultural-Psycological Approach to Assessment and Treatment

by

Lee Ann Hoff, RN, PhD
Norteastern University
College of Nursing
Boston, Massachusetts
U.S.A

ABSTRACT

The author points out that the suicidal behavior of many adolescents in the United States has sociocultural origins and is not best addressed by individual psychotherapy alone. American society is biased toward individualism, and there is a need for balancing psychological with social and cultural perspectives on teenage suicide.

The author explains her social-psychological-cultural crisis paradigm and illustrates its implications for teenagers experiencing isolated traumatic events, transition states, and alienation from their social settings. The nature of the adolescent's crisis should determine the nature of the help provided, and the sociocultural origins of much suicidal behavior among young people imply a need for preventive social action.

INTRODUCTION

During a recent workshop on suicide, a woman presented the case of her 16-year-old foster daughter, Leah. After suffering years of sexual abuse by her father and the painful secrecy that surrounds this crime, Leah finally went to her pastor for help. The pastor apparently did not believe her. He said, "Your father is a respected member of the community; go home and do as you're told." Some weeks later the father turned himself in to the police. The police said, "You know, some members of the community might be upset by what you've done, so why don't you leave town for a while until things cool down?"

Who cares? Certainly, the pastor and the police officer in this case did not seem to care. One result of such indifference from society was Leah's life-threatening suicide attempts, which were treated routinely through hospital emergency facilities and referrals to social service agencies. This treatment was not adequate for Leah, however, so her foster mother came to a teen suicide workshop to obtain additional help for Leah.

During the workshop group work, a participant suggested that Leah needed psychotherapy for her depression. In response, Leah's foster mother practically screamed at the audience, "She's had that, and it hasn't stopped her from wanting to kill herself! How can my daughter ever be healed as long as people ignore what her father has done?"

This foster mother seems to affirm what some suicidologists, including myself, claim: To treat a suicidal adolescent only with individual psychotherapy, without complementary family and group work, borders on malpractice. To do so in Leah's case, for example, implies that the meaning of her self-destructive behavior is not understood. The sociocultural source of her despair—abuse by her father—is ignored.

In this paper, I will propose a framework for understanding suicidal adolescents (based on epidemiological data and using Leah's case for illustration) that balances psychological with sociocultural approaches to their treatment. The context of my analysis is the United States and the cultural values and social problems in American society that offer partial explanations of the epidemic of adolescent suicide (see Endnote 1 for a summary of epidemiological data).

CASE ANALYSIS

First, what Leah's foster mother effectively said is that the community, which by definition has a mandate to care for its young and for others with special needs, had washed its hands of this crime of incest. The mother's desperate search for help on Leah's behalf is dramatized by her presence at a workshop intended primarily for professionals. The mother was a layperson whose attendance at the workshop signified a failure to get what she and her daughter needed from the professional community of care givers.

Second, in this case we observe continuity between the kind of service Leah had already received after her suicide attempts and that proposed by the workshop participants; that is, the focus was on Leah's depression, a symptom of a much deeper problem that was really a social problem—i.e., child sexual abuse. The essential ingredient lacking in Leah's treatment was attention to the sociocultural origins of suicidal behavior. By its very nature, individual psychotherapy traditionally focuses on personal behavior and responses to various events and life problems. By implication individual psychotherapy suggests that the causes and answers to one's problems lie essentially within the individual, rather than in the social structure and cultural values. Certainly, there are exceptions to this generalization, which I will discuss shortly. Also, I do not hereby suggest that individual therapy is not necessary. Rather, it simply is not enough in most cases of suicidal adolescents.

A fact of life is that people naturally belong to groups, and, traditionally at least, people have looked to group members for support. When this individual-group dynamic breaks down, we have the potential for alienation, despair, and possibly, suicide. A century ago, Durkheim (1966[1897]) categorized suicidal persons into anomic and egoistic (along with altruistic). Anomie, as an explanation for suicide, suggests that a person at one time felt socially integrated but now feels abandoned by social network members from whom she or he might have sought support. The concept of eogism suggests that the person was never well-integrated into a social group in the first place, with the consequence that everything revolves in excess around oneself, the ego.

In the United States, the deeply embedded cultural value of individualism adds power to this century-old explanation of suicide. The young person says in effect, "My father made it with hard work and sacrifice, but now, no matter what I do, I'll never be able to buy a house...and, besides, what's the use, anyway, when the whole world may be blown up before I even get started?" If such a young person belongs to a minority racial group, the potential for despair is even greater. Among young black males, for example, the suicide rate is twice that of young white females. A sociocultural interpretation of adolescent suicide includes recognition of the legacy of racism in the United States and its potential for breeding despair among the young.

Even this brief review of classical sociology, applied to suicide, suggests that we have known for a long time the importance of social factors in understanding and assisting distressed people. Meanwhile, research from many fields supports a shift from individual to social approaches to helping distressed people. That is, despite the prevalence of individual intervention techniques, overwhelming evidence from sociology, anthropology, epidemiology, and social psychology now shows that social networks and support are primary factors in

- one's susceptibility to disease,
- the process of becoming ill and seeking help,
- the treatment process, and
- outcomes of illness—either rehabilitation and recovery or death, including death by suicide.

(See Hoff, 1984a, chapter 5, for extensive references on social factors in health and illness and on social network intervention strategies.) Works by clinical practitioners from social work, nursing, and medicine support the social science literature. Hansell (1976), for example, a psychiatrist, cast his entire description of mental health and distressed people in a social framework.

Yet, nearly 100 years after Durkheim, and reams of research findings notwithstanding, the bias of individualism in treating suicidal adolescents and others in crisis is still evident. Why? An already suggested reason is the culturally embedded value placed on individualism in American society—the "I made it with hard work! What's wrong with you?" mentality. Another reason for the individualistic bias is the emphasis on the individual rather than sociocultural aspects of any problem whatsoever, stemming from medicine's—and, by extension, psychiatry's— focus on a person's internal system and biological and psychological anomalies.

The profound influence of medical model and individualism in policy decisions and practice is evident in the practice of many mental health professionals. For example, it is difficult to convince legislative funding and insurance groups that anything of value has been done unless something resembling a 50- minute therapy hour has been documented.

Telephone work, social networking, and time spent traveling into a home for family sessions to prevent crises and hospitalizations get short shrift in comparison to the 50-minute hour.

Individualistic models prevent the development of more holistic approaches to treatment and care, based on social realities. In the case of suicidal adolescents, for example, the most fundamental reality is that the young person is still dependent on the family, and regardless of the trigger for a particular suicidal episode—failure in school, divorce, physical abuse—the family is central to treatment and prevention. Therefore, individual psychotherapy alone for a depressed and suicidal adolescent is only a symptomatic response to the problem, while antidepressant drugs for such a youngster are definitely contraindicated, as in the case of any reactive depression.

Another reason to question dominant individualistic models encompasses race, class, and gender issues. Sexism, racism, and classism are the bases of the alienation and disengagement experienced by many in American society. Leah's case has introduced this issue in a general way. To support this claim, I will expand on the implications of her case and suggest a model that provides understanding of Leah and her foster mother and implies more comprehensive service to Leah, her foster mother, and anyone who feels alienated or in suicidal despair.

A CRISIS PARADIGM: SOCIAL-PSYCHOLOGICAL-CULTURAL

I have already noted Durkheim's categorization of anomic and egoistic suicide. Such social alienation, combined with personally traumatic events, such as school failure, is central to the current epidemic of teen suicide in the United States. In effect, many American young people are telling us that they are not interested in remaining in the world we have created for them and that there is no real chance for them to create an alternative, a more desirable one. The conclusion for many young people, therefore, is that they have no reason to continue living in this world, that they must either enter a fantasy world of alcohol and other drugs or resort to death because death is better than life. This suggests the need for balancing psychological factors, such as depression, with a social and cultural perspective on teenage suicide.

First, let us consider how individual, family, and societal factors work together in the lives of particular adolescents. For example, the divorce of an adolescent's parents is undoubtedly very stressful. But it need not lead to despair or suicide. Another youngster may fail in school or be left handicapped by an accident. As isolated events, they will probably not lead youngsters to suicide unless social support in such crises is gravely lacking. Some teens may feel pessimistic about their futures because of nuclear threat. But, by themselves, these individual, family, or societal situations are not usually the causes of despair for young people. For example, while many know that the threat of nuclear holocaust exists, by itself nuclear threat cannot be construed as an immediate cause of suicide. What seems to make the difference is the interaction between personal (including psychological), family, and societal factors.

For example, if couples who divorce each other do not also divorce themselves of their parenting roles or use their children as weapons between them, their divorce need not be a source of despair for an adolescent, even though it is certainly stressful. In one large U.S. secondary school, it was found that teens felt less hopeless about nuclear threat and their future when their parents took a stand on the issue and became overtly involved. It did not seem to matter whether the parents were left or right on the political spectrum so long as they acknowledged the reality of nuclear threat and were willing to discuss it openly. Similarly, teens may be confused with changing sex roles during an era of increasing civil rights for women, and when family and community supports are not available through this developmental transition, the potential for crisis is increased.

These examples present an overview of the usual ingredients for alienation or despair among young people. This interpretation of critical events is illustrated in a new research-based crisis paradigm (Hoff, 1984a) (see Figure 1 and Endnote 2).

Figure 1

CRISIS PARADIGM

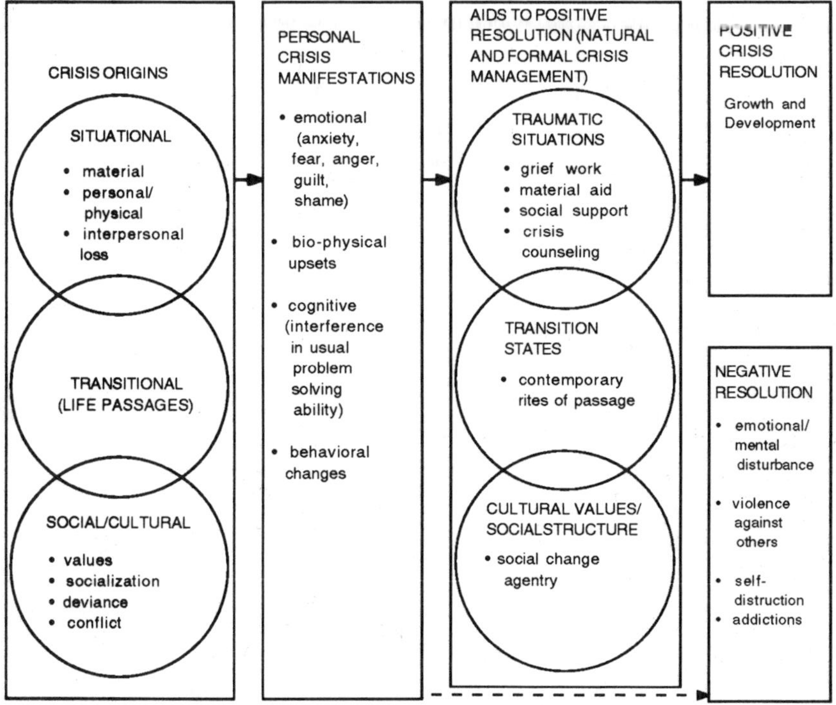

1. This paradigm presents a way to understand the process of the total crisis experience of people like Leah from the origin of a crisis to its resolution. This is depicted by the arrows showing the stages of the crisis process, moving from the left to the right of Figure 1.

2. The paradigm emphasizes the interactional relationship between crisis origins (the first box), personal crisis manifestations (the second box), and the outcomes of crisis for various individuals (the fourth box).

3. The paradigm also highlights the process of what needs to be done—either by the person experiencing the crisis or by health professionals—to manage the crisis effectively.

4. This model illustrates the need to tailor crisis intervention and follow-up strategies to the distinct origins of the crisis in order to foster positive crisis resolution and avoid the possible negative outcomes of crises, such as suicide, homicide, addiction, or emotional breakdown. The intertwined circles represent distinct yet interrelated origins of crisis and aids to positive resolution, but personal manifestations are often similar. In general, this paradigm emphasizes previously neglected social and cultural aspects of emotional crisis. It also presumes a social and cultural interpretation of crisis without, however, neglecting the psychological.

With this overview of the model, let us return to transition-state crises, which are central for young people, and examine more closely the second circle, Aides to Positive Resolution—specifically, contemporary rites of passage. Here the concern is not with acute crisis situations, but with normal transition states. The key issue here concerning suicidal adolescents is their ordinary need for social supports, they struggle with the tasks of growing up, achieving independence, and getting comfortable with a sex-role identity. When social support is not forthcoming from adults during crucial life transitions, such as puberty, young people will nevertheless seek it out through ritualistic behaviors with their peers. One of the most dramatic negative examples of this for college-age young people in the United States is the hazing (initiation) rituals on college campuses. Some hazing rites are so destructive and lacking in adult direction that they end in death. They also dramatize the need of young people for peer support and for a sense of belonging to a group. When such groups lack adult leadership, destructive rituals will be there to fill the vacuum. The challenge for caring adults, then, is to find some contemporary substitutes for what young people could count on in traditional societies through elaborate puberty rites. For example, in contemporary U.S. society, such an adult-supervised ritual could focus on the important adolescent event of receiving a driver's license. In other words, if young people sense their parents' lack of interest in or lack of time for events that are important to them, they will be more prone to abuse their new privilege of driving by drunk driving, etc.

Another example of contemporary rites of passage might be peer support groups concerned with changing sex roles. This kind of activity would not only help to get away from mother blaming for such contemporary problems as latchkey children but would help change traditional sex role stereotyping, which often leads to violence, unwed motherhood, divorce, and numerous other problems.

The focus in the paradigm thus far is various situational and transition-state crises—i.e., the unexpected traumatic events in the first circle and normal transition states in the second circle. Let us now consider the potential for despair and suicide when the source of the youngster's distress is not the normal challenge of growing up or the everyday misfortunes that befall human beings. Such situations and events can be traced to cultural values and to one's particular position within the social structure, including the family (see the last circle of Crisis Origins in the paradigm).

Here we return to the example of Leah and her foster mother. This facet of the paradigm allows elaboration on what happened to Leah and what might be done for Leah and mothers like her, who feel alienated from society, their families, and themselves.

With the paradigm as a guide, we note, for example, that a young person like Leah may be homeless (first circle) not because she is behaviorally disturbed but because she has escaped from an abusive situation. She may be facing a change in status from young girl to single parent (second circle) not because she wants to be a parent but because of incest, rape, or a perception that her most useful or only function in society is to bear children. These two sources of crisis for Leah, however, are really only secondary to the third category of origins: the social structure and cultural values in the lower circle. That is, the primary origin of Leah's crisis is deeply embedded values about women, marriage, and the family, the social inequality of women and children, and the deviant behavior of another person—in this case, her father. And if social action is not taken to stop such abuse or to hold abusers accountable for their behavior, victims might perceive such inaction or silence as collusion in the abuse. The same basic principle applies to victims of rape, battering, or other violent acts and to many runaway teenagers in the United States who are victims of abuse. Large numbers of runaway teens are also suicidal.

When dealing with crises that originate from such sociocultural sources, the emotional healing process takes on a tone that is different from that in cases where one can explain the crisis as an act of God or fate, as, for example, in losses from natural disaster. This is because part of the process of crisis resolution includes whatever people do to explain to themselves why certain terrible things happen to them. That is, the event somehow must fit into one's meaning system. Antonovsky (1980) referred to this as a sense of coherence. For example, if a young person loses a limb because of a car accident that was no one's fault or even loses a parent through cancer (traumatic situations, as noted in the first circle of Origins in the crisis paradigm), the person can explain the event as an act of God, bad luck, or fate. In such cases, barring extraordinary bungling by helpers or lack of social support, one can only predict that the crisis resolution will be fairly straightforward and will proceed to positive outcomes if necessary aids to resolution are present.

In stark contrast, when a young person suffers abuse, violence, and neglect rather than nurture and support from parents and network members, this represents a reversal of the moral order. Thus, the process of emotional healing for a person whose crisis stems from a social source demands some kind of social response either by that person or by social network members and others on the person's behalf. This is precisely what Leah's foster mother seemed to be saying to her fellow workshop participants.

Ideally, a social response includes victim compensation of some kind. Unfortunately, however, instead of compensation, many victims are victimized again through inadequate treatment or outright blame for their victimization. Compensation, along with linkage to a peer support group and knowledge that public action is being taken to stop abuse and violence, helps a victim in crisis make sense out of the traumatic experience. It inspires hope and therefore helps victims like Leah to know that their suffering has not been in vain, that something is being done to change the circumstances contributing to victimization by incest, rape, battering, etc. In this respect, victims of sexual assault and other forms of violence have something in common with survivors of the Holocaust and atomic bomb explosions and other victims of man-made disaster. The social responses corresponding to the sociocultural origins of certain crises are illustrated in the lower circle of Aids to Positive Resolution in the crisis paradigm—basically, it consists of social change strategies.

A word of caution is in order here. Crisis intervention alone is not a panacea for suicidal adolescents or all of life's problems. This crisis paradigm, however, goes well beyond the traditional crisis model by including social action and follow-up work as an integral part of comprehensive service for some of our most troubled young people and others. The paradigm illustrates this by showing that, if a problem is social, cultural, or political in origin, a strictly psychological or psychiatric approach alone will not do. This point is dramatized by the following story, quoted by McKinlay (1979) in Patients, Physicians and Illness: My friend, Irving Zola, relates the story of a physician trying to explain the dilemmas of the modern practice of medicine: "You know," he said,"Sometimes it feels like this. There I am standing by the shore of a swiftly flowing river and I hear the cry of a drowning man. So I jump into the river, put my arms around him, pull him to shore and apply artificial respiration. Just when he begins to breathe, another cry for help. So back in the river again, reaching, pulling, applying, breathing and then another yell. Again and again, without end, goes the sequence. You know, I am so busy jumping in, pulling them to shore, applying artificial respiration, that I have no time to see who the hell is upstream pushing them all in."

The "upstream" in the health and mental health fields can be interpreted as the social, political, and economic ills that are the root causes of personal and emotional pain and of the alienation of millions of young people and others. What seems essential, therefore, is a tandem approach: while continuing to rescue people and provide follow-up counseling and other service, mental health workers might reserve at least a portion of their time for looking "upstream" and working on preventing so many adolescents and others from falling into the stream of emotional crises. Basically this is the social action noted in the crisis paradigm.

These root causes vary between communities and between countries. In the United States, children, especially children of color and those in families headed by women, are the new poor. There is increasing evidence that the social/cultural roots of personal crises and despair can often be traced to social problems, which leave children, women, the poor, and people of color particularly vulnerable to crisis. It is sobering that it is among these groups that the U.S. suicide rate is increasing most dramatically. The tandem approach I have suggested not only should create hope for the alienated and despairing but can also protect health workers from burnout. When dealing with suicidal people, workers must see some light at the end of tunnel. A vision, plus a strategy for changing the sources of so much despair and alienation, is such a light.

ENDNOTES

1. Following is a brief summary of statistics on suicide and suicide attempts in the United States (Frederick, 1978; Peck et al., 1985; Shneidman, 1985; Vital Statistics of the United States, 1978). Between 1955 and 1979, the rate of suicide in males aged 10 to 24 increased by 200%; in males between ages 10 and 14, the rate triples. Suicide is the second leading cause of death among college students. Among Native Americans the rate is 64% higher than for whites and 254% higher than for blacks. The male-female ratio of completed suicides is between 2:1 and 2:7. Firearms and explosives are the most common means of suicide in the United States. Among suicide attempters, the female-male ratio is 2:1. Ages 20 to 24 are the peak years for suicide attempts; 50% of suicide attempters are under the age of 30, and self- poisoning is the most common method among this age group. Between 1955 and 1970, there was an increase of 1,104% in suicide attempts, and 15% of psychiatric visits are for suicidal ideation or behavior.

2. This paradigm is grounded in research (Hoff, 1984b) and builds on the seminal work of Caplan (1964) and my own extensive experience in the crisis field. My book People in Crisis (Hoff, 1984a) illustrates the application of this paradigm to a wide range of crisis situations.

REFERENCES

Antonovsky, A.: Health, Stress and Coping. San Francisco, U.S.A., Jossey-Bass, 1980

Caplan, G.: Principles of Preventive Psychiatry. New York, U.S.A., Basic Books, 1964

Durkheim, E.: Suicide, 2nd ed. (1897). Translated by Spaulding, J. A. and Simpson, G. New York, U.S.A., Free Press, 1966

Frederick, C.: Current trends in suicidal behavior in the United States. American Journal of Psychotherapy 32:172-201, 1978

Hansell, N.: The Person in Distress. New York, U.S.A. Human Sciences Press, 1976

Hoff, L. A.: People in Crisis: Understanding and Helping, 2nd ed. Menlo Park, California, U.S.A., Addison-Wesley, 1984

Hoff, L. A.: Violence Against Women: A Social- Cultural Network Analysis. PhD dissertation, Boston University, Boston, U.S.A., 1984b

McKinlay, J. B.: A case for refocusing upstream: the political economy of illness, in Patients, Physicians and Illness, 3rd ed. Edited by Jaco, E. G., New York, U.S.A., Free Press, 1979

Peck, M., Farberow, N., Litman, R. (eds.): Youth Suicide. New York, U.S.A., Springer Publishing,1985

Shneidman, E.: Definition of Suicide. New York, U.S.A., Wiley-Interscience, 1985

Vital Statistics of the United States, 1978, vol.29, no. 6, supplement 2: Final Mortality Statistics. Hyattsville, Md., U.S.A., National Center for Health Statistics, 1978

Wexler, L., Weissman, M.: Suicide attempts 1970-1975: updating a United States study and comparisons with international trends. British Journal of Psychiatry 132:180-185, 1978

Commentary 3.1

Child Psychiatry in Kenya

by

Anonymous Reviewer

Njenga and Ndirangu report the results of a study involving 71 children during a period of 7 months. Their introductory cursory review of the literature, as well as the findings from their exploratory study, point to a number of similarities with the West. For example, a 1976 study of ten-year-old children with psychiatric disorders in England show a prevalance rate of 10-15% , 10% in 10-year olds and older in two villages in Ethiopia, and 12% in adolescents in rural Kenya. The investigators also pointed out that Kenya is experiencing social changes (such as increase in broken families and single parent families) that were reported previously in the United States and Britian. So, along with the differences between the West and Africa, a number of similarities are prominent.

A number of specific findings of the study are highlighted: l) no referrals of children below five years of age; 2) 23% of children referred were from troubled families; 3) a great number of children at risk; 4) number of trained personnel very small .

Commentary 3.2

Black Children in Psychiatric Outpatient Treatment

by

Anonymous Reviewer

The authors report the findings of an examination of the use of public health services by families of Black adolescents. A major significant finding is underscored: a growing increase in the number of Black children referred for services, but a decided underrepresentation of Blacks in treatment. The investigators suggest several factors as underlying causes: l) racism; 2) misdiagnosis; 3) staff composition. In the opinion of the reviewer, these factors are often, if not usually, interrelated

Several statements warrant emphasis, and should be addressed in all mental health training and service programs: l) "A comprehensive assessment requires a basic understanding of the social cultural context from which the child comes," In addressing the matter, the evaluator must be cautious lest he/she not attend to myths as facts; 2)"...race and ethnicity may play a major role in determining how a patient seeks help, what he defines as a problem, and what he views as a useful intervention." The reviewer adds that it is imperative that the diagnostic/therapist refrain from imposing her/his definitions on the patient.

Case vignettes illustrate well the aforementioned factors that serve as barriers to the treatment of Black children. Suggestions for the removal of barriers must be heeded.

Commentary 3.3

Innovations in Mental Health Care for Children and Adolescents in the United States and Britain

by

Anonymous Reviewer

Earls introduces this presentation with a statement that a review of innovations in mental health care for children and youth in the West has bearing on the growth of child psychiatry in Africa. The author's reference to the limited effect (modest or none) of therapeutic intervention, as practiced in the United States, and his supporting data, is likely to provoke concern, if not pain, for many practitioners in the West. However, as Earls points out, this is not a new impression and such impressions have stimulated research and the development of innovative therapeutic practices.

Three innovative projects are described: 1) delivery of comprehensive health care to adolescents; 2) school-based interventions; 3) prevention of conduct disorders in high-risk infants through use of a day care program. Each of the undertakings was designed as a research project rather than demonstration. The prevention of isolation of the field of child psychiatry is a common thread. For example, the focus on integrating mental health care into primary health care for adolescents underscores the need/value of expanding child psychiatry into a primary care specialty. The other two projects demonstrate methods for incorporating mental health care into other community service programs.

Certainly, the benefits of this paper are not limited to our African colleagues. Our American colleagues will also find it of considerable value in evaluating existing programs and developing new programs.

Commentary 3.4

Suicidal Adolescents in the USA: A Sociocultural-Psychological Approach to Assessment and Treatment

by

Anonymous Reviewer

Epidemiological data and a case vignette are used for a framework for the development of a model that would be useful in understanding suicidal adolescents. As indicated in the title, sociocultural and psychological factors are considered. Hoff's presentation provides several pragmatic lessons: l) tailoring of crisis intervention to the specific origins of the crisis; 2) utilization of the author's "crisis paradigm" in understanding and responding to adolescents' troubled responses to normal transition states; 3) the need to inquire about a history of sexual abuse and to address the matter, if it is a history of such abuse, in the course of therapeutic intervention.

The author's repeated reference to sociocultural issues and the interweaving with psychological factors warrants practitioners' constant attention. The reviewer adds the need to also address culture as a changing, rather than static phenomenon.

Commentary 3.5

Child Psychiatry

by

Anonymous Reviewer

As a pioneering venture, the Nairobi conference succeeded admirably. In particular, the quality of the formal presentations and the level of discussion on topics of children and adolescents were very high.

As reflected in the four papers making up this section, no great insights or breakthroughs were achieved, but a surprisingly large amount of common turf was mapped out. The paper by Njenga and Ndirangu from Kenya illustrates how the development of child psychiatry outpatient services is just beginning. On the other hand, according to Wright and Cole of the United States, relatively well established clinics in South Carolina are still struggling to accommodate the needs of their black patients. A common note is heard in both places. The authors acknowledge how critical it is to understand the role of the family in children's lives in order to formulate diagnosis and treatment plans. In Kenya, the primary problems appear to be the manpower shortage and the need to educate parents, physicians and school personnel in the recognition of mental disorders in children and adolescents. In South Carolina, the problems are a shortage of black mental health professionals and the need to improve training of white professionals in terms of cultural sensitivity.

The papers by Earls and by Hoff go beyond traditional medical settings into a variety of community contexts and involve the social structure and indigenous values of the United States itself. Both authors address the need to expand concepts and clinical approaches to children by describing how institutions provide a structural basis for creating problems in children that individual and drug therapies can not influence. While this kind of thinking has long beeen a part of the established sociological wisdom in the United States, it has been only slowly and with difficulty incorporated into practice and into restructuring of health care institutions.

Although Africa and the United states are at different stages in their respective histories, they should continue the dialogue on child mental health started at this conference. A critical need is to share and refine methods of evaluating children and their families until common knowledge and a consistent language are developed. But equal attention must be directed at prevention and health promotion in both settings. In the African context this may seem like a challenge far beyond even the foreseeable future, since attention must first be given to creating and sustaining a base of operation in medical settings. Nevertheless, the greatest impact on a developing society, rich in the potential of its human resources, is most likely to occur with a public health approach that emphasizes education, early detection and prevention. A balance between clinical and public health approaches must be vigorously pursued. If this is not done, it becomes all too easy to sink resources in clinical services because demand is so high. It should be anticipated that as the pressures of modernization and schooloing continue to increase in Kenya, Nigeria, and many other developing societies of Africa, the demand for psychiatric services will also increase. Now is the time to plan services aimed at preventing mental disorders and promoting the competence of families and young children (Earls, 1987).

REFERENCES

Earls, F.: Child psychiatry in an international context: with remarks on the current status of child psychiatry in China, in The Role of Culture in Developmental Disoder edited by Super, C.M., San Diego, Calif., U.S.A., Academic Press, 1987, pp. 235-249

SECTION IV:

Substance Abuse

Chapter 25

Cannabis Psychosis: Facts and Myth

by

R. Onyango Sumba, MBChB, MRCPsych
Department of Psychiatry
Faculty of Medicine
University of Nairobi
Nairobi, Kenya

ABSTRACT

Much of the research on the deleterious effects of cannabis has relied on subjective reports. Rottanburg et al., however, analyzed urine samples from 117 psychotic male hospital patients and administered the Present State Examination (PSE). The percentage of positive urine tests was 59.8%, and the patients with unequivocally high levels (30.8%) had significantly more hypomania and agitation than matched cannabis-free patients and significantly less affective flattening, auditory hallucinations, incoherence of speech, and hysteria. The author studied 25 consecutive hospital patients of both sexes, with a variety of diagnoses and found positive urine samples in only four (16.0%); only one appeared to have cannabis psychosis. Cannabis psychosis may occur only after heavy cannabis use, which is more likely in persons who have abnormal personalities or life styles or have underlying psychotic illnesses. True cannabis psychosis is therefore probably less frequent than indicated by the many unverified reports.

INTRODUCTION

For centuries, many cultures and communities have assumed cannabis to be a causative agent in mental illness. Most countries have laws prohibiting the cultivation, sale, and consumption of cannabis. This paper is subtitled Facts and Myth because the concept of cannabis psychosis is entangled in a web of controversial facts and myths.

That cannabis has harmful effects has not been conclusively proven. It is ironic that some drugs with well-demonstrated deleterious effects on health, such as alcohol and tobacco, continue to be officially sanctioned. The economic benefits governments derive from the alcohol and tobacco industries must contribute to this double standard.

This paper examines the current evidence linking cannabis with mental illness to determine how realistically this evidence can be viewed. The earliest works on cannabis came primarily from North Africa. They were written mainly by French investigators during the pre-World War II era. Among others, they include papers by Bouquet, Meunier, Porot, Racine, Gautier, and Pascal (Bouquet, 1950).

The next large body of works originated from the Indian subcontinent. The most notable of these were by Chakraborty (1964 & 1966), Bhaskaran and Saxena (1970), Thacore et al. (1971), Varma (1972), Chopra and Smith (1974), and Thacore and Shukla (1976).

The third group comprises works by Americans, including Halikas et al. (1971), Kolansky and Moore (1971), Tennant and Groesbeck (1972), Linn (1972), Annis and Smart (1973), and Treffert (1978).

Little has been published by investigators from other parts of the world. British researchers have largely ignored the subject, and I could find little from sub-Saharan Africa, apart from the survey on drug use in Nairobi done by Yambo and Acuda in 1983.

The common element of the North African (or French), Indian, and American studies—indeed, the bulk of the research on cannabis—is that too much reliance is placed on subjective reports. Few objective measures have been used to reduce the bias of the subjects and researchers. Too many of these papers are no more than anecdotal descriptions of cases of presumed cannabis psychosis. Scant attention has been given to subject's past psychiatric history or personality. Laboratory methods, although long available, have not been incorporated into the research design. In short, from many of these works it is impossible to determine whether the described phenomenology was due primarily to cannabis or to an ongoing psychotic illness in which cannabis played an incidental role.

STUDIES:

South African Study

A different approach was taken by Rottanburg et al. (1982). They systematically analyzed urine samples of 117 psychotic male patients admitted to psychiatric hospitals in South Africa. They also administered the Present State Examination (PSE) to the psychiatric hospitals in South Africa. They also administered the Present State Examination (PSE) to the patients shortly after admission and one week and related these results to the urine findings. A surprising finding was the high percentage (59.8%) of men with cannabis-positive urine.

Rottanburg and associates found that if they only considered samples with unequivocally high levels of cannabinoids—i.e., those with more than 79 ug of cross-reacting cannabinoids per gram of creatinine— then the percentage was 30.8% (N-36). Table 1 shows the PSE scores of 20 of these patients and 20 cannabis-free patients matched for age and clinical diagnosis. The 20 patients with high levels of cannabinoids showed significantly more hypomania and agitation at the first testing and significantly less affective flattening, auditory hallucinations, incoherence of speech, and hysteria. The patients with high levels of cannabinoids tended to improve fairly quickly. This improvement coincided with a fall in the level of cannabinoids in their urine.

Table I
PSE-1 AND PSE-2 PROFILES OF CANNABIS AND CONTROL GROUPS[1] (15)

PSYCHOPATHOLOGY	CANNABIS GROUP (N=20) PSE-1	CANNABIS GROUP (N=20) PSE-2	CONTROL GROUP (N=20) PSE-1	CONTROL GROUP (N=20) PSE-2
Hypomania	16	8	7	7
Agitation	10	3	3	6
Self-Neglect	10	2	10	7
Sexual and Fantastic Delusions	14	3	13	13
Delusions of Reference	11	4	13	13
Grandiose and Religious Delusions	11	4	13	13
Delusions of Persecution	8	2	9	8
Irritability	16	7	15	9

1. PSE-2 done seven days after PSE-1

This was the only study I could find that clearly linked the presence of cannabinoids in the body with a particular symptom pattern. I was also intrigued by the high percentage of cannabis-positive urine samples in that study, and I decided to replicate the study, albeit modified, with a sample of British patients at the hospital I was working in at the time.

Current Study

I collected urine samples from 25 consecutive hospital patients who were younger than 35. Patients of both sexes and all diagnoses were included. About 48% of the subjects admitted ever using cannabis, but traces of cannabis were found in only four (16%) of the urine samples.

The patients' past psychiatric histories were taken. Three of the four patients with cannabis-positive urine had long psychiatric histories. Two were clearly schizophrenic, and they had a total of nine previous admissions between them. They were floridly psychotic on admission and were only marginally improved 1 month later. The third patient had a personality disorder and was not at all psychotic. He was released from the hospital after a week.

The fourth patient, however, was quite interesting. He was a 23-year-old West Indian of the Rastafarian faith who had had no previous psychiatric contact. His personal history disclosed eccentricity and an inability to form stable relationships or hold down a steady job. He was on probation at the time, having been charged with possession of cannabis. He was admitted to the hospital after his behavior attracted notice. He was walking about half-dressed, trying to drag girls off the street to his apartment for sex, taking goods from neighborhood shops without paying for them, and trying to urinate on people from the balcony of his apartment, which was one floor above the street. His electricity and gas had been disconnected by the authorities because the bills had not been paid, and he had lit a fire in the middle of his living room to keep warm. His probation officer described him as labile in affect; he occasionally cried abruptly but most of the time he was elated and jovial.

On admission, this man was disheveled and dirty, restless, and disinhibited; he cracked jokes and giggled. He appeared to be hearing voices, although he denied this. He called himself King John and, at times, God, and felt he could communicate with God. He did not know where he was, the date, or the day of the week.

He was treated with haloperidol (10 mg/day), and after a few days he became less elated, although he remained disoriented up to the fifth day. His urine was strongly cannabis-positive. By the seventh day of hospitalization, the patient was sufficiently improved and the medication was stopped. He remained well and was discharged on the twelfth day.

This was the only case I could identify that could remotely be called cannabis psychosis. The fact that one was found at all in a study of this size could be ascribed more to luck than to any other factor.

The percentage of cannabis-positive samples found in the South African study was much higher than in mine (59.8% vs. 16.0). I can think of a few possible explanations. All subjects in the South African study were male and psychotic. In my study, samples were collected from all patients, of either sex, and with any diagnosis. The diagnoses were schizophrenia(N=9), personality disorder (N-5), depression, (N=5), schizoaffective disorder (N=3), manic-depressive disorder (N=1), situational reaction (N=1), and drug psychosis (N=1).

Secondly, the laboratory methods were different. The South African study used immunoassay, which is said to be up to 50 times as sensitive as the chromatography used in my study.

Actually, if one examines only the 11 subjects in my study who were comparable to those in the South African study—i.e., male and psychotic—the percentage with cannabis-positive urine (27.3%, N=3) is similar to that for the 36 patients in the South African study who had unequivocally high levels of cannabinoids in their urine (30.8%).

So, to come back to my original question, Does cannabis psychosis exist? I would say that it does but not with the frequency that one would be led to believe by the many unverified reports.

OBSERVATIONS

It has been documented (Treffert, 1978) that cannabis can exacerbate schizophrenia, so it is possible that many of the described cases involve schizophrenic patients who happen to abuse cannabis, which triggers the acute episode. It is also probable that cannabis-related psychosis occurs only after heavy use of the drug. A person who abuses cannabis heavily is also likely to have an abnormal personality or life style or to have an underlying psychotic illness. Cannabis is used to achieve psychedelic effects, which have a special attraction for people predisposed to inner fantasies, such as schizophrenic individuals.

Alcohol can produce a psychotic syndrome, the so- called pathological drunkenness or mania a potu. However, we cannot argue convincingly that alcohol should be banned because it produces mental illness. The psychotic syndrome related to alcohol seems to occur in susceptible individuals, and the same could apply to cannabis.

Cannabis is often blamed for producing a steady deterioration of personality. It is seldom pointed out that heavy cannabis use could be a result of deviance rather than its cause.

REFERENCES

Annis, H. M., Smart, R. G.: Adverse reaction and recurrences from marijuana use. British Journal of Addiction 68:315-319, 1973

Bhaskaran, K., Saxena, B. M.: Some aspects of schizophrenia in the two sexes. Indian Journal of Psychiatry 12:117-184, 1970

Bouquet, J.: Cannabis. Bulletin on Narcotics 2(4), 1950

Chakraborty, A.: An analysis of paranoid symptomatology. Indian Journal of Psychiatry 6:172- 179, 1964

Chakraborty, A.: Visual hallucination. Indian Journal of Psychiatry 8:21-25, 1966

Chopra, G. S., Smith, J. W.: Psychotic reactions following cannabis use in East Indians. Archives of General Psychiatry 30:24-27, 1974

Halikas, J. A., Goodwin, D. W., Guze, S. B.: Marijuana effects: a survey of regular users. Journal of the American Medical Association 217:692-694, 1971

Kolansky, H., Moore, W. T.: Effects of marijuana on adolescents and young adults. Journal of the American Medical Association 216:486-492, 1971

Linn, L. S.: Psychopathology and experience with marijuana. British Journal of Addiction 67:55-64, 1972

Rottanburg, D., Robins, A. H., Ben-Arie, O., et al.: Cannabis-associated psychosis with hypomanic features. Lancet 2:1364-1366, 1982

Tennant, F. S., Jr., Groesbeck, G. J.: Psychiatric effects of hashish. Archives of General Psychiatry 27:133-136, 1972

Thaecore, V. R., Saxena, R. C., Kumar, R.: Epidemiology of drug abuse in Lucknow with special reference to methaqualone. Indian Journal of Pharmacology 3:58- 65, 1971

Thacore, V. R., Shukla, S. R. P.: Cannabis psychosis and paranoid schizophrenia. Archives of General Psychiatry 33:383-386, 1976

Treffert, D. A.: Marijuana use in schizophrenia: a clear hazard. American Journal of Psychiatry 135:1213-1215, 1978

Varma, L. P.: Cannabis psychosis. Indian Journal of Psychiatry 14:241-255, 1972

Yambo, M., Acuda, S. W.: Epidemiological Study of Drug Problems in Kenya: Final Report of a Pilot Study. Nairobi, Kenya, University of Nairobi, 1983

Chapter 26

Specific Problems of Drug Abuse in Kenya

by

S. W. Acuda, MD
Kenyatta National Hospital
and
Department of Psychiatry,
Faculty of Medicine,
University of Nairobi,
Nairobi, Kenya.

ABSTRACT

Like most other countries, Kenya has experienced a considerable increase in drug abuse during the last decade, especially among young people. The major drugs of abuse are tobacco, alcohol, cannabis, khat, and, to a lesser extent, tranquilizers and volatile solvents. The author reviews three important epidemiological studies of drug use among the young and describes the effects of the major drugs of abuse. Kenya is unlike developed countries in that khat is used widely, tobacco use continues to increase, the prevalence of alcohol abuse in rural and urban areas are similar, and opioids and cocaine are rarely used.

INTRODUCTION

Over the last decade or so, there has been a considerable increase in the use and abuse of various types of drugs in most parts of the world, especially among youths. Kenya has not been an exception. Indeed, nearly every day an article appears in one of the country's newspapers expressing concern about the drug problem. Court cases involving drug-related offenses are equally common. According to a recent paper from the Ministry of Education, Science, and Technology, drug use and drug abuse have been recognized by the Ministry as among the major reasons children do not take full advantage of the free educational opportunities provided by the government. Additionally, the use of drugs by students in some parts of the country is so widespread that it constitutes a public health problem, (Kenya Ministry of Education, 1985).

STUDIES

Several studies have assessed the nature and extent of drug abuse in the country. Virtually all of them confirm that a drug problem exists and that action should be taken to reduce it (Acuda, 1982 & 1985; Dhadphale et al., 1982; Owino, 1982; Yambo and Acuda, 1983). These studies have identified the major drugs of abuse in Kenya as alcohol, tobacco, cannabis (marijuana, bhang), khat (miraa, gat) and, to a lesser extent, tranquilizer and volatile solvents (gasoline, glue, and plastics). Other drugs of abuse that are responsible for the most serious health and socioeconomic problems in other parts of the world (opium, cocaine, and heroin) are rarely encountered in Kenya. However, they may pose problems in the future.

In the first major study on the use of drugs by youths (Dadphale et al., 1982), 4,450 secondary school pupils were surveyed. They were between the ages of 12 and 20 and attended 10 secondary schools in different rural and urban parts of the country. The study was carried out with a simple questionnaire designed by the authors. The questionnaire asked about the student's knowledge, attitudes, and practices involving alcohol, cigarettes, and cannabis.

During the 3 month study, two of the authors visited the selected schools and administered the questionnaire with the help of teachers.

The schools had been informed of the study's aim and methods well in advance. Moreover, on the day of the exercise the students were assembled in their classrooms and the purpose of the exercise was explained to them again. They were assured of confidentiality and anonymity. Of the 4,450 students given the questionnaire, 2,870 (64%) completed it. The major findings were as follows:

- 10.0% of the respondents reported drinking alcohol three or more times a week (the amount and type of alcohol were not specified)
- 16.3% reported smoking cigarettes more than three times a week
- 13.3% smoked cannabis at least once a month
- 16.8% reported using other (specified) drugs in order to feel high
- 28% said they knew of or had seen cannabis being grown
- 35% knew someone else in their neighborhoods or families who frequently smoked cannabis

Drug use was most common in the urban areas and least common in the rural schools. The study had two major drawbacks. The questionnaire consisted of only six items, which did not inquire into the amount of drug used, whether the drug use reported was recent or in the past, or whether there were any problems associated with the use of drugs. Also, teachers assisted in the study and were present while the questionnaires were completed. Although the students had been assured of confidentiality, quite a large number of them (36%) choose not to complete the questionnaire.

The next study, which was more comprehensive in scope and methodology, also focused on students in secondary schools and teacher-training colleges but also included teachers and parents. Owino (1982) surveyed 246 students and138 teachers and parents in five different schools in three provinces. The results showed both similarities to and differences from the first study.

- Up to 32% of the students regularly drank alcohol three or more times a week
- 20.6% smoked cigarettes regularly

- Only 2% reported ever trying cannabis
- Only 1.9% occasionally chewed khat (miraa)
- 42.1%, mostly females, had never used any of the drugs mentioned

The study identified the most common drugs used as alcohol, tobacco, cannabis, and khat, in descending order. While the male students tended to use nonmedical drugs, the female students tended to use medical—i.e., prescription or over-the-counter—drugs. The students reported that their major sources of information on drugs were friends or relatives (70.7%) and newspapers or books (25.0%). The major sources of drugs were bars, social gatherings, drugstores, schools, laborers, and the black market. The drugs most frequently used by their parents and teachers were, in descending order, alcohol, cigarettes, cannabis, and khat. According to the teachers, the main reasons the students took drugs were, in descending order, influence of friends, easy availability of drugs, and bad parenting.

The main weaknesses of this study were in flawed data-gathering instruments and the hurry with which the study was done; active data collection started in July 1982, and the report was dated August 1982. The questionnaire was also administered in schools with the permission and knowledge of teachers, so influence by other students and teachers cannot be ruled out.

In perhaps the most sophisticated study on the epidemiology of drug use and abuse performed in Kenya to date (Yambo and Acuda, 1983), 563 youths and 235 parents and guardians were interviewed in a household survey in Nairobi and in one rural district. The youths were between 10 and 29 years of age. A slightly modified version of the World Health Organization (WHO) questionnaire for student drug surveys (Smart et al., 1980) was used. The objectives of the study were to determine the prevalence of drug use and abuse in the two areas, identify the drugs involved, specify the population at risk, outline community attitudes to drug use, and recommend prevention measures.

In Nairobi, a random-sampling procedure was used. The population was stratified for income and socioeconomic status to determine which households to survey. In the rural district 50 kilometers away, a cluster random-sampling procedure was used for the same purpose. In each household selected, two youths, one in school and one out of school, and the head of the household were interviewed. A separate questionnaire was used for heads of household. The sample of respondents included in the final analysis were as follows:

- Nairobi, high-income households—59 youths and 30 heads of household
- Nairobi, middle-income households—149 youths and 90 heads of household
- Nairobi, low income households—239 youths and 115 heads of household
- Rural district—116 youths and 58 heads of household

In the final sample, 70.7% of the youths were male and 29.33% were female.

The results of this study, like those of the previous two studies, confirmed that drug use by youths is quite prevalent in Kenya, although the prevalence was not as high as had been feared. A drug abuser was defined as someone who had used one drug on three or more occasions during the previous week. The main drugs of abuse were tobacco (30.0%), alcohol (11.2%), khat, (3.6%) and cannabis (33.6%).

The tendency toward drug abuse was related to age; the greatest number of abusers of tobacco, alcohol, and cannabis were in the 25-to-29 age group. A striking exception here was the use of khat, which was significantly more prevalent among the 10-to-14 age group. Other drugs the respondents reported taking frequently were cocaine (0.4%), amphetamines (1.6)%, inhalants (1.6%), and tranquilizers and sedatives (2.0%). The study further shows that polydrug use was much more common than of a single drug use. For instance, 65% of those who smoked regularly also abused alcohol, and vice versa. Polydrug use most frequently involved tobacco, alcohol, khat, and tranquilizers, but cannabis abusers tended to confine themselves to cannabis. The study also showed that over 30% of regular users of a given drug also turned out to be abusers.

Tobacco abuse, although widespread in all Nairobi income groups and in the rural area, was most prevalent among the low-income group and those out of school. Next to tobacco, alcohol was the most frequently abused drug, affecting 11.0% of boys and 4.1% of girls. The highest percentage of alcohol abusers was in the low-income group (14.0%) and the lowest rates were in the high-income group (5.0%) and the group from the rural area (3.6%). Student status was also important in alcohol use; only 5% of those still in school could be classified as alcohol abusers, compared with 17% of those no longer going to school.

Socioeconomic background, therefore, seemed to be a major factor in drug use or abuse, but it was probably mediated by the wide availability of drugs. The attitudes of the household heads were a better predictor of the youths' drug use than the attitudes of the youths themselves. Given these findings, any campaign against drugs should focus primarily on tobacco, alcohol, cannabis, and khat and only secondarily on tranquilizers, amphetamines, and inhalants. The major thrust of the campaign should be reducing the availability of or access to these drugs and changing the attitudes of young people towards drug use. The campaign could, therefore, include police action and health education.

SUBSTANCE PROPERTIES AND EFFECTS

Khat (Miraa, Qat, Catha, Edulis)

This drug deserves special mention because it is hardly known in other parts of Africa even though it has been widely used in parts of East Africa since the beginning of this century (Bally, 1945; Carothers, 1945; East African Medical Journal, 1945).

When chewed, khat produces mild to moderate euphoria, suppresses the appetite, sustains alertness, and eliminates fatigue. It is therefore used as a means of relaxing, bringing people together and facilitating communication during social events, and suppressing sleep and fatigue. It has also been used in work situations that require sustained alertness.

Traditionally, it was chewed by adults who did not use alcohol for religious reasons. Few problems were associated with its use in this context. In the studies just reviewed, khat was the third most frequently used drug, and it is the drug most preferred by 10-to-14-year olds. Unlike the adults who used it in the traditional setting, who chewed it alone, Kenyan youths frequently use it concurrently with alcohol, cigarettes, or cannabis, which could increase the likelihood of associated problems.

In addition to case histories describing khat use related to mental illness (Dhadphale et al., 1981), two recent studies have addressed the socioeconomic and public health problems associated with khat use in Kenya. A major study in Garissa, a town where khat chewing is almost part of the normal way of life, showed that heavy khat users displayed evidence of dependence and tolerance (Haji, 1985). They spent a considerable amount of their working and leisure time, an average of 6 hours per day, chewing khat and spent over half of their salaries on the drug. The families of heavy khat users were emotionally disturbed, were economically deprived, and faced marital problems, including divorce.

Delinquent behavior was much more common in their children than in the children of parents who did not chew khat. Elsewhere in this collection, Omolo (1985) summarizes his study in a khat-growing district of Kenya. He found that heavy khat users had more medical and psychological problems than non users of khat. Their main health problems included frequent constipation, tooth decay, sexual problems, poor appetite, weight loss, irritability, and depression.

Cannabis (Marijuana, Hashish, Bhang)

Next to alcohol and tobacco, cannabis is the most frequently abused drug in Kenya. The studies reviewed earlier indicate that up to 25% of young people have used it regularly. Whereas 40 to 50 years ago the use of cannabis was confined to a few middle-aged or elderly individuals living in rural areas, in recent years there has been a marked change in its use pattern. The drug is now being used overwhelmingly by young people aged 15 to 25 years.

A considerable amount of current evidence shows that excessive use of cannabis can be harmful, although most of its harmful effects have so far been observed mainly in animals (Meyer, 1978). Regular cannabis use by humans is known to produce dependence and tolerance, although the withdrawal symptoms are mild. Cannabis use also can distort perception of time and other sensory perceptions. Furthermore, heavy use can interfere with attention, concentration, memory, and logical thinking and can grossly impair the ability to perform complex actions, such as driving a car or formulating sound judgements. Some heavy cannabis users are known to have developed psychotic illnesses characterized by confusion, excitement, paranoid delusions, and hallucinations (Meyer, 1978). It is not yet clear whether this psychosis is a direct toxic effect of the drug on humans or whether the drug simply unmasks a psychotic process in individuals predisposed to psychosis. A small proportion of chronic heavy users of cannabis may also develop the amotivational syndrome, which is characterized by slow, progressive loss of energy and drive, apathy (loss of emotional reactivity), poverty of ideas, loss of memory, and deterioration in personal hygiene.

Other harmful consequences of cannabis abuse (so far observed mainly in animals), include production of abnormal chromosomes, teratogenicity, carcinogenic effects, suppression of the body's immune systems, and interference with male reproductive functions (Meyer, 1978).

Tobacco

Smoking of tobacco is such a common sight in many parts of the world that few people outside the health professions are aware that nicotine can cause some of the most serious health problems, which could be prevented by cessation or reduction of smoking.

Although no major studies on smoking and health have been done in Kenya, there is now overwhelming evidence that tobacco smoking is responsible for up to 30% of all cases of cancer, at least 80% of the cases of lung cancer, 75% of the cases of other chest diseases, and 25% of the cases of myocardial infarction. Furthermore, it has been estimated that each year over one million babies are born prematurely and die shortly afterwards as a result of their mothers' smoking tobacco during pregnancy. Perhaps even more serious was the discovery that the spouses of heavy smokers or other persons who stay close to smokers for prolonged periods—e.g., co-workers—also stand a greater than normal chance of developing these diseases (WHO, 1983).

In developed countries, increased awareness of the hazards of smoking, due to health education, has recently led to a sharp fall in the rate of tobacco smoking. But the habit continues to rise in developing countries at an estimated rate of 2% each year (WHO, 1983). The three Kenyan studies I reviewed earlier indicate that tobacco is the drug most widely abused by youths in Kenya.

Alcohol

Alcohol is the next most widely consumed drug in Kenya. It also produces the most serious health and socioeconomic problems. Several studies done in Kenya have shown that between 50% to 60% of the young people aged 12 to 24 use alcohol regularly and that approximately 12% of them show features of alcohol dependence (Yambo and Acuda, 1983). In other studies, 11% of patients attending primary health clinics in various parts of Kenya were suffering primarily from alcoholism (Dhadphale,1985) and 21% of patients admitted to Mathari Hospital had alcoholic psychosis (Badia, 1985). Unlike the situation in industrialized countries, where alcohol problems are more acute in the urban areas, in Kenya the problem seems to be equally widespread in rural and urban areas (Bittah et al., 1979; Wanjiru,1979). Elsewhere I have reviewed the nature and extent of alcohol problems in Africa (Acuda, 1982, & 1986).

Prescription Drugs

Surprisingly little has been written about the abuse of psychoactive prescription drugs in Kenya, although it is well known that they are widely prescribed and widely consumed.

Major tranquilizers (neuroleptics, or antipsychotics) are usually prescribed for long periods—e.g., in the treatment of schizophrenia—but have little or no tendency to produce tolerance and dependence. However, many of them produce nasty side effects, even in small doses. The minor tranquilizers, especially the benzodiazepines, which are widely used for treatment of anxiety and sleep disturbances, do produce dependence, tolerance, and withdrawal syndromes. Numerous cases of benzodiazepine dependence have now been reported worldwide.

In Kenya, however, there has been only one publication on diazepam addiction so far (Acuda and Muhangi, 1979). One of the patients described was a middle-aged man who had developed such high tolerance and dependence on diazepam over several years that by the time he was referred for treatment he was taking between 40 and 60 mg/day of diazepam intravenously, together with large doses of nitrazepam at night.

Another patient described in that paper was a young man who presented at the emergency department of the Kenyatta National Hospital in status epilepticus. It was later learned that he had been taking 100 to 150 mg of diazepam daily and had developed severe withdrawal symptoms, including status epilepticus, when he failed to get the drug that weekend.

In one of the epidemiological studies referred to earlier (Yambo and Acuda,1983), up to 15% of the youths had taken tranquilizers at least once in the preceding 12 months and 3% to 5% had taken them at least once that week. The use and abuse of these drugs may be quite widespread in Kenya, particularly among health personnel, who have easy access to them. However, no study has been done to date to confirm or alleviate this fear.

Similarly, cases of abuse of the dangerous drugs of addiction, such as asmorphine and pethiadine, occasionally come to the attention of psychiatrists or hospital administrators, but the magnitude of the problem in Kenya remains unknown. Heroin and opium dependence are still rare in Kenya.

REFERENCES

Acuda, S. W.: Drug and alcohol problems in Kenya today: a review of research. East African Medical Journal 59:642-644, 1982

Acuda, S. W.: Drug and alcohol problems research—international review, I: East Africa. British Journal of Addiction in Kenya today: a review of research, East Africa. British Journal of Addiction 80, 1985

Acuda, S. W.: Alcoholism: Developing a drinking habit. Africa Health 8:13-15, 1986

Acuda, S. W., Muhangi, J.: Diazepam addiction in Kenya. East African Medical Journal 56:76-79, 1979

Badia, P.: Alcoholism among inpatients in Mathari Hospital. M Med dissertation, University of Nairobi, Nairobi, Kenya, 1985

Bally, P. R. O.: Catha edulis. East African Medical Journal 22:2-3, 1945

Bittah, O., Owola, J. Oduor, P. A.: A study of alcoholism in a rural setting in Kenya. East African Medical Journal 56:577-579, 1979

Carothers, J. C.: Miraa as a cause of insanity. East African Medical Journal 22:4-6, 1945

Dhadphale, M.: Psychiatric morbidity among patients attending rural district hospital outpatient clinics in Kenya. MD thesis, University of Nairobi, Nairobi, Kenya, 1985

Dhadphale, M., Mengech, A., Chege, S. K. W.: Miraa (Catha edulis) as a cause of psychosis. East African Medical Journal 58:130-135, 1981

Dhadphale, M., Mengech, H. N., Syme, D., et al.: Drug abuse among secondary school students in Kenya: a preliminary survey. East Africa Medical Journal 59:152-156, 1982
East African Medical Journal: The need to control miraa (editorial) East African Medical Journal 22:1, 1945

Haji, A.: The socio-economic problems associated with use and abuse of khat in Kenya. MA thesis, University of Nairobi, Nairobi, Kenya, 1985

Kenya Ministry of Education: Behavioral and psychological problems in Kenyan schools and colleges. Presented at the Intercountry workshop on Mental Health in Kenya, Nairobi, Kenya, August 1985

Meyer, R. E.: Behavioral pharmacology of marihuana, in Psychopharmacology: A generation of progress. Edited by Liptom, M. A., DiMascio, A., Killam, K. F., New York, U.S.A., Raven Press, 1978, pp. 1639-1652.

Omolo, E.: Medical and psychological problems among miraa users in Meru District, Kenya. M. Med dissertation, University of Nairobi, Nairobi, Kenya,1985

Owino, G.: Report on the problem of drugs among Kenyan students in secondary schools and teacher training colleges. Presented at the IV ICPA World congress, Nairobi, Kenya, August 1982

Smart, R. G., Hughes, P. H., Johnson, L. D., et al.: A Methodology for Student Drug Surveys. World Health Organization off-set publication no. 50 Geneva, Switzerland, WHO, 1980

Wanjiru, F.: Alcoholism: Effects on man and his integration into society. BA thesis University of Nairobi, Nairobi, Kenya, 1979

World Health Organization: Technical reports series no. 695. Geneva, Switzerland, WHO, 1983

Yambo, M., Acuda, S. W.: Epidemiological Study of Drug Problems in Kenya: Final report of a pilot study. Nairobi, Kenya, University of Nairobi.

Chapter 27

Medical and Social Aspects of Khat Use in Kenya

by

O.E. Omolo, MD
Specialist Psychiatrist
and
Chief Administrator,
Coast Province General Hospital,
Mombasa, Kenya

ABSTRACT

Khat leaves are a major source of income in Kenya and are in demand both abroad and locally. Khat has a stimulant effect and is often used in social settings, but it has many adverse physical and psychological consequences. The author reviews the literature and describes his own study of the prevalence of khat use in randomly selected hospital outpatients. The prevalence was higher among patients younger than 20, but young users consumed only moderate amounts of khat. There was a strong association between khat use and use or abuse of tobacco or alcohol. The study confirms earlier findings of psychological dependence and lack of tolerance. Health workers are advised to emphasize khat in their health education talks and to look for alcoholism in khat chewers. Because of the economic benefits of growing khat, an alternative cash crop is needed before khat can be banned.

INTRODUCTION

The plant khat obtained its scientific name Catha edulis Forsk, in the 19th century from the Danish botanist Peter Forskaal. It is known under many names in the countries where it is produced. Khat is an evergreen that grows in highlands and may live up to 200 years. It is a native of Ethiopia and the Arabian peninsula. Early Moslem literature refers to it as a flower of paradise because of its mood- elevating properties. In its native home it is used in various ceremonies and medicaments. The colonial governments of Kenya and Somalia banned it because it was regarded as a drug of addiction.

Khat is a major cash earner in Kenya, although this is not common knowledge because it is grown in a circumscribed area. It is exported to Somalia, Djibouti, Sudan, Uganda, Zaire, and Middle Eastern countries. There is a substantial and ever increasing local demand.

Khat leaves are consumed in a variety of ways. They may be smoked, brewed, kneaded into a paste and mixed with honey, or simply chewed. The consumption generally occurs in a social setting.

Khat is sold in bundles of various sizes. Fresh green khat is preferred, so it is transported by fast cars or planes to its destination. Most of the adult male population of Somalia, Yemen, and Djibouti use khat regularly. This leads to the importation of large quantities from Kenya and Ethiopia.

There are two major groups of compounds in khat: phenylalkylamine derivatives and the basic alkaloids. The main psychoactive substances in khat are cathine (CNE), and cathinone, which are found in the amine fraction. Levo-cathinone is a potent amphetamine- like compound and is the constituent of khat that is mainly responsible for its central nervous system effects. It produces a stimulant effect by increasing dopamine turnover at the central dopaminergic terminals and noradrenaline at the peripheral noradrenergic nerve endings. Cathinone has various effects on body systems, such as mydriasis, logorrhea, euphoria, excitation, hyperactivity, insomnia, lack of fatigue, anorexia, and constipation.

REVIEW OF THE LITERATURE

Psychiatric symptoms have been reported to follow the use of khat (Carothers, 1945; Dhadphale et al., 1981; Elmi, 1983; Heisch, 1945; Peters, 1952). However, toxic psychosis is rarely seen among khat users (Bulletin on Narcotics, 1980). Tolerance or physical dependence has not been observed. Khat is associated with moderate but often persistent psychic dependence.

A survey of khat chewers in Kenya (Maitai, 1973) showed that they experienced systemic symptoms and the socioeconomic consequences of drug abuse. The 1980 report of a World Health Organization (WHO) advisory group (Baasher, 1983) enumerated the medical consequences of khat chewing: periodontal disease, stomatitis, esophagitis, gastritis, malnutrition, cirrhosis of the liver, constipation, and anorexia. Chronic khat users have a high frequency of spermatorrhea and, in later stages, impotence. Adverse psychological effects are insomnia, reactive depression when the drug effects wear off, and irritability the following morning. These may result in lateness for work and diminished work performance among chronic users.

In her work on the pharmacology of khat, Guatai (1982) found the effects of cathinone have a more rapid onset and shorter duration than the actions of CNE, and she suggested that this may explain the continuous chewing observed among khat users. Concurrent abuse of alcohol or hypnotics has been observed among khat chewers (Peters, 1952). Multiple drug abuse has been observed among secondary school students in Kenya (Dhadphale et al., 1982). In his review of the pharmacology of khat, Kalix (1984) noted that the social environment appears to influence the chewer's response, and the effect is said to be more readily perceived by the habitual users.

A study on the socioeconomic aspects of khat use (Haju, 1985) showed that most chewers were young single males who had some formal education and were employed. The lack of alternative leisure activities, the nature of their jobs, and socializing were some of the reasons given for khat chewing. Problems arising from this habit were financial mismanagement, family discord and divorce, poor health, poor work performance, an increase in sexual activity due to heightened desire, and multiple drug abuse.

A STUDY IN MERU

I carried out a small study to identify the sociodemographic characteristics of khat users, their physical and psychiatric symptoms, and the pattern and extent of simultaneous drug abuse.

METHOD

The study was conducted at the Meru District Hospital's outpatient department. The subjects were randomly selected. They were all given physical examinations. A locally validated version of the Self-Rating Questionnaire (SRQ) was used. A drug use/abuse questionnaire was used to elicit the use/abuse of khat, alcohol, cannabis, or any other drug or chemical. Another questionnaire was used to determine demographic and personal data and medical and psychiatric histories.

The modified Standard Psychiatric Interview (SPI) was used to assess the mental state in subjects found to be khat users. The non-users of khat were designated as a control group for the khat chewers as they were similar in all respects except the use of khat.

RESULTS

Khat use was more frequent among the subjects aged 19 or below and less frequent among those aged 50 and above. Among the khat chewers, people who were 19 or younger were moderate users, while those aged 50 and above were heavy users. Most khat users had never been married, and the users who had never been married were more likely to be moderate users, while married people were generally heavy khat users. Questions about knowledge, attitudes, and practice showed that non users were more aware of the adverse effects of khat than the users. Some symptoms suspected to arise from chronic or excessive use of khat were found to be significantly more frequent among khat users than among nonusers.

A very significant finding of this study was the strong association between khat use and the use or abuse of tobacco and alcohol.

Multiple drug abuse among khat chewers was also noted. More neurotic symptoms were observed among heavy khat users, especially those khat chewers who also abused alcohol. According to the SRQ and SPI, 50% of the whole sample had psychiatric disorders and 3% were psychotic.

There was no difference in the prevalence of neurotic symptoms between moderate khat users and nonusers. However, there were more neurotic symptoms among heavy khat users than among nonusers. There were also significantly more neurotic symptoms among heavy khat chewers who also used alcohol than among chewers who did not use alcohol.

Educational level was not significantly related to the use of khat. No particular job was associated with khat use, but there was an excess of students in the user category. Most of the khat users were in the lower socioeconomic group. But the degree of khat use was not associated with income. Only one-third of the sample had ever chewed khat, and 72% of this group chewed it daily. All heavy users chewed khat daily, which can be interpreted as a manifestation of psychic dependence.

The age at first use—i.e., duration—is not related to the amount of khat used. This indicates that tolerance does not develop with time. Most of the khat chewers used it for ease of communication during social interactions. Those who cited increased work performance as a reason for using khat were farmers. In this respect, khat fulfills a useful function, for it is well known that it alleviates hunger and fatigue. In general, the sample knew about khat's wide range of side effects.

MANAGEMENT OF KHAT USERS

Khat use is a community problem and should be approached accordingly. Health workers must first of all be taught and made familiar with the psychological, medical, and other problems caused by chronic khat use. In the khat-growing areas, medical workers should always emphasize various aspects of khat use during their health education talks. Individual tailored talks should also be given to khat chewers with medical or psychological problems related to khat use. The medical worker must also be on the lookout for signs and symptoms of alcoholism among khat chewers. If present, appropriate advice and treatment should be given.

THE CONTROVERSY REGARDING KHAT USE

From time to time, local newspapers are full of arguments for and against khat chewing. The dangers of excessive khat chewing are no longer in dispute, at least among medical personnel. What remains unclear is the degree of khat chewing that constitutes abuse. In economic terms, an alternative cash crop must be introduced before khat growing can be banned. The exportation of khat brings badly needed foreign money into Kenya. At this stage, the country may not be able to afford to lose this source of income. In any case, no local study has addressed all the undesirable aspects of khat use. Such a study is urgently needed; the results may help the government to define its position vis-a-vis the cultivation, trade in, and use of, khat. In the meantime, heavy khat chewers should be identified and informed of the deleterious effects of their habit.

REFERENCES

Baasher, T.: The Epidemiology of Khat: Report of the WHO Intercountry meeting on the Health, Social and Economic Aspects of Khat(Mogadishu,Somalia).Geneva, Switzerland, WHO 1983 Bulletin on Narcotics 32(3), 1980

Carothers, J. C.: Miraa is a cause of insanity. East African Medical Journal 22:4-6, 1945

Dhadphale, M., Mengech, A., Chege, S. W.: Miraa (Eatha edulis) as a cause of psychosis. East African Medical Journal 58:130-135, 1981

Dhadphale, M., Mengech, H. N., Syme, D., et al.: Drug abuse among secondary school students in Kenya: A preliminary survey. East African Medical Journal 59:152-156, 1982

Elmi, A. S.: Khat: spreading epidemiology and problems in Somalia. Presented at the I.C.K., Antananarivo, Madagascar, 1983

Guantai, A. N.: Cathe edulis forsk (miraa): Occurrence, active constituents, and pharmacological activity. MSc thesis, University of Nairobi, Nairobi, Kenya, 1982

Haju, A. R. J.: Study on the socioeconomic aspects of khat use and abuse in Garissa Town. MA thesis, University of Nairobi, Nairobi, Kenya, 1985

Heisch, R. B.: A case of poisoning by Catha edulis. East African Medical Journal 22:7-9, 1945

Kalix, P.: The pharmacology of khat. General Pharmacology 15:179-187, 1984

Maitai, C. K.: A toxicological investigation of catha edulis forsk. Ph.D. dissertation, University of Nairobi, Nairobi, Kenya, 1973

Peters, D. W. A.: Khat: Its history, botany, chemistry and toxicology. Pharmacology Journal 169:16-18, 36- 37, 1952

Chapter 28

Trihexyphenidyl in Zimbabwe

by

Myrl R. S. Manley, MD
Lecturer,
Department of Psychiatry,
University of Zimbabwe,
Harare, Zimbabwe

ABSTRACT

After arriving in Zimbabwe, the author noticed use of trihexyphenidyl by many psychiatric patients for whom it was not prescribed or clinically indicated. He presents observations from his ongoing study of the patterns of trihexyphenidyl use, its subjective efffects, and associated DSM-III diagnoses. The patients' psychiatric diagnoses and histories of substance abuse are quite varied, but the patients agree that standard doses of trihexyphenidyl make them happy, more sociable, and better able to concentrate and work. The author points out the widespread medical availability of trihexyphenidyl and many patients' belief that the euphoria produced by trihexyphenidyl is part of medical treatment.

INTRODUCTION

When I came to Zimbabwe from New York, I began seeing what I subsequently found out had long been recognized by the staff at Harare, that some of our psychiatric patients were abusing trihexyphenidyl.

They demanded it in clinics, took lots of it, and took it when it was not prescribed or clinically indicated.

Trihexyphenidyl is an anticholinergic, antiparkinsonian drug that is most commonly used in psychiatry to treat extrapyramidal side effects caused by antipsychotic drugs. Although trihexyphenidyl abuse has been recognized and described in the United States and England, (Bolin, 1960; Goggin and Solomon, 1979; MacVicar, 1977; Marriott, 1976; Rubinstein, 1978, Saran, 1986; Smith 1980), it seemed much more common at the clinics in Harare.

I was deeply impressed, not just with the numbers, but with the extraordinary lengths to which people would go to get the drug. One man walked 10 kilometers from one hospital to another when told that the first was temporarily out of trihexyphenidyl. In another incident, a young woman brought her infant son to the outpatient clinic and, in front of staff, began screaming and beating the child. She complained of auditory hallucinations and, not surprisingly, was admitted and given antipsychotics. She demanded trihexyphenidyl and, when she did not receive it, absconded.

My curiosity aroused, I began studying patterns of trihexyphenidyl use.

METHODS

To call any person's drug-taking habits abuse indicates a number of presuppositions, which are particularly unwarranted given how little we know about the issues I shall be presenting to you. I use the phrase trihexyphenidyl abuse for the sake of semantic convenience. Extra medical use would probably be more accurate. I have arbitrarily defined a trihexyphenidyl abuser as any patient who repeatedly asks for trihexphenidyl, has no clinically detectable extrapyramidal symptoms, and has taken trihexyphenidyl at least some time in the past while not taking neuroleptics. Because of the possibility of subclinical extrapyramidal side effects, it may be necessary to limit the study eventually to only patients who are not taking any antipsychotic medication at the time they demand trihexyphenidyl.

I asked for referrals from all inpatient and outpatient services of the medical school in Harare. I interviewed each patient referred to determine the pattern of trihexyphenidyl use, the subjective effects of the drug, other substance abuse, and the psychiatric diagnosis according to DSM-III criteria. Each patient is also referred for testing with the Minnesota Multiphasic Personality Inventory (MMPI), administered by a clinical psychologist working with them, Margaret Henning.

Neither Margaret nor I is fluent in Shona, the primary language of most of our patients, and so much of our work must be done through translation.

We are not able to say how much this confounds our investigation other than that it makes it more laborious and that we are certainly missing considerable richness and subtlety in what we are told. Additionally, the MMPI has not been standardized for Zimbabwe, and we may ultimately not be able to use these results. However, we are mostly interested in how much our patients resemble or differ from one another rather than in interpretations of specific test items. It was our initial impression and our working hypothesis that a large proportion of patients suspected of being trihexyphenidyl abusers had fairly severe personality disorders with borderline and antisocial features.

I have interviewed six patients to date, and formal testing is complete on five out of the projected group of 30. Consequently, the observations I am presenting here are tentative and anecdotal, although my confidence in them is strengthened by informal talks with many more patients not yet admitted to the study. I will raise more questions than I can answer in this paper, but I hope the questions will be provocative and will stimulate some of my colleagues in Africa and elsewhere to look at this issue more closely with me.

RESULTS

Our most striking finding so far is the lack of homogeneity among our patients, which weakens our initial hypothesis that they shared certain personality features. The psychiatric diagnoses and MMPI profiles are quite varied. The diagnoses range from schizophrenia to mixed personality disorder with hysterical features to no psychopathology. This is even more striking in light of the fact that, for all our patients, trihexyphenidyl was initially given as an adjunct to an antipsychotic, consequently skewing our population strongly toward severe psychotic illnesses.

The history of other substance abuse also varies considerably, even within our small sample. Some patients have histories of heavy daily use of alcohol and marijuana. Others have no history of substance abuse. One patient, for example, has not drunk any beer for several years; hc tricd smoking marijuana once, found the effect unpleasurable, and was never tempted again. This story was independently corroborated by several family members.

Two points on which our patients agree are the pattern of use and the reported subjective effects. All trihexyphenidyl users appear to get the drug from hospitals and clinics. There do not seem to be any black market or street sales of trihexyphenidyl, unlike the situation in the United States. There is, moreover, a resounding chorus of unanimity in the reported subjective effects. All of my patients say trihexyphenidyl makes them feel more happy, more sociable, better able to concentrate, and better able to work. One patient, a 28 year old man with a diagnosis of schizophrenia, has had only one full time job in his life; he worked as a newspaper vendor for 3 months, and then only while taking trihexyphenidyl. Although it is, of course, impossible to establish cause and effect retrospectively, in his own mind he emphatically links being able to work with his taking trihexyphenidyl. Repeatedly, patients say trihexyphenidyl makes them feel normal. One patient said trihexyphenidyl improved his appetite. All patients deny that trihexyphenidyl improves sleep or increases libido.

In the very small literature on trihexyphenidyl abuse in the United States since the first reported case in 1960, two patterns of drug use have been described. One is intentional overdose to create a toxic delirium with hallucinations. This use seemed to be especially frequent among people also taking LSD, mescaline, or peyote, particularly during the late 1960s and early 1970s, when use of hallucinogens was common in the United States.

The other pattern reported in the literature is sustained use of lower doses for a prolonged euphoric or antidepressant effect. The latter use is seen in all of our patients. Typically, patients will take 10 to 15 milligrams per day, which is also the standard prescribed dose. Patients acknowledge occasionally taking higher doses and inadvertently causing a toxic delirium with amounts ranging from 20 to 30 milligrams per day. In each case, this was felt to be undesirable, so the person carefully titrated his use to subtoxic doses. As stated by one patient, a schizophrenic whose psychotic symptoms were in remission, 30 milligrams made the illness come back; made the voices start again.

DISCUSSION

If it is true, as I believe it is, that the prevalence of trihexyphenidyl abuse is higher in Zimbabwe than in the United States, what are some of the possible reasons?

One may be the absence of other drugs of abuse. Alcohol and marijuana are the only two drugs widely available. There is no heroin. Cocaine is rumored to be used by a few wealthy people, but I have never been able to substantiate this. A miniscule number of narcotic addicts in Harare use morphine and synthetic narcotics, and a moderate but uncounted number of middle-class patients are addicted to anxiolytics or barbiturates prescribed by their private physicians. For the vast majority of the population, however, alcohol and marijuana are the only drugs widely available. Someone inclined to drug abuse might exploit whatever becomes available.

In other words, there may be a higher prevalence of trihexyphenidyl abuse because it is there and nothing much else is. However, our preliminary data show that a significant number of our patients have no history of other substance abuse.

Probably of greater importance is the widespread medical availability of trihexyphenidyl. For many years, Zimbabwe has had a desperate manpower shortage in mental health care, and it is still not fully alleviated. The tremendous demand for extremely limited services has necessitated some flexibility and adaptation. Many patients are maintained on long-acting neuroleptics, and often an antiparkinsonian drug will be started concurrently with an antipsychotic. Nurses are empowered to dispense and refill prescriptions without consulting physicians, and many rural clinics are staffed only by nurses. A result of all this is that a relatively large number of patients are given trihexyphenidyl initially, and once they receive it they find it fairly easy to obtain and to stockpile by going from clinic to clinic and asking for more. If, out of all the patients for whom trihexyphenidyl is prescribed, a certain percentage continue to use the drug when it is no longer medically indicated, then the prevalence of trihexyphenidyl abuse will increase when the drug is widely prescribed.

A third factor is that many of our patients do not make the same distinction between therapeutic effects and unanticipated or unwanted side effects as do we physicians. The euphoria and sense of well-being that accompany the use of trihexyphenidyl are seen as an intended part of medical treatment. One patient was asked if, given his choice, he would rather have beer, marijuana, or trihexyphenidyl, and he quickly answered trihexyphenidyl. When asked why, he answered (a little disingeniously, I think) that although all of them made him feel good, trihexyphenidyl is given by doctors and is therefore good for you and a part of medical treatment.

It must seem very perverse to some patients when we insist on compliance with drugs that make them feel tired, heavy, stiff, dizzy, and, sometimes impotent, and then insist they stop taking a drug we have given them that actually makes them feel better.

PROPOSED PROGRAMS

Where do these observations lead us? It would be easy to close with the usual call for heightened vigilance in dispensing and prescribing antiparkinsonian drugs because of their abuse potential. But this ignores the more interesting question of what conditions are our patients treating by their determined continued use of trihexyphenidyl? It is widely recognized that trihexyphenidyl and other anticholinergic drugs have a central psychoactivating effect. In fact, it was this observation, among others, that led some researchers to propose a central cholinergic-adrenergic imbalance in the etiology of certain affective disorders (Janowsky et al., 1972 & 1973). According to this theory, some depressions are the result of a central functional hypercholinergic state. If we can document what our patients are telling us—that trihexyphenidyl results in increased work performance, greater sociability, and enhanced sense of well-being—and if self-medication does not result in increasing doses with toxic sequelae, are there any justifications for calling it abuse? Clearly, we need additional information. When I have finished the initial survey, I hope to begin controlled trials with a few select patients to observe the effects of trihexyphenidyl on work performance and mood over time. In the meantime, I am eager to hear of other peoples' experience and solutions to these clinical issues.

REFERENCES

Bolin, R. R.: Psychiatric manifestations of Artane toxicity. Journal of Nervous and Mental Disorders 131:256-259, 1960

Goggin, D. A., Solomon, G. F.: Trihexyphenidyl abuse for euphorogenic effect. American Journal of Psychiatry 136:459-460, 1979

Janowsky, D., El-Yousef, M. K., Davis, J. M., et al.: A cholinergic adrenergic hypothesis of mania and depression. Lancet 2:632-635, 1972

Janowsky, d., El-Yousef, M. K., Davis, J. M., et al: Parasympathetic suppression of manic symptoms by physostigmine. Archives General Psychiatry 28:542-547, 1973

MacVicar, K: Abuse of antiparkinsonian drugs by psychiatric patients. American Journal of Psychiatry 134:809-811, 1977

Marriott, P.: Dependence on antiparkinsonian drugs. British Medical Journal 1:152, 1976

Rubinstein, J. S.: Abuse of antiparkinsonism drugs. Journal of the American Medical Association 239:2365- 2366, 1978

Saran, A. S.: Use or abuse of antiparkinsonian drugs by psychiatric patients. Journal of Clinical Psychiatry 47:130-132, 1986

Smith, J. M.: Abuse of the antiparkinson drugs: a review of the literature. Journal of Clinical Psychiatry 41:351-354, 1980

Chapter 29

Special Aspects of Alcoholism Among American Blacks

by

Roy W. Menninger, MD,
Director,
Department of Preventive Psychiatry,
and
The Menninger Foundation,
Topeka, Kansas, U.S.A.

ABSTRACT

The prevalence of alcoholism among blacks is difficult to determine, but it is an important social and medical problem. Alcohol use by blacks is characterized by two major patterns—heavy drinking and abstinence; the latter is common among black women. Excessive drinking by blacks may be associated with several cultural factors, including the availability and visibility of liquor in black communities and the widespread acceptance of excessive drinking as a normal part of life. The lack of encouragement and support for blacks who want treatment contributes to postponement of treatment, so many of those who do seek help are in the late stages of the disorder and have a poor prognosis. Many blacks do not know where to go for help or have limited trust in the existing services, which are generally run by and for whites. Suggestions for improving alcoholism treatment for blacks include locating access points where black alcoholics spend time (e.g., bars, pool halls, barber shops) and improving mental health professionals' appreciation of cultural issues.

INTRODUCTION

As a white psychiatrist, I am addressing this issue because it is important and most American psychiatrists are relatively ignorant about it. The task of preparing this paper has substantially increased my awareness of this problem and its seriousness. My remarks are intended to share some of what I have learned, but they are not a definitive discussion of the problem. From my review of the subject, four impressions stand out.

1. According to Peter Bell, Executive Director of the Minnesota Institute on Black Chemical Abuse (personal communication), chemical dependence may be the number one social problem of black Americans and the black community in the United States.

2. Most blacks come to treatment late, when the disorder is already severe, and they commonly come without much encouragement or support from either the community or the family.

3. When they do come for help, blacks are typically treated in systems organized by whites, administered and staffed by whites, and used by a largely white clientele. As a result those providing treatment lack knowledge and empathic understanding of the special cultural needs of the black alcoholic.

4. Because white mental health professionals in the United States outnumber black professionals, whites have a special responsibility to understand what the problem is, what knowledge is required, and, in particular, how

to provide better preparation in bicultural psychiatry for mental health trainees of all kinds.

Such factors as prevalence, accessibility, and cultural patterns and attitudes contribute to making alcoholism a major psychosocial issue for blacks and the black community.

PREVALENCE

Although the prevalence of alcoholism is difficult to determine among whites and blacks, deaths from cirrhosis of the liver among American blacks are nearly twice as common as in whites (Williams, 1985). There are also higher rates of pancreatic disorders (Ng-A-Qui, 1984) and other alcohol-related diseases, including esophageal cancer (Williams, 1985). In one study of 225 urban black drinkers (King et al., 1969), it was estimated that 62% of those in their early 30s were heavy drinkers and that some 17% demonstrated recent serious difficulties secondary to alcohol use. Among this group, the absence of a father in the childhood home and failure to graduate from high school predicted heavy drinking and alcohol problems.

Alcohol plays a prominent role in criminal behavior in many cultures, but particularly in the black community. In one study (Peter Bell, personal communication), it was found that one-third of black felons in prison had been under the influence of alcohol at the time they committed their crimes. Alcohol was involved in the crimes of 70% of the black men and 67% of the black women who had committed homicide, and alcohol was a factor in 11 of 12 stabbings and 8 of 10 arrests for crimes involving weapons.

One of the factors promoting alcoholism among blacks is the accessibility and the visibility of liquor. It is estimated that there are three times as many liquor stores in the residential areas of black communities as in white neighborhoods. There are five times more advertisements for liquor in black communities than in white communities. It is estimated that, for blacks, some 10% of earnings are spent on alcohol—some 7 billion dollars—and $125 more per capita per year is spent on liquor than on food (Bailey et al., 1965; Dawkins et al.; Harper, 1980; Sterne and Pittrman, 1972).

DRINKING PATTERNS

The patterns of drinking among blacks are noteworthy in several respects. Typically, urban blacks drink more than rural blacks, perhaps reflecting the greater visibility and accessibility of alcohol in the urban setting.

Alcohol plays a role in bringing people together and enhances the sense of community participation, especially among blacks. As a result, there is relatively less solitary drinking among blacks than among whites. As in other cultures, drinking carries a certain macho quality with it. Heavy drinking is a means of obtaining peer approval. Staying cool while drinking to excess is acceptable evidence of manhood. In contrast to many other cultures, blacks do not have a tradition of using alcohol during religious ceremonies, which may contribute to the absence of black cultural sanctions controlling its use.

The prominence of such enormous social problems as racism, economic frustration, unemployment, underemployment, and poverty lend superficial support to their etiologic role in alcoholism among blacks. There is reason, however, to question an assumption of simple causation. Most American blacks have experienced the oppressive aspects of racism, but only a few are alcoholic. Peter Bell has pointed out that contemporary racism is less malevolent now than it was 100 years ago, and yet alcoholism has vastly increased since that time. As Brisbane (1986) has put it, alcoholism is a clear example of an equal opportunity disease. The complex etiology of alcoholism is beyond the scope of these remarks, but it is relevant to call attention to a recent review (Donovan, 1986) suggesting that alcoholism is probably a heterogeneous disorder whose etiology involves a mixture of psychological, genetic, biological, and sociologic factors. Racism alone is an insufficient explanation.

In general, blacks either drink heavily or not at all. Moderation is not the rule. This is especially true for women; in one study (Dawkins and Harper, 1983), 51% of the black women and 39% of white women were abstainers. It seems particularly important to note that many blacks do not distinguish abuse from use. Those who use alcohol excessively do not think of their drinking as abuse or even excessive. Others do not recognize them as abusers or see them as persons who should receive treatment. As Dawkins and Harper

(1983) write, "The black community has yet to realize, or to admit, that alcohol abuse has been an integral source in the destruction of black people, black families, and black communities." Those are harsh words, but they reflect this cultural failure to distinguish between abuse and use.

The relative abstinence of black women is particularly noteworthy (Cahalan and Cisin, 1968; Cahalan et al., 1969). They are less likely than white women to drink heavily for such psychological reasons as loneliness, lack of hope, and personal misfortunes, (Dawkins and Harper, 1983). Observers have noted the importance of religion for blacks generally and for black women especially pointing out "the close association [of black women] with the church as a source of strength and comfort from ... everyday stress and strain; religion ... provides clear and consistent values that conflict with substance abuse practices....Typically, the female is more apt to remain closely associated with church services and special [religious] functions as she grows older" (Shalom, Inc., 1983). Brisbane and Womble (1985) suggested that the strength of spiritual beliefs among black women may contribute to their lower rate of drinking. The recognition of spiritual power as a force greater than the self is congruent with the philosophy of Alcoholics Anonymous (AA), a powerful peer-related treatment method. One should add, however, that AA was initially organized by whites and is therefore not perceived as freely available to blacks, the philosophical parallels notwithstanding.

TREATMENT ISSUES

Treatment of alcohol abuse is difficult under optimal circumstances, but especially so for blacks. As noted earlier, a major impediment is the widespread reluctance among blacks to acknowledge that excessive drinking is not a normal pattern of living. Typically, neither the family nor the friends of an alcoholic encourage treatment, and neither gives much support to those who seek it. On the contrary, such people may be seen as deviants. Such denial or lack of awareness of a need for treatment means that those who finally do come for help tend to be in the late stages of the disorder and have a poorer prognosis as a result. Broadly successful intervention will require a shift in social attitudes away from the present acceptance of abusive drinking to recognition of it as a disorder in need of treatment.

No treatment system works unless the community is also involved. Brisbane and Womble emphasized the importance of such community involvement—the family, church, and local businesses. Bell (personal communication) has observed that the lack of recognition of alcohol abuse as a serious problem points to an absence of community definitions of behavior—what kind and how much drinking is acceptable and what is not? For this reason, there is a vital role for educational efforts that use the media, public service announcements, bill boards, posters, pamphlets, and newspaper articles to develop stronger social sanctions and minimal community standards limiting the use of alcohol. These same efforts can bring the black community to see that alcoholism is a primary disorder, not just a secondary symptom of racism. There is a great need to teach the dynamics of the addiction process, to talk about the importance of treatment and the ways it can be accomplished, and to involve the black alcoholics who might otherwise seek treatment but do not know how to get help. They do not know how to work the system. They do not know where the point of entry is or how to find it, and there is no one to show them. Consequently, some have suggested that points of ready access to the treatment system should be located where the black alcoholics are—i.e., in bars, barber shops, beauty parlors, jails, and pool halls—as well as in the churches and social service agencies (Peter Bell and Frances Brisbane, personal communication). Unless accessibility is substantially increased, particularly in the face of considerable cultural resistance, it is clear that many who need treatment will never get it. At this time, most of the black alcoholics who are referred to treatment come from the courts, where the crime-related nature of the referral is an additional problem. There are few referrals from family, friends, work places, or schools, where they ought to be coming from.

Blacks are much more reluctant to use treatment services. They have only limited trust in existing services, especially if these services are run by whites, as most are. There are few models of successful treatment, since most recovered black alcoholics do not go back to the communities from which they came.

An approach that appears to address some of these accessibility problems is the community Minority Alcoholism Program (MAP), described by Maypole and Anderson (1983). This model successfully combines ethnic values and minority participation with more traditional models of service delivery. The MAP, controlled by the minority group and physically located in the minority group neighborhood, provides a program of outreach, information and referral, community education, and counseling services that focus on the total family. Clients with severe problems are referred through them to the appropriate agencies. By serving as both the entrance and exit point for the system, the MAP maintains an ongoing relationship with the community, buffers the unwelcoming reception of the majority- culture service agency, and constructs a link between the client and the services he/she needs.

Effective intervention is also impeded by the lack of an adequate appreciation of cultural issues by those providing the treatment, whether they are black or white. Such an understanding is imperative.Treatment methods are not simply transferable from one culture to another; they must incorporate the relevant values of the minority culture. Without working knowledge of special cultural and social problems, service providers are likely to be ineffective and are quite likely to lose patients.

There is a great need for more and better treatment programs that are adequately funded, carefully designed, and run by culturally sophisticated professionals.

TRAINING CENTERS AND EDUCATIONAL PROGRAMS

Psychiatric training centers must put greater emphasis on providing mental health trainees with a thorough understanding of the impact of cultural values on behavior. Mental health professionals ought to have a good grasp of the cultures their patients live in and understand how culturally reinforced attitudes not only interfere with access to and utilization of treatment, but also limit therapeutic effectiveness when the minority patient does finally arrive for help.

Since 1982, The Menninger Foundation has cosponsored a succession of conferences on issues involving substance abuse and the black family. Involving a range of scholars, clinicians, and experienced laymen, these conferences have sought to provide students and practicing professionals with useful information and a sophisticated perspective. The effectiveness of this format suggests it may be useful as a model for other academic centers interested in imparting a bicultural perspective on treating substance abuse to trainees and practitioners.

There is a great need for educational programs to enhance the clinical effectiveness of those working with minorities throughout the country. The mental health professions share the responsibility for meeting that need.

REFERENCES

Bailey, M. B., Haberman, P. W., Alksne, H. The epidemiology of alcoholism in an urban residential area. Quarterly Journal of Studies on Alcohol 26- :19-40, 1965

Brisbane, F. L. Alcoholism and the black church presented at the "Action for a Better Community" conference, Rochester, N.Y., U.S.A.,. May 16, 1986, pg. 5

Brisbane, F. L., Womble, M.: After thoughts and recommendations, in Treatment of Black Alcoholics. Edited by Brisbane, F. L., Womble, M. New York; U.S.A., Haworth Press, 1985, p. 249-270

Cahalan, D., Cisin, I. H., Crossley, H. American Drinking practices: summary of findings from a national probability sample. Quarterly Journal of Studies on Alcohol 29(1):130-151, 1968

Cahalan, D., Cisin, I. H., Crossley, H.: American Drinking Practices. Rutgers Center for Alcohol Studies, monograph no. 6. New Brunswick, N.J., U.S.A., 1969

Dawkins, M. P., Farrell, W. C., Johnson, J. H.: Spatial patterns of alcohol outlets in the Washington, D.C., black community. Proceedings of the Pennsylvania Academy of Science 53:89-97, 1979

Dawkins, M. P., Harper, F. D.: Alcoholism among women: comparison of black and white problem drinkers. International Journal of Addictions 18:333-349, 1983

Donovan, J. M.: An etiologic model of alcoholism. American Journal of Psychiatry 143:1-11, 1986

King, L. J., Murphy, G. E. Robins, L. N., et al.: Alcohol abuse: a crucial factor in the social problems of Negro men. American Journal of Psychiatry 125:1682- 1690, 1969

Maypole, D. E., Anderson, R.: Minority alcoholism programs: issues in service delivery models. International Journal of Addictions 18:987-1001, 1983

Ng-A-Qui, M.: Drugs — problems for blacks. Texas Black Alcoholism Council Newsletter 1(1):1, 1984

Shalom, Inc.: Substance Abuse Prevention with Black Families - A Manual for Implementing an Epidemiological Approach. Harrisburg, Pa., U.S.A., Pennsylvania Department of Health, Division of Information Services, p. 17 1983

Sterne, M., Pittman, D. J.: Drinking patterns in the ghetto. St. Louis, Washington University, Social Science Institute, Mo., U.S.A., 1972

Williams, M.: Blacks and minority health. (1982), Blacks and alcoholism: issues in the 1980s, Alcohol Health and Research World 6(4):1331, 1985

SECTION V:

Training, Education and Service Delivery

Chapter 30

Problems in Psychiatry Services in Sub-Sahara African Countries

by

G. Mustafa, MD, MB, BS, DPM, FRCPsych
Chief Consultant Psychiatrist
Mathari Hospital
Nairobi, Kenya

ABSTRACT

Insufficient facilities, poor care, and lack of qualified staff are responsible for the inadequate treatment of many psychiatric patients in sub-Saharan countries. Psychiatric services received low priority for many decades, and it was long thought that psychiatric disorders were less prevalent in Africa than in developed countries. The problems confronting psychiatrists in Africa have included cultural factors affecting diagnosis, lack of trained personnel, centralization of services, isolation from other medical facilities, lack of organized rehabilitation programs, and discontinuity of care and responsibility. Services are now being decentralized and extended to the community, and the importance of the family and social context is being recognized in development in inpatient and rehabilitation services. Training programs for mental health workers are receiving increased attention, although there are still too few qualified personnel. Despite the many obstacles still remaining, however, the image of psychiatry in Africa has taken a more definite shape.

INTRODUCTION

In all sub-Saharan countries, thousands of psychiatric patients are treated inadequately as a result of insufficient facilities, poor care, and lack of qualified staff. To improve psychiatric care, these problems must be alleviated.

The main object of health planners is to provide means for meeting patients' needs and preventing disease. Psychiatrists in sub-Saharan countries trying to achieve these goals encounter many difficulties caused by a number of factors. Psychiatry was given low priority by health planners for a long time, and psychiatric services tended to take second place behind other branches of medicine. Attention was at first focused more on infections, parasitic, and other crippling organic diseases.

Besides, it was thought that the prevalence of psychological disorders was low compared to that in developed countries. Therefore, psychiatric disorders were not considered major medical problems and were given low priority.

Only in the last three decades have data revealed the true dimensions of psychiatric problems (Baasher, 1961; Boroffka, 1964; Diop, 1967; German, 1972; Giel and Van Luijk, 1969; Leighton et al., 1963). Psychiatrists in sub-Saharan countries have encountered the various psychiatric disorders seen in other parts of the world. None are particular to these other countries, although cultural factors may influence some external manifestations. Epidemiological studies have been done, but more organized studies are required.

SERVICE DEVELOPMENT

Establishing correct clinical diagnoses has been one of the problems confronting psychiatrists. Some psychiatric disorders may hide under various physical disguises. Depression, for example, may present with dominant psychophysical symptoms; crying, feelings of guilt, and self-reproach may not figure prominently in the clinical picture of depression in the African subject, whereas somatic complaints are extremely frequent. This difference in both thought content and expression of the illness can be regarded as a cultural coloring of the same disease. Such problems of diagnosis are, of course, overcome by experience and awareness of their existence. One of the major problems in the development of psychiatric services in sub-Saharan countries has been the gross lack of trained and skilled personnel. Not long ago many African psychiatrists had the unpleasant experience of being the one-man staff responsible for rendering psychiatric services to an entire country. The number of psychiatric personnel in many African countries has increased gradually but is far from being the number required for minimal care. The mammoth task of overcoming the problems in mental health services, which are handled by a handful of psychiatrists in each country, needs an exceptionally bold approach.

In many countries all the psychiatric services have been restricted to one large mental hospital, and there are no facilities for community services and no active work outside the hospital walls. The disadvantages of centralized services are obvious, but such systems are difficult to change. Rates of admission to these hospitals are influenced by economic factors and by the patients' distance from the hospitals. The urban population is growing not only because farmers and their families are attracted by the diversions, glamour, and services in the cities, but also because of the steady influx of traders and daily laborers. Young people leave their rural homes and come to the cities in search of education, jobs, and a better standard of living. The pressure on the psychiatric hospital's beds and outpatient centers, which are usually located in urban areas, is therefore always increasing. The services are still too limited and centralized. The obvious need is to establish adequate peripheral services.

During the sixties, small psychiatric units were built in many countries. These units faced a great deal of difficulty. The number of beds was inadequate, maintenance was neglected, sufficient qualified staff was not available, etc. It is hoped, however, that with more training programs, which will turn out more psychiatrists, psychiatric nurses, enrolled nurses, and psychiatric social workers, the manpower problem will ease gradually.

Developing a workable system to integrate psychiatric services with other medical facilities is difficult. Recent advances in psychopharmacology, the time-honored physical methods of treatment, the more effective psychotherapeutic techniques, and the progressive approaches to mental illness have positively affected the structure and organization of psychiatric services. For one thing, it is now possible to treat mental patients in open psychiatric wards of general hospitals. This is surely of great significance in countries where the image of mental illness has been colored by witchcraft and demons. Apart from having economic advantages allowing access to and the technical facilities of a general hospital, the psychiatric ward is a good medium for coordinating psychiatry with general medicine. Furthermore, it is a useful place for professional training and research.

In the countries where such wards exist, life for the psychiatric patients is easy, simple, and relaxed. No rigid restrictions are laid down. Indeed, patients are encouraged to conduct their lives as normally as possible. Since admission to these wards is voluntary, patients can leave the hospital at their convenience. The presence of relatives makes social relations easy. Accompanied by relatives, patients can visit their homes, movie theaters, and other public places. Psychiatrists have to seize every opportunity to break abnormal patterns of behavior in which patients have become fixed. Socialization of psychotic patients must start at the very beginning of treatment. Including psychiatric wards in general hospitals seems to be one of the best means for avoiding hospital dependency and preventing social withdrawal. Unfortunately, many countries lack such psychiatric wards. It seems as though certain health planners think of psychiatric services in terms of psychiatric hospitals and nothing else.

It is well known that the families in developing countries, especially in rural areas, are closely knit. In case of need or disease, much familial help and support is given. One good example is mental retardation, which is relatively common in many African countries. Most of the mentally retarded are absorbed into the community, and the family provides care and protection for them.

Unfortunately, providing the same comprehensive community care for psychiatric patients is not possible because of the lack of manpower and resources. Maintenance of therapy and follow-up, especially for chronic psychotic patients, are essential elements in treatment and rehabilitation. Relapses and chronicity are often the sequelae in cases where the follow-up system is poor or when there are social difficulties, poor communication, inadequate qualified personnel, or a lack of services for patients whose homes are far from psychiatric clinics and institutions. Social education, involvement of the family, and participation of general health workers would be of great help.

The focus of mental health has shifted from the psychiatric hospitals, usually remote and isolated, to the center of the community. Organized rehabilitation services for patients are lacking in many sub-Saharan countries. Since the social context varies from country to country, the success of rehabilitation services depends on originality, appropriate working conditions, and the right approach. The ultimate goal is to prevent permanent hospitalization of psychotic patients. This implies early, active treatment. A short stay in the hospital may be necessary for administration of physical treatments, drugs, or psychotherapy, but it should be followed as soon as possible by outpatient care to minimize the patient's absence from the family or usual social environment. Whenever possible, of course, the patient should be cared for at home and should continue to work.

Achievement of these aims implies an extensive range of treatment, rehabilitation, and inpatient and outpatient facilities, corresponding to all stages of the disease. Transfer from one environment to another, particularly from hospital to community, should be carefully supervised not only to avoid an excessive stay in the hospital, but also to prevent any abrupt change, which might threaten progress. To meet this need, continuity of care and responsibility is essential. Unfortunately, in most countries, this chain of outpatient services, along with the patient passes, is completely absent. There are no facilities for partial hospitalization (day hospitals). Occupational rehabilitation—e.g., industrial rehabilitation, sheltered workshops in the community, sheltered employment, and substitute homes—is totally absent. This means that care and rehabilitation can not be shifted effectively from hospital to the community. In other words, the patient remains cut off from his natural environment over long periods, as his life in the psychiatric hospital is under highly artificial conditions.

It is often difficult for the mental patient to make social contacts. Because of this, the relationship he develops with the psychiatric team while in the hospital should not be broken. The psychiatric team should have at its disposal treatment centers and joint facilities in the community, but at present they are lacking. Opportunities should be provided for the psychiatric team to establish contacts with members of the community—e.g., social workers, families, teachers, magistrates, general practitioners. Because of the lack of resources, chronic patients have usually been denied community services and have been confined to ill-equipped institutions without the prospect of active treatment.

FUTURE TRENDS

Despite the acute shortage of manpower, the difficulty of recruiting and training personnel, the inadequacy of medical facilities, the high cost of drugs and equipment, and the challenge of introducing new ideas and new techniques, the image of psychiatry has taken a more definite and clear shape.

Past experience is very illuminating. Preliminary exploration has shown the importance of the broader aspects of psychiatry. Most important is the shift of emphasis to the community and mobilization of social and cultural potential. Another pivotal development is the current stress on training programs for mental health workers. They will eventually reinforce the front line of psychiatric care and help cover peripheral areas.

The need for hospitalization of mentally ill patients will continue, and one type of psychiatric care should not be developed while another is neglected.

However, the future of extramural services does look brighter. Many times progress is made after the proper buildings are provided. Mental health workers, therefore, should go to the politicians, governments, authorities, and nongovernmental organizations and insist on proper surroundings for the treatment of psychiatric patients.

Finally, the inpatient setup should be a miniature of society as much as possible. With more imagination, better psychiatric models will be designed to meet the growing needs of the community. In our present era, opportunities for original work are plenty, and there are reasons to have hope for the future.

REFERENCES

Boroffka, A.: Psychiatrie en Nigeria. Zentralblatt fur Neurologie und Psychiatrie, 176:103-104, 1964

Diop, M.: La depression chez la noir african. Psychopathologie Africaine 3:183-194, 1967

German, G. A.: Aspects of clinical psychiatry in sub- Saharan Africa. British Journal of Psychiatry 121:461-479, 1972

Giel, R., Van Luijk, J. N.: Psychiatric morbidity in a small Ethiopian town, British Journal of Psychiatry 115:149-162, 1969

Leighton, A. M., Lambo, T. A., Hughes, C. C., et al.: Psychiatric Disorder Among the Yoruba, Ithaca, N.Y., U.S.A., Cornell University Press, 1963

Wood, J. F.: A half century of growth in Ugandan psychiatry, in Uganda Atlas of Disease Distribution. Edited by Hall and Langlands, Kampala, Uganda, , 1968

Chapter 31

Postgraduate Psychiatric Education in Africa

by

Ayo Binitie, MD(Lond) MRCPsych, FNMCPsych
Professor
Department of Mental Health
University of Benin
Benin City, Nigeria

ABSTRACT

The considerable prevalence of mental illness in Africa and the large numbers of patients seen by psychiatrists there argue for the training of more psychiatrists. Because organic psychiatric disorders are so common in Africa, a strong medical background is necessary; the existing African psychiatry training programs emphasize neurology, immunology, and virology. Classical psychotherapy, group psychotherapy, and child psychiatry are less prominent. Psychiatrists in Africa fill many roles, and training must also cover local culture, psychology, and sociology, but no African training program has yet recognized traditional healing. The author believes that the emphasis on the organic basis of psychiatry will continue and, as the population becomes more sophisticated, training in psychotherapy will probably receive more attention.

INTRODUCTION

When we think about postgraduate psychiatric education in the African context, we have to ask certain fundamental questions:

- Is this the time for training in psychiatry as a medical specialty?
- Why should we train psychiatrists in Africa?
- Is the community prepared to use the services of psychiatrists?
- What services does the community want from psychiatrists?
- Do psychiatrists provide what the community wants, or should we do more and educate the community?
- Finally, having decided on what psychiatrists do and what they ought to do, how do we train to meet these requirements?

An additional issue is the importance, in this day and age, of being able to communicate across national boundaries and to speak to an international audience. Graduates must, therefore, serve not only the local community, but the international community as well.

THE NEED FOR PSYCHIATRISTS

The prevalence of mental illness in Africa has been estimated in various epidemiological studies. Leighton et al. (1963) found a 15% prevalence in a rural area of Nigeria and a 19% prevalence in a Nigerian city. In my own study of rural Nigeria (1981), the prevalence was 35.7 per 1,000 population. Whichever figure is considered, it can be seen that there is considerable psychiatric morbidity. In the face of such large numbers of mentally ill persons, there is sufficient justification for training psychiatrists in Africa. However, it is one thing to determine that there is a need for service and quite another for people to come forward and use these services. Examples abound of facilities that have been provided in African communities but not used for one reason or another. This question is particularly relevant in the African setting, where alternative systems of care exist. Local communities appreciate services provided by traditional healers because the healers understand thoroughly the life of their people and can relate to and empathize with their patients. Therefore, it is possible that the role of psychiatrist is being more than adequately filled by local healers.

It is not easy to answer directly the question of whether additional psychiatric services would be used. There is, however, indirect evidence. Most African nations now have trained psychiatrists, who have formed an association for the exchange of information. Psychiatrists all over Africa report that they are very busy. They complain not about a lack of patients but, rather, about the lack of facilities to adequately treat the large numbers of patients under their care. There is evidence that more psychiatrists are needed to provide mental health services in African communities.

Organic psychiatric disorders are common and may account for anywhere from 10% to 40% of psychiatric disorders. The actual rates in Uselu Psychiatric Hospital during 1969 and 1970 were 18.7% and 20.8%, respectively. These figures do not include patients who went to the hospital for purely physical ailments; if these were included, the percentages would be higher still. These figures show that the practice of psychiatry in Africa should be firmly based in medicine and practitioners should know the fundamentals of general medicine.

Psychiatrists in Africa are usually found in large urban centers and frequently work in relative or total isolation. It is unusual to find six psychiatrists in any one center. Psychiatrists, therefore, must cover large distances to communicate with colleagues. Staying up to date is not easy either; journals are frequently not available in many places and more often than not arrive months after they have been mailed.

THE PHILOSOPHY OF PSYCHIATRIC EDUCATION

My survey showed that a psychiatrist working in Africa is required to act in a number of roles, such as clinician and medical practitioner, scientist, anthropologist, psychologist, sociologist-psychotherapist, interpreter of local culture, and most important, pharmacologist. The goal of psychiatric education should be to train a person to satisfy all these needs. We should aim to produce someone grounded in medicine and psychiatry who can understand local culture and has enough psychological and sociological background to understand many of the psychological problems in the community. He should be able to see his patient through both African and European eyes. He should have the capacity to look objectively at his clinical activity, scientifically record the findings, and explain his ideas to both the local and international communities.

So much for philosophy and theory. What actually exists? There is a training program in Egypt, one in East Africa, one in Nigeria, and one for English-speaking West Africa. Having served on both the Nigerian and West African boards, I know that the requirements of the two bodies are more or less the same. Moreover, the examiners are interchangeable.

DIFFERENCES BETWEEN TRADITIONAL AND AFRICAN TRAINING

The general requirements for training follow the traditional patterns. There are requirements for knowledge of anatomy, physiology, biochemistry, and pharmacology as it relates to the nervous system. In addition, the ability to understand local culture and local beliefs is also required. The traditional clinical subjects are also similar, but there is greater emphasis on neurology, immunology, and virology. There is also a medical component related to the most common medical disorders, especially hypertension and infectious and parasitic disorders, since the psychiatrist is frequently called on to treat and recognize common medical ailments, such as trypanosomial malaria and other gastrointestinal disorders.

On the other hand, classical psychotherapy and group psychotherapy are less prominent in the training program. Child psychiatry is a requirement but, on the whole, poorly taught. Probably this is due to a dearth of trained child psychiatrists among the teachers. Only a handful of the teachers specialize in child psychiatry. One area that training programs need to look into and incorporate is the broad area of traditional indigenous practices. No training program as yet recognizes the role of traditional medical practice in Africa. This failing is due to a lack of systematic knowledge about the subject. Teachers of psychiatry need to accumulate information and develop means of including much of this knowledge into training programs.

The trend for the future seems likely to be an emphasis on the organic basis of psychiatry, since organic psychiatric syndromes are so prevalent. It also seems likely that, as the population becomes sophisticated, a division for psychotherapy will emerge and that this area will be handled both by psychiatrists and by the related professions of psychology and the social sciences.

REFERENCES

Binitie, A.: Psychiatric disorders in a rural practice in the Bendel State of Nigeria. Acta Psychiatrica Scandinavia 64:273-280, 1981

Leighton, A.M., Lambo, T. A., Hughes, C. C., et al.: Psychiatric Disorder Among the Yoruba. Ithaca, N.Y., U.S.A., Cornell University Press, 1963

Chapter 32

Training of Mental Health Nurses in Kenya: Challenges and Problems

by

C. M. Mbugua,
Psychiatric Nurse,
Senior Nursing Officer,
Ministry of Health,
Nairobi, Kenya

ABSTRACT

After passage of the Nurses Act in 1949, many nursing schools were established in Kenya. The first nurses training were practical, or enrolled nurses, and they provided hospital nursing care. In 1952 the first program for training registered nurses began, and in 1966 programs for enrolled nurses began to focus on community nursing. Psychiatric nursing has been established slowly because of the lack of students, but 343 enrolled psychiatric nurses have been trained since 1977, and 174 registered psychiatric nurses have been produced since 1979. Shortage of qualified teaching staff, unavailability of suitable textbooks, and lack of equipment and teaching aids are continuing educational problems.

Registered psychiatric nurses, nonetheless, are equipped to provide patient care, supervise other nursing staff, and coordinate mental health services in hospitals, psychiatric units, and the community. General nursing programs are now covering mental health care, and Kenya has adopted mental health as one of the essential elements of primary health care.

As psychiatric care shifts to rural areas, appropriate training and retraining will be necessary. Also, with the present increase in psychosocial stresses in Kenya, counseling skills need to be further developed, but new programs are limited by the same problems that affect existing training.

HISTORICAL BACKGROUND

Psychiatric nursing—indeed, the mental health field—is a noble profession to be associated with. Before we look at the training of mental health nurses in Kenya, a quick look at the historical background of nursing education in Kenya will help bridge the gap between the past and present trends in mental health education. Although the early missionaries to Kenya established programs as early as the end of the nineteenth century, it was not until the beginning of this century that any form of nurse training was established.

In 1910, the Presbyterian Church of East Africa, then known as the Church of Scotland, started a nurse training school at Kikuyu Hospital, which is about 15 kilometers from Nairobi. This was soon followed by establishment of a school of nursing by the Roman Catholic Mission at Mathari, Nyeri, and another by the Anglican Church at Maseno in western Kenya. Around the same time, the government opened a school in Nairobi near the present site of the College of Health Professions.

In 1949, an act of Parliament provided for training of enrolled and registered nurses. This was the same year the Mental Treatment Act was passed. The Nurses Act was revised several times, and a new act took effect in 1982. The Mental Treatment Act has remained almost the same, however, although plans are under way to establish a new one.

With the passage of the Nurses Act, schools of nursing were established in most mission hospitals and in government institutions.

Initially, the nurses trained were practical nurses, or enrolled nurses, who are the second-level nurses in this country. Their main function at the time was hospital-based nursing care. In keeping with the changing needs of our society, a more comprehensive syllabus was introduced in 1966. The nurse graduating from the new program becomes an enrolled community nurse. On completion of her training, this nurse is well equipped for general nursing, midwifery, and community nursing. She is, however, still deficient in mental health nursing. All government institutions that used to train nurses at the enrolled level have not converted to enrolled community nursing training.

In 1952, the first registered nurses training in Kenya started at the present College of Health Professions. Later, the school began offering postgraduate courses, which currently include midwifery, community nursing, intensive care nursing, and surgical nursing.

EVOLUTION OF TRAINING PROGRAMS FOR PSYCHIATRIC NURSES

Although Mathari Hospital opened in 1910, the nursing care of patients was left in the hands of unskilled patient attendants supervised by a few foreign nurses. The care was mainly custodial. The first formal training of psychiatric nurses in Kenya was in 1962, when enrolled nurses were recruited to join a 1-year postbasic course leading to a certificate in enrolled mental health nursing. Because of a shortage of enrolled nurses, this program was discontinued in 1965. In 1964, a 3-year basic training program for enrolled psychiatric nursing was established. This course continued until 1978, when it was discontinued in favor of the 1-year postbasic enrolled psychiatric nursing course, which had been reintroduced in 1977. Since psychiatric nurses receive no special privileges, recruitment tends to be slow.

The enrolled psychiatric nurse is a very useful member of the psychiatric team. Before we produced enough registered psychiatric nurses, the enrolled psychiatric nurses manned the psychiatric units around the country, and it is no secret that they were the managers and mental health consultants in those units. Since 1977, we have trained 343 enrolled psychiatric nurses. With this increase in numbers, the deployment pattern has changed greatly. These nurses can now be seen in most nursing situations, including general hospitals and the health centers.

In 1979, a 1-year postbasic course in registered psychiatric nursing began at the Mathari Hospital School of Nursing. Before that, all registered psychiatric nurses had received their training outside Kenya. Although this program was implemented with enthusiasm and dedication, it has met with several difficulties, mainly shortages of students and qualified teaching staff, unavailability of suitable textbooks (Kenya does not publish psychiatric nursing textbooks), and lack of equipment. The program, however, continues to produce high-caliber psychiatric nurses.

The course offers a variety of experiences, so the psychiatric nurses who graduate are suited to coordinate psychiatric nursing activities wherever they are posted. The training offers a variety of theoretical and practical experiences, e.g., study of human behavior and interpersonal relationships, psychiatry, sociology, and mental health nursing. Besides their day-to-day work with the mentally sick, these nursing students research psychosocial problems affecting the community. The training also encourages thinking positive about professional psychiatric nursing activities and fosters development of capable, unique, and responsible individuals.

Continuous self-evaluation makes it easier for students to understand their patients' needs and, therefore, plan appropriate care. Upon graduation, the registered psychiatric nurse is expected to be deeply involved in patient care and coordination of mental health services at the hospital, ward, unit, and community levels. She has the ultimate responsibility for supervising other nursing staff in a given clinical setting. She, therefore, has to be well prepared and skilled in handling the various problems encountered in day-to-day work. Since 1979, Kenya has produced 174 registered psychiatric nurses, who are employed in psychiatric hospitals, psychiatric units, schools of nursing, and general hospitals.

INVOLVEMENT OF NURSES IN MENTAL HEALTH CARE

The advanced nursing program at the University of Nairobi includes psychiatry and mental health nursing in its curriculum.

This gives mental health experience to all the nurses in that program.

As early as 1974, the Kenyatta National Hospital School of Nursing at the Medical Training Centre saw the need to expose all nurses to mental health care. All students undergoing general nursing training pass through Mathari Hospital, where they hear lectures on psychiatric nursing and spend time with mentally ill patients in the clinical areas.

The Nursing Council's requirements for enrolled community nurses also include some experience in mental health care. Although the exposure to mental illness is rather brief (8 weeks), the knowledge gained is invaluable because nurses work in strategic positions in the community, where promotion of mental health and prevention of mental illness begin. Mental health experience is also offered in the postbasic community health nursing course.

CHALLENGES AND PROBLEMS

A few years ago, mental health workers, including psychiatric nurses, were regarded as odd by the community and, surprisingly, some other health professionals. Even mentioning that you worked at Mathari Hospital cast doubt in people's minds. These negative attitudes toward the mentally ill and mental health workers are gradually changing, and communities have started to recognize the value of mental health workers.

Since Kenya has adopted mental health as one of the essential elements of primary health care, there is hope that mental health activities will be much more tolerated than in the past. If mental health is discussed along with such issues as immunization, family planning, water, environmental sanitation, etc., the community is likely to give it more support than in the past. There is also likely to be an increase in nursing students.

The inclusion of mental health in primary health care calls for a shift from the present hospital- based psychiatric care to community-based care. In keeping with the changing needs of society and government policy on rural development, it is inevitable that the current psychiatric nursing programs will need to be revised to reflect this shift in emphasis. At the same time, it may be necessary to develop an entirely new syllabus for providing retraining in community mental health to the psychiatric nurses already working in the field. However, qualified trainers for this extra program are lacking. We are already experiencing difficulties in procuring textbooks and manuals, getting adequate transportation, and hiring personnel, and it seems likely that the situation would only be worse if a new course is introduced. Nevertheless, if we produce community psychiatric nurses, they would operate in the community, give mental health education, strengthen the follow-up of discharged psychiatric patients, and ensure consistency and continuity of care.

To cope with the increased psychosocial stresses that our society is exposed to, psychiatric nurses also need to further develop their counseling skills. Kenya has no facility for courses in such specialized subjects such as psychotherapy, crisis intervention, and family therapy. We need to establish short-term courses in these areas. This involves either engaging a few nurses in established programs to take on extra training or obtaining a trainer from another country who would teach a core group of trainers. Both alternatives are expensive. But if nurses have to be developed in this area, the long- term benefits would be invaluable.

Obtaining training materials for teaching psychiatric nursing is a constant source of frustration.We would like to publish psychiatric nursing manuals and textbooks, but funding is not available. There is also a need for films and facilities for producing our own slides of local subjects. Currently, we borrow films from drug companies and embassies, but we cannot always get the types of films we want.

Chapter 33

The Role of Voluntary Agencies in the Development of Mental Health Programs in Kenya

by

Lawrence E. Banta, MD
School of Medicine,
Department of Psychiatry,
Creighton University,
Omaha, Nebraska, U.S.A.

ABSTRACT

Christian institutions and other voluntary agencies have always played a major role in effective health care systems in Kenya. The major thrust of health care in developing countries has so far been primary care, and mental illness and psychosocial issues are often overlooked. Cultural changes and natural disasters have increased the vulnerability to mental illness in rural areas of Kenya, and mental health needs should become an integral part of primary health care. The author states that the ultimate objective of a cooperative program by government and voluntary agencies should be a model rural mental health center, which would provide care, train personnel, and send mobile teams into bush areas. More mental health technicians are needed and should be trained by transcultural or local psychiatrists. Voluntary agencies could help conduct field studies, recruit personnel, promote awareness of mental illness among professionals and in the community, and develop mobile mental health clinics. Mental illness is still avoided in Kenya, and cooperative ventures might increase awareness of treatment and rehabilitation possibilities and bring effective, humane care to the thousands of mentally ill persons there.

HISTORICAL BACKGROUND

Since early in the history of health care programs in Kenya and other developing countries, Christian institutions and other voluntary agencies have played a major role in the development of effective health care systems. Initially, that role was to relieve the immense suffering in areas of high disease prevalence. Particular diseases, such as tuberculosis and leprosy, have also been the subject of intense work. The involvement of voluntary agencies in the research, treatment, and control of these diseases has been of tremendous benefit.

Currently, the major thrust of those involved in health care in the developing countries is primary health care. This concept emphasizes public health practices, including nutrition, education, and immunization. This is coupled with the treatment of the major diseases in particular areas, control of epidemics, provision of clean water, and, in general, promotion of a better standard of living.

MENTAL HEALTH CARE PROBLEMS

In the process of promoting good health, some problems may be inadvertently overlooked. Certain problems do not often come to the attention of a primary health center for a variety of reasons. Examples are physical disabilities, mental illness, deformities, and ostracism. In my experience, the entire community often feels that such a case is hopeless. Often this is true, as the primary health centers generally have no facilities for rehabilitation.

In India and Africa, elders in the tribal community can relate story after story of severely mentally ill persons who wander from village to village pursued by spirits that no shaman can banish. Some inadvertently kill themselves, some die of malnutrition or disease, some commit suicide, but very few of the severely ill live long lives.

Much about mental illness is shrouded in mystery even in our sophisticated Western culture, but it may be more so in animistic cultures. The mentally ill are less likely to come to a primary health center or hospital than the physically ill. However, many are seen for physical illness, and the mental disturbance is missed.

In discussions with mission agencies and hospital staff, a general lack of awareness of mental illness is consistently seen. As the mentally ill often remain hidden from the clinic, their actual needs are very difficult to see.

During my own 20-month stay in Kenya, I lived in rural villages and was able to see the impact of mental illness. With the encroachment of westernization into these more rural areas, there has been less tolerance of deviant behavior and some increase in psychophysiologic and affective disorders. In many areas, the trauma of war has disrupted traditional cultural standards and practices.

Famine has destroyed self-respect. The frequency of death due to illness or natural disasters has further increased the vulnerability of these areas to mental illness.

Thus, mental illness is already a problem in many areas. In many other areas it is not quite so visible, yet risk factors for its development are clearly obvious. We need to formulate ways to cooperatively develop an effective program for the identification, prevention, and treatment of mental disorders. Clearly, mental health care needs to be an integral part of primary health care.

COOPERATIVE PROGRAM APPROACHES

There are many ways in which a cooperative program could be developed. Of course, the primary issue would be the willingness to work together and take advantage of the resources each party has to offer. Voluntary agencies are generally able to recruit and retain well-trained motivated personnel. They can also often obtain funding.

The eventual objective would be the development of a model rural mental health center, perhaps in association with a mission hospital. This could be used to train personnel to work with the mentally ill. Mobile teams that would travel into bush areas and provide screen and treatment could be developed gradually.

In a World Health Organization (WHO) collaborative study (Murthy and Wig, 1983), it was shown that village mental health workers in India were effective in reaching out into underserved areas and providing quality mental health care. Kenya is training mental health technicians, but many more are needed. Transcultural psychiatrists are also needed to train the technicians. Very few Western psychiatrists have the training or experience necessary for effectively training local workers.

REQUIREMENTS FOR COOPERATIVE VENTURES

Currently, the following seem to be the major needs of cooperative ventures:

- More awareness of mental health problems by churches and voluntary agencies.
- Cooperation between government and voluntary agencies in developing a rural mental health center pilot program.
- Cooperative field studies using existing primary health centers.
- Recruitment of local individuals by churches, etc., to be trained as mental health technicians. Many of those involved in pastor training or primary health care training might be willing and able to work as mental health technicians.
- Adequate exposure of primary health care workers to mental illness to improve recognition, referral, and treatment.
- Recruitment by voluntary agencies of trained mental health professionals to work in mission hospitals and elsewhere to promote awareness of mental illness,

provide training, and develop programs to reach out to rural areas.

- Work with local religious leaders, village elders, and other community leaders to promote awareness of mental illness and the possibilities of treatment.
- Mobile clinics staffed by mental health technicians for evaluating and providing ongoing treatment to the mentally ill in particular areas. A physical therapist and a mental health technician could also work with a nurse or other professional to provide services to the physically disabled.
- Training of physicians in the diagnosis and treatment of mental disorder.

Mental illness is one of the many major problems confronting the developing world. Even within the developed countries mental health care has not been adequate. Major advances have been made in the identification and treatment of various disorders. Some of these treatments can be easily transported and used in developing countries. In previous times, leprosy and tuberculosis were largely avoided because they had no cures. Today, mental illness is still viewed in the same light. Because of effective treatment programs, rehabilitation centers, and cooperative ventures in many countries, the battle against leprosy is gradually gaining ground. Such cooperative ventures might provide humane care for the thousands in Kenya who suffer silently and often needlessly from chronic debilitating mental illness.

The purpose of this paper is not to suggest a better way to manage mental health problems, but to suggest a meaningful way in which more resources might be developed and used effectively to reach more of those who are suffering. We need a unified front and a cooperative attitude to accomplish more.

REFERENCES

Murthy, R. S., Wig, N. N.: The WHO collaborative study on strategies for extending mental health care, IV: a training approach to enhancing the availability of mental health manpower in a developing country. American Journal of Psychiatry 140:1486-1490, 1983

Chapter 34

Community Mental Health Services in Nairobi, Kenya

by

M. M. O. Okonji, MD
Nairobi, Kenya

ABSTRACT

Until recently, mental health services in Nairobi, Kenya, were predominantly institution-based and involved virtually no community follow-up or rehabilitation. In 1984 the Department of Community Mental Health was established. It is staffed by a multidisciplinary team and concentrates its efforts on the most economically and socially disadvantaged part of Nairobi. The department is engaged in five specific programs:

- Mental health education
- Domiciliary visit

- Strengthening of mental health components in primary health care
- Identification of community resources
- Training of students and village health workers

Among the future activities planned by the Department of Community Health are epidemiological studies, establishment of a day hospital, and establishment of more psychiatric clinics in primary health centers.

INTRODUCTION

As in the rest of Kenya, mental health services of Nairobi have been predominantly institution-based. The two institutions that provide most of the psychiatric care for the residents of Nairobi are Mathari Mental Hospital, with an average of 800 inpatients, and the psychiatric outpatient clinic at Kenyatta National Hospital. The former admits patients with major psychoses, whereas the latter caters to patients with less severe disorders, mainly psychoneuroses and affective disorders. The few patients who can afford it obtain private psychiatric treatment in private clinics and hospitals.

Until recently, there has been virtually no community follow-up of patients seen in the above institutions. Furthermore, the various community resources potentially available for patients have never been identified. When identified, they could be used to improve mental health or to support and rehabilitate mentally ill patients.

The Nairobi City Commission health centers, which are the primary health care units for the majority of city residents, do not provide any mental health care and do not stock basic psychotropic drugs. The implied policy is that provision of mental health services is the responsibility of Mathari Mental Hospital.

DEPARTMENT OF COMMUNITY MENTAL HEALTH

Because of the dissatisfaction with these institution- based services, the Department of Community Mental Health was formed in

October 1984. The overall objective of the department was to initiate community- based mental health services for Nairobi. The department currently comprises:

- One consultant-psychiatrist as coordinator
- One psychiatric registrar on a 3-month rotation basis
- Two Kenyan registered community nurses
- One enrolled (practical) community nurse
- Two psychiatric social workers
- One occupational therapist
- One clinical psychologist

In practice, the roles of the members of the department overlap. The department's catchment area is the area covered by the Nairobi City Commission. The population is slightly over 1,000,000. However, because of limited resources, the Department of Community Mental Health has concentrated on the eastern half of Nairobi, which has a population of 600,000. This area is the most economically and socially disadvantaged part of the city. Most of the slums are in this area. The rate of unemployment is highest here. Those employed work as laborers in industries or are self-employed as hawkers, tinkers, welders, etc. The area is also known for brewing and distilling illicit types of liquor, locally known as Chang'aa. Alcohol and drug abuse are rampant. There are, however, also a few middle-class residential neighborhoods.

The primary health facilities in this area are seven dispensaries, seven health centers, 19 maternal and child health clinics, and four maternity units. The primary health workers employed in the primary health facilities are 13 physicians, 34 clinical officers, 26 Kenyan registered nurses, 221 enrolled nurses, and 30 social workers.

SPECIFIC PROGRAMS

Mental Health Education

Members of the team devote part of their time to mental health education. It is hoped this will improve community knowledge about mental health and change negative attitudes toward mental illness. Health education is directed at the following groups:

- Chiefs, party leaders
- Patients and relatives waiting at primary health facilities
- Patients and relatives seen during home visits

Village health committee members and village health workers in collaboration with the Department of Health Education of the Ministry of Health are in the process of producing appropriate visual aids and charts for mental health education.

Domiciliary Visits

Members of the department visit an average of 300 homes every month. The many reasons for domiciliary visits include:

- information gathering
- getting to know family dynamics and family support
- providing mental health education
- advising families on services available in the community
- supervising patients who receive long-term medication

Strengthening Mental Health Aspects of Primary Health Care

Our objective is to strengthen the mental health component in the Nairobi City Commission health centers. For example, a multidisciplinary psychiatric clinic was established at the Kariobangi Health Center in March 1985. The patients are referred to the clinic by medical officers, clinical officers, social workers, and traditional healers. Health Center staff and the multidisciplinary psychiatric team meet regularly.

We hope that, by including psychiatric care at the primary health care unit, we shall increase recognition of mental health problems presenting in this setting and teach general health workers to manage them or make referrals to specialize personnel if necessary.

Identification of Community Resources

Mental health, like general health, is very much affected by multiple factors now directly under the control of the Ministry of Health. Mental health services should not only be integrated into the general health care system, but should also be linked to the social support services provided by sectors not directly concerned with health matters.

We are conducting a survey to identify all governmental and nongovernmental organizations operating in the catchment area. This will enable us to compile a directory of the organizations and services they offer. Furthermore, the department intends to hold regular meetings for representatives of these various organizations to discuss areas of cooperation. One such meeting was held and was attended by 50 participants representing 20 organizations.

Training

We have participated in the community mental health training of members of village health committees, village health workers, and several groups of students—i.e., in the third year postgraduate of psychiatry, postenrolled mental health nursing, and postregistered mental health nursing. Also, the Undugu Society and the Redeemed Gospel Church have begun training village health workers in the slums of our catchment area. So far, we have taken part in training 60 village health workers.

PROBLEMS

Some of the many problems the Department of Community Health has encountered are lack of transportation, lack of drugs, lack of mental health knowledge among the general health workers, and lack of appropriate occupations for discharged patients.

FUTURE ACTIVITIES

Among the many future activities we plan to undertake are:

- Conducting community epidemiological studies
- Providing in-service mental health training for general health workers
- Establishing three psychiatric clinics at other strategically placed health centers
- Establishing a day hospital

Chapter 35

Providing Mental Health Services with Meager Resources in Tanzania

by

G. Bugaisa, TRN, RMN (UK), CPN (UK)
and
N.L. Rugeiyamu, TRN, RMN (UK)
Muhimbili Medical Centre
Dar es Salaam, Tanzania

ABSTRACT

Between the 1890s and 1960, when Tanganyika (now Tanzania) attained independence, psychiatric services were centralized and provided through hospitals. Since 1961, local personnel have been trained and psychiatric care has become less centralized. Psychiatric units have been established in seven regional hospitals and are complemented by regional and district mental health centers, rehabilitation villages, home visits, and seminars for general health care workers. In the 1970s Tanzania launched the National Mental Health Program to extend mental health services to the village level and integrate them into general medical services. In 1980 the World Health Organization and the Danish International Development Agency agreed to provide technical and financial assistance. Psychiatric services in the Dar es Salaam region are described to illustrate mental health care nationwide, and the role of traditional and spiritual healers is discussed.

HISTORICAL OVERVIEW

In Tanzania, as in many other developing countries, mental illness was regarded in the early days as a curse, hence incurable or untreatable. Relatives, friends, and others tended to fear and reject mental patients. As a result, no efforts were made to provide any degree of psychiatric care. Instead, people resorted to witchcraft and traditional healers, who were believed to have supernatural powers to drive away curses or ghosts. In the event that such patients were not cured, they were in most cases abandoned, rejected, or expelled from their immediate communities.

However, after the 1880s, concrete steps were taken to provide psychiatric services for mental patients in Tanzania. These steps were initiated by foreigners, particularly Christian missionaries and, later, colonial rulers, such as the Germans and British. Early psychiatric services were centralized in other mental hospitals or specific institutions.

In the late 1890s, when Tanzania (then Tanganyika) was under German rule, Lutheran missionaries converted a small institution of about 50 beds (originally a home for slave orphans) into a mental hospital. This small mental hospital was situated at a beautiful place called Lutindi in the Korogwe District in the Usambara Mountains. The Lutindi Mental Hospital was a forerunner of psychiatric services in Tanzania and has continued to provide psychiatric services under Lutheran missionaries until today. It now accommodates up to about 200 patients and has improved services and mental rehabilitation programs for people in the immediate area (see Figure 1).

Figure 1
LOCATIONS OF PSYCHIATRIC SERVICES IN TANZANIA.

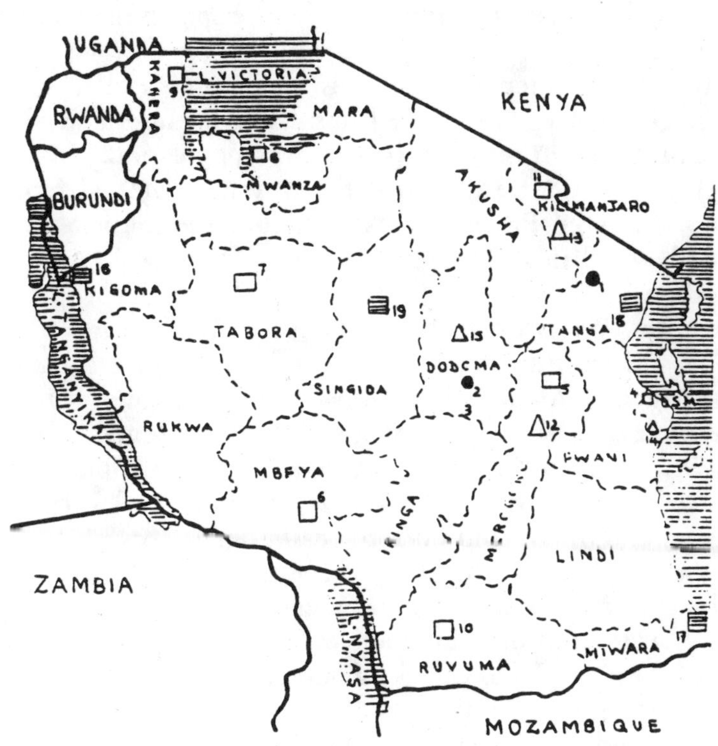

KEY:

PSYCHIATRIC INSTITUTIONS
1. Lutindi
2. Mirembe
3. Broadmoor

COMMUNITY PSYCH. SERVICE
12. Meregere Zone
13. Kilimanjaro Zone
14. Dar-el-Salaam Zone
15. Dodoma Zone

PSYCH. SERVICES WITHOUT UNIT
16. Kigoma
17. Mtwara
18. Tanga
19. Singida

PSYCHIATRIC UNITS
4. Dar-es-Salaam
5. Meregere
6. Mbeya
7. Tabora
8. Mwanza
9. Buboka
10. Songeli
11. Moshi

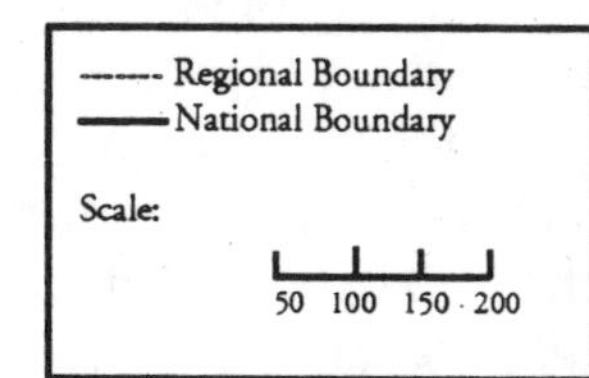

Located more or less on the northern periphery of the country, the Lutindi Mental Hospital was not easily accessible to most people from the southern, central, eastern, and western parts of Tanzania. The vast distances to Lutindi discouraged most people. Hence, the Lutindi Mental Hospital primarily served people in the northern part of the country.

In the 1920s, when Tanzania was under British rule, the Lutindi Mental Hospital was considered unsuitable because it was located a great distance from most of the country's population. In 1925, the British government established the Mirembe Mental Hospital at Dodoma, Central Province, which attained the status of a national mental hospital in 1927 and 1928. The Mirembe Mental Hospital was progressively developed and expanded in order to provide full psychiatric services for the entire country. In the early 1970s, this hospital was accommodating up to 2,000 civilian mental patients.

The Mirembe Mental Hospital had the advantage of being located more or less in the center of the country. Hence, it was more accessible than Lutindi and could serve more people. However, because of the country's great size, distance and varying tribal behaviors and beliefs continued to be limiting factors.

In the early 1950s, the government also recognized the need for psychiatric services for criminal mental patients. So in 1951 an institution to provide these services was established near Mirembe Mental Hospital. It was called Broadmoor Institution. At that time, it could accommodate about 300 patients. Since then it has been expanded, and now it can accommodate over 600 criminal patients.

DEVELOPMENT OF SERVICES

For about 70 years, between the 1890s and 1960, when Tanganyika (Tanzania) attained independence, psychiatric services were provided on a centralized basis through large institutions, as already outlined. This arrangement also helped make individual patients and the population in general aware that mental illness is common and is curable or treatable, like many other diseases. By 1960, the demand for psychiatric services had grown so great that the three existing institutions were inadequate, and the limitations of distance and varying environmental factors were still evident. For instance, the Mirembe Mental Hospital, with 800 beds, was accommodating over 1,600 patients by 1962.

Because of the growing demand for psychiatric services and the limitations of the existing facilities, the newly independent Tanganyikan government, in spite of its limited resources, decided to address the urgent need to extend psychiatric services on a much broader scale. Therefore, in subsequent government programs from 1961 to the present, development, expansion, and decentralization of psychiatric services have been featured substantially in medical services. In spite of the meager resources, particularly financial, the government has taken tangible steps to train specialized personnel in the psychiatric field and to establish psychiatric units in regional hospitals, regional and district mental health centers, and rehabilitation villages and community psychiatric services at the district and village levels.

TRAINING

At the time of independence, in 1961, there were no qualified local psychiatric personnel in the country. Hence, for the government to implement its program of developing, expanding, and decentralizing psychiatric services to eventually cover the entire country, it was imperative to train local personnel. There were no local training institutions in the country, and the situation was further aggravated by limited financial resources. The government secured technical financial assistance from the British government for training local personnel in Great Britain. Between 1961 and 1970, medical and nursing personnel underwent intensive training in Great Britain. By 1970, three psychiatrists and 13 psychiatric nurses had qualified and started working in psychiatric institutions and units. This group was the nucleus of the future development and expansion of psychiatric services in Tanzania.

The training of psychiatric personnel has since continued both overseas and locally. Training schools for nurses have been established at Dar es Salaam and Dodoma. These schools are turning out 40 to 50 nurses every year. Also, psychiatric orientation courses are given by the psychiatry department of Muhimbili Medical Centre to students and workers at all levels.

REGIONAL PSYCHIATRIC UNITS

With the increased availability of qualified local psychiatric personnel in the country, the government embarked on a program to decentralize the psychiatric services of the Mirembe Mental Hospital. The decentralization program was aimed at taking the services closer to the communities, thus minimizing the distances traveled by patients and eliminating tribal differences. At the same time, it reduced the congestion at the Mirembe Mental Hospital.

Between 1965 and the late 1970s, psychiatric units were established in the regional hospitals at Dar es Salaam, Tabora, Mwanza, Mbeya, Morogoro, Moshi, Bukoba, and Songea. With the exception of the Dar es Salaam unit at the Muhimbili Medical Centre, which is also a teaching unit for the Faculty of Medicine, each of these units is manned by about 10 locally trained medical and nursing personnel and several junior workers. On the average, each unit has the capacity to treat about 50 inpatients and an unlimited number of outpatients.

The services provided by the regional psychiatric units are complemented by mental health centers and rehabilitation villages. In these centers and villages, patients are treated and rehabilitated through training in occupational skills and preparation for normal lives in their communities.

The establishment of regional psychiatric units helped achieve the national objective of increasing the population's access to psychiatric services. This stage, however, mostly benefitted those who lived in urban centers and adjacent areas. Because of the great distances from rural areas to regional hospitals, it fell short of achieving the ultimate objective of reaching the entire population, down to the village level.

NATIONAL HEALTH PROGRAM

To facilitate the development of psychiatric services and their extension to the entire population, Tanzania joined the African Mental Health Action Group in 1970. This was in response to World Health Assembly resolution 30.45, which called on developing countries to launch national mental health programs aimed at providing and improving such services in their respective countries.

Hence, in the 1970s, Tanzania launched a national mental health program to extend psychiatric services from the regional to the village level by the year 2000. However, financial constraints delayed the implementation of this program until the late 1970s, when technical and financial assistance was secured. In 1980 the World Health Organization (WHO) and the Danish International Development Agency (DANIDA) agreed to provide technical and financial assistance for this program. A three-phased joint implementation plan was agreed on by the Ministry of Health, WHO, and DANIDA.

PHASE I, to be implemented over 3 years, involved the following:

- Training of mental health workers
- Developing relevant curricula and producing appropriate manuals and other teaching materials
- Formulating the necessary administrative mechanisms
- Implementing at least one regional mental health care model in one selected region
- Setting up regional mental health coordinating committees and a national mental health coordinating group
- Creating a mental health resources center and setting in operation its consultative and training components
- Conducting an evaluation study of program development at the end of the 3-year period to assess progress, identify problems, and propose appropriate adjustments in the program.

PHASE II was also designed to be implemented over 3 years. It involved opening mental health centers at the regional and district levels. As part of this phase, the country was divided into four geographical zones:

- Zone1— Dar es Salaam, Coast, Lindi, and Tanga
- Zone 2 — Morogoro, Mbeya, Iringa, Rukwa, and Ruvuma
- Zone 3 — Dodoma, Singida, Tabora, Shinyanga, and Kigoma

- Zone 4 — Kilimanjaro, Arusha, Mara, Mwanza, and Kagera

The proposed deadline for PHASE III is the year 2000. Its goals are the establishment of mental health centers covering the whole country, from the regional down to district and village levels, and the integration of mental health services into other medical services.

Community Psychiatric Services

In pursuit of the ultimate objective of taking psychiatric services as close as possible to the people and to ensure as much psychiatric care and follow-up care as possible, a program to develop community psychiatric services has been initiated to complement the mental health centers. Community psychiatric services will aim to:

- establish mental health clinics at every possible place close to the communities
- set up more rehabilitation villages
- provide domiciliary services
- disseminate mental health information to the general public through publications, posters, radio broadcasts, seminars, and workshops.

To date, community psychiatric services have been started in eight regions—Dar es Salaam, Morogoro, Dodoma, Kigoma, Mtwara, Tanga, Kilimanjaro, and Singida. In these regions, community services have been extended from the regional level to the district level and, in some cases, such as Morogoro, to the village level.

Considering the prevailing conditions and limitations, particularly in financial and human resources, the development of psychiatric services in the country at present can be considered satisfactory. Eleven psychiatric institutions or units have been established in 10 regions, covering 55% of the country. Community psychiatric services have been established in eight regions at the district level and, in some of them, at the village level. This represents about 40% coverage of the country. Rehabilitation villages have been established in four regions, which is about 20% coverage of the country.

PSYCHIATRIC SERVICES IN THE DAR ES SALAAM REGION

The preceding sections summarize the historical development of psychiatric services in Tanzania, the current objectives, plans, and methods for further development of psychiatric services in the country, and the stages reached so far. Here we wish to describe in detail, as a case study, the status of psychiatric services in the Dar es Salaam region, where we have worked for over 10 years.

In 1965, a psychiatric unit was established in Dar es Salaam at the then Muhimbili Hospital to provide psychiatric services in the eastern region. This region has since been divided into the three regions of Dar es Salaam, Coast, and Morogoro. At that time the unit had 50 beds for inpatients and was divided into three wards for males, females, and grade I care. It was staffed by one foreign psychiatrist and the following local personnel: one assistant medical officer with psychiatric experience, three trained psychiatric nurses, and three trained nurses and several nursing auxiliaries. Besides the usual psychiatric treatments for both inpatients and outpatients, the unit had other sections, such as occupational therapy, EEG, and the psychiatric social workers' sections. The unit also ran a rehabilitation village at Mwera, about 30 kilometers away.

In 1977, the Muhimbili Hospital incorporated the Faculty of Medicine of the University of Dar es Salaam. The psychiatric unit was converted into a distinctly specialized department of psychiatry. Between 1977 and 1980, the unit was expanded. A ward for acute psychiatric patients was added, and three research sections, a community mental health nursing unit, and a laboratory were started. The Department of Psychiatry also offered orientation courses of psychiatry for medical and nursing students from the Faculty of Medicine and the nursing school. These orientation courses were also offered to medical staff from regional and district hospitals.

During this period, the Department of Psychiatry secured technical and financial assistance from DANIDA through the Ministry of Health. This assistance, which still continues, enables psychiatric staff to receive overseas training and upgrading and provides vehicles, equipment, materials, drugs, etc. DANIDA's assistance has been supplemented by assistance from WHO and countries other than

Denmark, such as Holland. Because of the expanded services, the department is currently staffed by five psychiatrists, one psychologist, nine psychiatric nurses, seven trained nurses, five psychiatric social workers, two psychiatric community nurses, and 28 nursing aides.

With the establishment of mental health and rehabilitation centers, the unit is now treating about 50 inpatients and 350 outpatients monthly. The main methods of treatment applied are group, relaxation, behavior, drug, and occupational therapy.

Between 1982 and 1983, the Department of Psychiatry at Muhimbili Medical Centre requested the Dar es Salaam city council to establish community psychiatric services in the district hospitals in order to decentralize the services and bring them closer to the communities, provide follow-up services to patients discharged from the Muhimbili psychiatric unit, and educate the communities in mental illness and involve them in the care of their patients. The city council agreed to the proposal and in 1983 started a 3-month orientation course for district health workers at the psychiatric unit at Muhimbili Medical Center. The first group trained under this program comprised of six nurses from the district hospitals. In 1984, these trained health workers helped to establish mental health centers in the district hospitals of Ilala, Temeke, and Kinodoni.

The Ilala Center has a catchment area with a 15- kilometer radius. It serves approximately 250 patients, of whom 60% receive oral medication and 40% receive injections of fluphenazine decanoate.

The catchment area of the Temeke Mental Health Center has a radius of over 20 kilometers. Because of its great size, a subcenter has been established at Kigamboni. The Temeke Center has an attendance of about 320 patients, of whom approximately 60% take oral medication and 40% receive fluphenazine injections.

The Kinondoni Mental Health Center has a catchment area with a radius of over 30 kilometers, and a subcenter has been established in Magomeni. It serves approximately 215 patients, of whom about 70% take oral medication and 30% receive fluphenazine injections.

Each mental health center is staffed by two community psychiatric nurses who have taken the orientation course at the Muhimbili psychiatric unit. However, the centers receive supervision and consultation from the Department of Psychiatry at Muhimbili Medical Center, where a team of three psychiatrists, three psychiatric social workers, and two psychiatric community nurses are assigned to assist these mental health centers.

Rehabilitation Villages

In its continuing efforts to promote regional psychiatric services, the psychiatry department has established two rehabilitation villages in the region. They were established to help patients live normal lives in their communities. Hence, in these villages, the patients are trained in such skills as farming, animal husbandry, carpentry, and sewing.

The Mwera Rehabilitation Village was started in 1960. It has accommodations and other facilities for 30 patients. It is run by a psychiatrist, one trained nurse, and four nursing aides. The major activities in the village include farming and raising poultry. The village currently maintains 500 chickens, assorted vegetable gardens, orange trees, and cassava and rice farms.

Construction of the Vicroute Rehabilitation Village began in 1976, and the village became operational in 1986. It has an area of about 77 hectares and accommodates 30 patients, or villagers. Major activities in the village include farming, poultry, animal husbandry, carpentry, masonry, and sewing. Although still in an early developmental stage, the village has already made a positive start. At present it has several hectares of pineapples, pawpaws, orange trees, cassava, and coconut trees. It also has two dairy cows, 15 pigs, and 900 chickens.

Between 1984 and February 1986, the Vicroute village realized about 186,000 Tanzania shillings from these activities. These funds are being used to develop the village further and to purchase equipment, development of fish ponds, pay incentive allowances to the villagers, and purchase a truck. The ultimate objectives are self-sufficiency and self-support for the villagers and creation of a model for rehabilitation villages proposed for other parts of the country.

The Vicroute Village is managed by a staff of five: one occupational therapist, one social worker, one farm manager, one trained psychiatric nurse, and one security guard.

Domiciliary Services

Domiciliary services have been initiated under the community psychiatric services program in the region. Each of the five mental health centers offers home visits to selected patients, particularly those who are in the immediate vicinity of the centers. About 30 patients receive domiciliary services from each center annually. Because of the lack of transportation, services are offered only to those within a radius of two to three kilometers—that is, those who can walk or use public transportation.

In most cases, the patients' relatives are receptive to these services. Only in a few cases do they show passivity or negative attitudes because of social stigma.

Seminars

Since 1984 the community psychiatric services section of the Department of Psychiatry at the Muhimbili Medical Center has held seminars on mental health for health workers; financial support is provided by the National Mental Health Program Ministry of Health. Three seminars, lasting 1-3 weeks, have been held in Dar es Salaam, Tanga, and Mwanza, to date. The main topics discussed in these seminars include identification of mental illness, signs and symptoms of mental illness, management of patients' drugs, and effects of alcohol, drugs, and tobacco.

In addition, the psychiatric staff from the psychiatry department give special lectures in community-oriented seminars, such as those organized by police, women's groups, schools, colleges, and youth clubs. Radio broadcasts on specific topics, particularly those related to community psychiatric services, have also been introduced.

TRADITIONAL AND SPIRITUAL HEALERS

As already mentioned, traditional and spiritual healers played a significant role in the case of psychiatric patients in Tanzania before the advent of modern psychiatric services. Even today, these healers care for many patients, depending on the nature of the illness. For example, they still play a vital role in the management of psychiatric patients, particularly those with psychological problems, who do benefit from consulting traditional healers. However, psychotic patients are not helped by traditional healers. Instead, their medical treatment is delayed and chronicity can result.

Spiritual healers are known to help neurotic patients who have feelings of guilt. Prayers, confessions, and meditation bring relief to such patients.

SUMMARY AND CONCLUSIONS

The development of psychiatric services in Tanzania can be grouped into three periods. Until the mid-1920s, psychiatric services were more or less nonexistent, except for a small mental hospital established and run by Lutheran missionaries in the 1890s. Between the mid-1920s and the early 1970s, psychiatric services were provided on a centralized basis by the two national mental hospitals established at Dodoma by the British government. These central mental hospitals were intended to provide psychiatric services for the entire country. Since the early 1970s, psychiatric services in Tanzania have developed rapidly. The National Mental Health Program was launched and is extending psychiatric services to the communities.

Since the National Mental Health Program was implemented, appreciable progress has been achieved. Psychiatric services have been extended to cover nearly 50% of the country through regional psychiatric units, mental health centers, rehabilitation villages, domiciliary services, and seminars. During this period, emphasis has also been put on training psychiatric staff at various levels to improve psychiatric services in the country. These efforts are well illustrated in the Dar es Salaam region, where services have been extended from the regional psychiatric unit to district-level mental health center to domiciliary services and rehabilitation villages. It is hoped that this trend will be maintained and extended to all regions so the whole country will be covered by the year 2000.

Some operational problems have been experienced in the program. The major problems are shortages of funds, reliable transportation, and lack of manpower. To a lesser extent, cultural factors, such as tribal beliefs, taboos, and religions, have sometimes hindered efforts to bring psychiatric services from the national level to the rural areas.

Inadequate financial resources are the central problem, however.

To implement the program fully, funds are required at all levels for the necessary development tools, such as buildings, equipment, drugs, transportation, teaching materials, field kits for community workers, establishment of rehabilitation villages, and training. Unfortunately, because of meager resources, particularly financial, the government has not been in a position to finance the program fully through its annual budgetary allocations. Hence, the pace of psychiatric service development has been dictated by the availability of funds. Support and assistance, both technical and financial, have been received from external agencies and governments, such as DANIDA, WHO, the Dutch government, and others.

Chapter 36

The Chronic Mentally Ill: What Do We Know, And Why Aren't We Implementing What We Know

by

John A. Talbott, MD
Chairman and Professor,
Department of Psychiatry,
School of Medicine,
University of Maryland,
Baltimore, Maryland,
U.S.A.

ABSTRACT

Since the deinstitutionalization of the mentally ill in the United States, many elderly chronic patients have been transferred to nursing homes, a large number of young chronic mentally ill individuals have appeared on city streets, and some of the latter group have entered the correctional system. The needs of the chronic mentally ill are met to varying degrees by the many settings in which they are treated and receive care, but continuity of care may be more important than any single tretment or care ingredient. The author reviews recent findings on community programs for chronic patients and the reasons successful programs have not been widely emulated. Governmental programs in the United States consist of parallel, nonintegrated services, and current reimbursement systems contain strong disincentives for better community care of the chronically mentally ill. The author predicts that the situation will get worse before it gets better but envisions an eventual reallocation of resources and redivision of labor among the disparate parts of the mental health system.

INTRODUCTION

Major reports on the chronic mentally ill were published in 1978 by the American Psychiatric Association (APA) (Talbott, 1978), the Group for the Advancement of Psychiatry, and the President's Commission on Mental Health. Since then, this population has been studied a great deal. This research provides us with much new information about treatment and care. In this paper, I will summarize what we now know, emphasizing what is new (Talbott, 1984) since the publication of the three pivotal reports, then discuss why we are not implementing what we know, and conclude with some predictions for the future.

Before I proceed, I wish to define the population I am talking about. Like APA's Committee on the Chronically Mentally Ill, I have found most useful the definition offered by Bachrach (1976): those people who are or might have been in public mental hospitals, especially state hospitals, 30 years ago. Therefore, I am not using the term for only those suffering from a particular illness, for only those who have been discharged from state facilities, or for only those in a specific age group. The chronic mentally ill include those suffering from severe episodic chronic mental illness—i.e., the 36% of patients admitted to programs in the community serving the chronically ill who have never been hospitalized—both children, who make up 4% of the population, and the elderly, whose rate of mental illness is exponentially higher than that for people under the age of 65. For reasons of simplicity, it does not include the mentally retarded or those suffering from alcohol or drug abuse.

WHAT DO WE NOW KNOW?

In 1978 we did know several important things about the chronic mentally ill (Talbott, 1980). We knew something about 1) their numbers, location, functioning, and needs, 2) a number of model programs for the mentally ill, 3) what factors ensured continuing treatment in the community, and 4) the economic factors that controlled treatment and care of the chronic mentally ill.

However, in the past 8 years, the amount of information we have accumulated about the chronic mentally ill is greater than that published over the entire past 80 years; for example, the appendix of the 1978 APA publication on the chronic mentally ill contained only 46 references. In this section, I will summarize some of the new data regarding the population, treatment and care, and program principles.

Population

In 1978, we knew that the number of chronic mentally ill persons in America was large. It was estimated to be between 1 and 7 million, but it took the National Institute of Mental Health (NIMH) study (Bachrach, 1976) to tell us specifically 3 million persons were suffering from severe mental illnesses, 2.4 million of whom had had these illnesses for a long time— i.e., were chronic—and 1.7 million of whom had not only suffered for a long time but were disabled as a result.

In what settings do these 1.7 million severely and chronically mentally ill and disabled individuals reside? The peak state hospital census nationwide occurred in 1955. Since then, it has steadily, and in the late 1960s, precipitously, declined. Now it has essentially bottomed out (Figure 1).

The patients currently in state facilities comprise two large groups: those 65 and over, who have been and will be hospitalized for long periods, and a much younger (30-ish) group, who came into the hospital for much shorter periods of time (Figure 2).

Figure 1
NUMBER OF RESIDENTS IN U.S. STATE MENTAL HOSPITALS 1900-1980

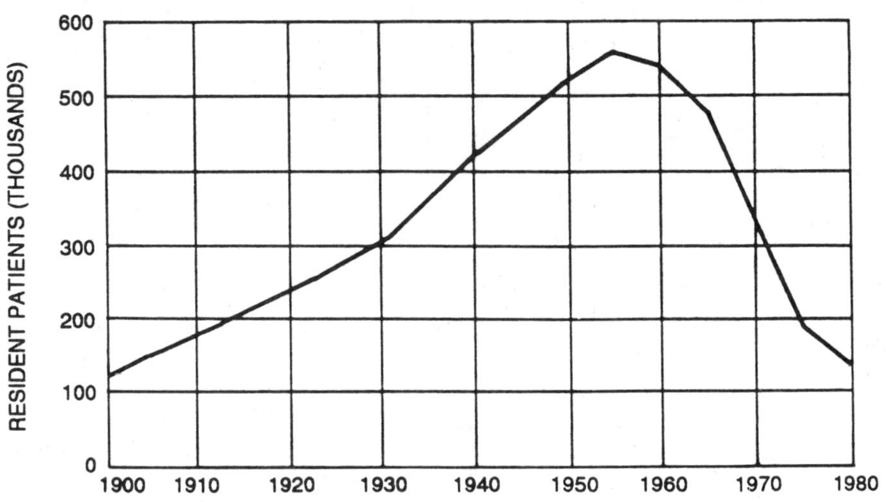

Figure 2
AGE PROFILE OF RESIDENTS OF STATE MENTAL HOSPITALS IN NEW YORK STATE, U.S.A.[1]

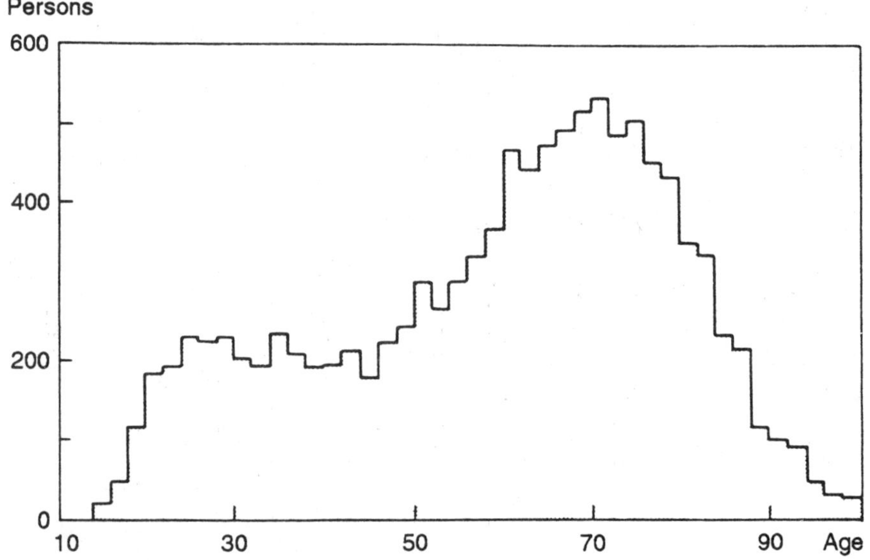

1. Source: New York State Office of Mental Health.

For these younger individuals, hospitalization is only one small facet of their treatment and living experience. Rates of readmission to state facilities have changed dramatically since 1955. Over 60% of all admissions now are readmissions, and discharged patients have about a 60% chance of being readmitted within 2 years.

If state hospitals contained 560,000 patients in 1955 and now contain only 130,000, where else do the chronic mentally ill reside? First and foremost, they live in other institutions, primarily nursing homes. Indeed, since the percentage of Americans in all types of institutions did not change between 1950 and 1970, it is apparent that what occurred could more aptly be termed transinstitutionalization than deinstitutionalization (Figure 3).

While the state hospital population declined to one-quarter of its

Figure 3

DISTRIBUTION OF PERSONS IN U.S. INSTITUTION BY TYPE OF INSTITUTION, 1950 AND 1970[1]

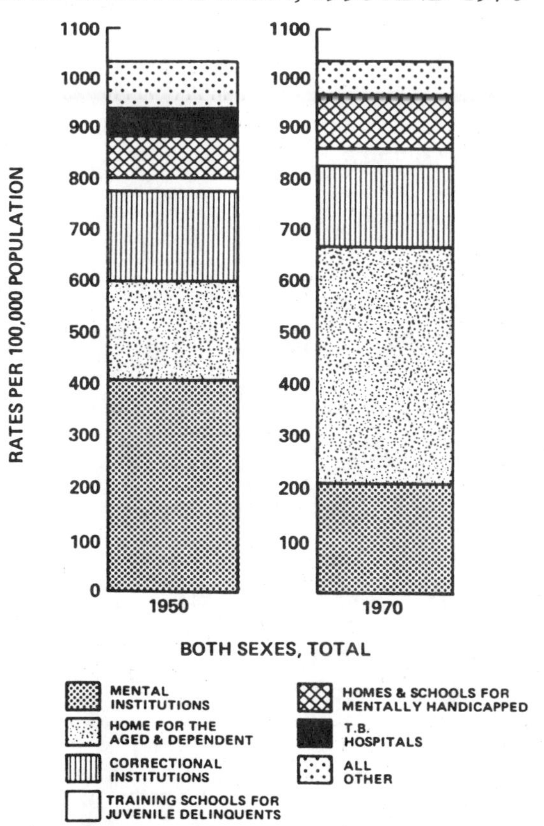

1. Source: U.S. Bureau of the Census.

former size, the nursing home population tripled. The graying of America will present us with a massive public policy problem in the next few years. The population of U.S. citizens over the age of 65 will double by the year 2030, the prevalence of mental illness is dramatically higher in this group, and 50% of nursing home beds are now occupied by persons suffering from mental illness. Thus, if states continue to freeze the number of new nursing home beds, there will be no logical institution in which to care for the elderly mentally ill who no longer need acute hospital care.

Aside from the vast numbers of persons who were transinstitutionalized to nursing homes, it is obvious, from the picture seen in all too many urban communities, that there is now a large number of young chronic mentally ill individuals who have seemingly overflowed into our city streets. They are the visible evidence of the huge post-World-War-II baby boom and are now entering the decades where they will either develop symptoms of schizophrenia or first come into contact with the health system for its treatment (Figure 4).

Figure 4
AGE PROFILE OF THE U.S. POPLUATION, 1970 AND 1980[1]

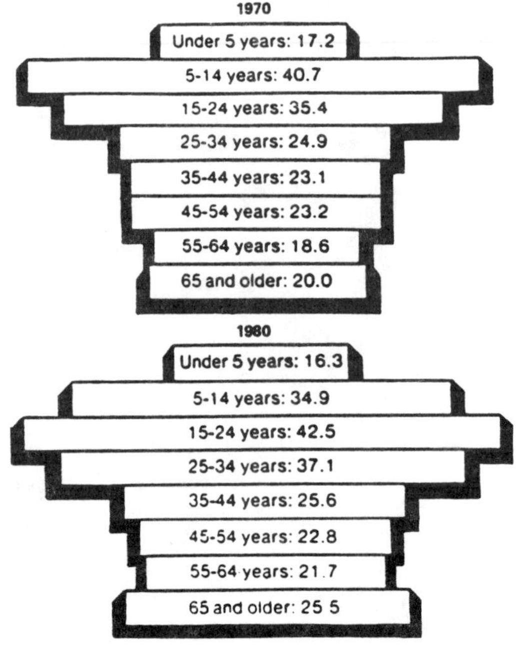

1. Source: U.S. Bureau of the Census

These new, or young, chronic mentally ill individuals have been the subject of great concern in the field, primarily because of their overwhelming numbers (up to 83%), their heavy utilization of services, and their noncompliance with treatment (Pepper and Rygiewicz, 1982 & 1984). They are generally described as young males, 20 to 35 years old, who have no permanent homes, abuse substances frequently, are often arrested (mainly for nuisance crimes or misdemeanors rather than felonies), and have a high suicide rate (4% in one study), poor social and vocational skills, and histories of violent behavior or poor impulse control.

Some have clearly entered the correctional system. The number of prison and jail inmates who are mentally ill and the number of patients who have been admitted to mental hospitals because of criminal behavior have both increased beyond the increase experienced by the prison system in general.

While the needs of the chronic mentally ill have been known for a long time, only relatively recently have we achieved a comprehenisve conceptualization of how those needs are met in different types of settings. Elizabeth Boggs has placed human needs along the horizontal axis and settings along the vertical axis, in order of restrictiveness, to give us a schema of the range of settings in which this population is housed. It is clear that, in moving from a totally institutionalized setting to independent living, ones needs in no way diminish and some means must be found to fulfill the needs not met in a particular setting (Figure 5).

It is important to remember that the number of chronically mentally ill persons who live in various types of residences in the community is nearly as large as the number who reside in hospitals or nursing homes.

Treatment and Care

Since 1978 there have also been advances in understanding how to best treat and care for the chronically ill. I have divided these areas of knowledge into systems of care, hospital versus community care, hospital care alone, disease processes, rehabilitation, and economic issues. We have learned two new important things about systems of care. First, it is clear, both from the Boggs schema and the existing program models, that a range of settings and services must be available for the chronic mentally ill (Figure 6).

Figure 5
NEEDS MET BY VARIOUS SETTINGS, IN ORDER OF RESTRICTIVENESS, FOR THE CHRONIC MENTALLY ILL[1]

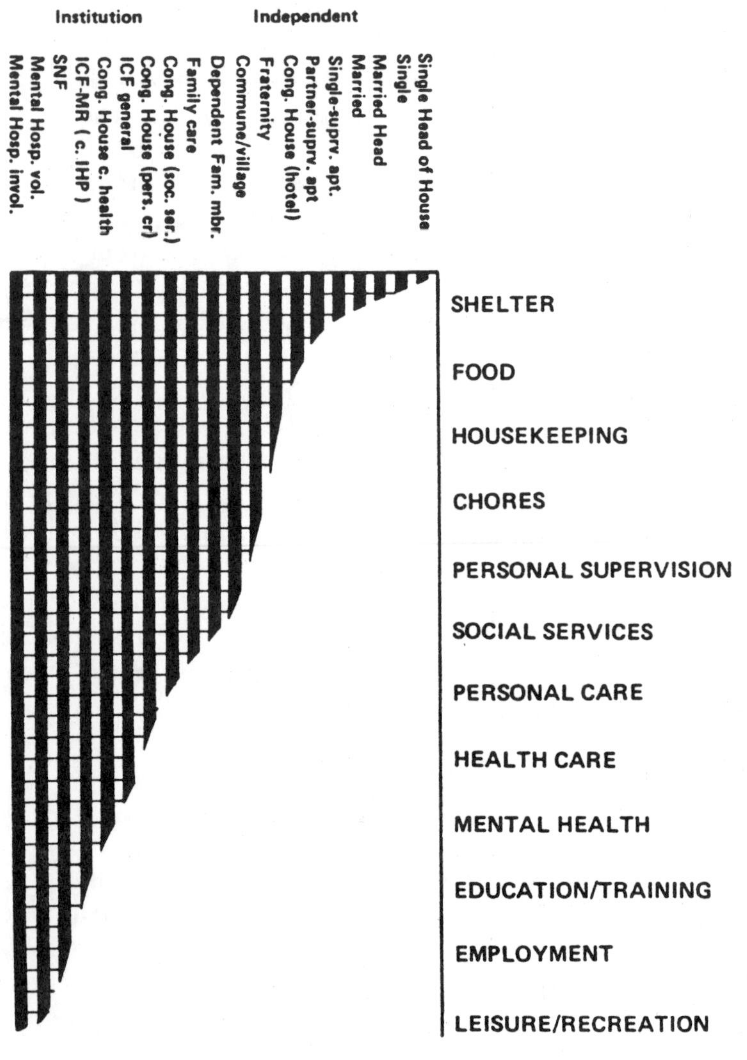

1. Source: Elizabeth Boggs, Ph.D., personal communication.

Figure 6
SPECTRUM OF OPTIMAL TREATMENT SERVICES AND LIVING SITUATIONS FOR THE CHRONIC MENTALLY ILL

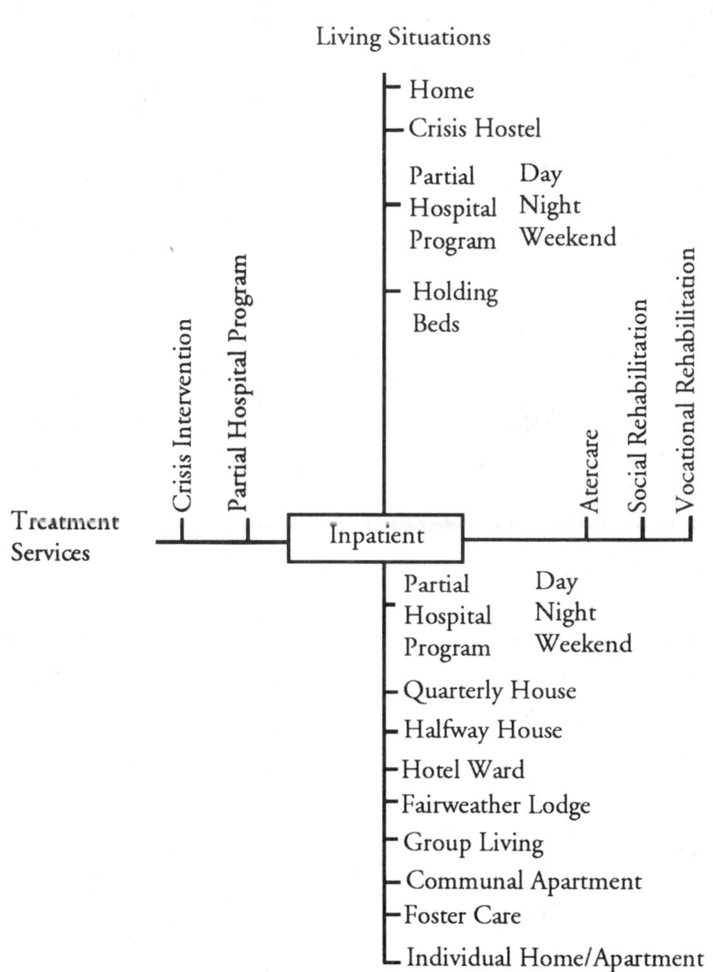

Second, as the Veterans Administration (VA) collaborative day hospital study (Linn et al., 1979) demonstrated, continuity of care may be far more important than any other single treatment or care ingredient. In addition, the pertinent studies on what prevents or forestalls both hospitalization and exacerbation of illness reveal that the two most potent weapons we have in our armentarium are continuing medication and continued personal contact—e.g., psychotherapy. If that is the case, then the facts that fewer than 50% of discharged patients continue to take their prescribed medication and only 25% continue in some form of outpatient care lead to the inescapable conclusion that few of the chronically mentally ill are receiving the few treatment elements that work (Minkoff, 1978).

There have been several reviews of the literature on whether it is better to treat the chronic mentally ill in hospital or community settings. Kiesler (1982) and Braun et al. (1981) reached essentially the same conclusion: there is no advantage to hospital care and, indeed, there is some advantage to community care—e.g., improvements in symptoms and quality of life as well as the fact that individuals like it better. This is not to say, however, that we will not always need hospitals for the mentally ill who need constant supervision, a high degree of structure, and limits on their impulsivity or wandering.

However, experts agree that the proportion of such individuals is probably only about 2% or 3% and that such settings, while offering asylum, in no way need to be traditional state-run asylums (Elpers and Crowell, 1982).

Indeed, they can be small locked facilities in the community, modeled along the lines of intermediary care facilities. Such settings, pioneered in California and called facilities, are considered by many experts to be far superior to either hospitals or unsupervised community residences for a specific subset of the chronic mentally ill (Lamb, 1980).

Regarding hospital treatment, Glick et al. (1984) concluded that, whereas long hospitalizations are preferable for first episode schizophrenic patients, for a chronic mentally ill patient the optimal strategy is brief readmissions for adjustment of medication and reformulation of the treatment plan, followed by prompt return to a community support system. Our training and thinking still, however, tend to dictate short-term hospital stays for those suffering from acute illnesses and longer-term stays for chronic patients.

Several states, notably New York and Texas, have conducted studies of their state hospital populations and concluded that one-third of the patients would not need that level of care if an adequate number of community alternatives were available and that one- third could live in the community if a good community support system were available. The hitch is the if's. We have neither enough alternatives nor enough good community support programs, despite the NIMH's 8 years of energetic activity in this arena.

Several developments in community care for the chronic mentally ill directly bear on better treatment and care for this population. First, it now appears that, while medication and psychosocial interventions are not additive, they are interactive and neither is sufficient in and of itself (Gunderson and Mosher, 1975). Second, while adequate doses of medication are essential for symptom suppression in the acute phase or during acute exacerbations of chronic illness, they are often detrimental after discharge, when patients' coping skills need honing (Segal and Aviram, 1978). Third, on the basis of May et al.'s work, it is reasonable to conclude that, for the chronically ill in the community, group therapy has the edge over individual treatment (May, 1975).

There have also been many new developments in what we now know about the serious diseases commonly found among the mentally ill. Foremost among these is the completion of several long-term follow-up studies of schizophrenics, both in the United States and elsewhere (Ciompi, 1980; Bleuler, 1979; Huber et al., 1980; Harding and Strauss, 1983). These studies are revealing in many ways. They demonstrate that 1) schizophrenia has many courses and most commonly results in either recovery or mild outcomes, 2) only 40% of persons afflicted will have bad outcomes, and 3) onset, course, and outcome are independent (Figure 7). These data are especially useful in advising the family of a schizophrenic that their relative's future is not necessarily bleak.

In addition, it has been demonstrated that early signs and symptoms of relapse can be identified both for schizophrenics as a group and for schizophrenic individuals (Herz, 1984; Carpenter et al., 1982). This is terribly important clinically, since with intermittent or low-dose medication schedules, patients and families can be taught to be on the alert for signs of exacerbations of illness, which permit prompt and aggressive reintroduction of psychotropic drugs.

Another terribly important therapeutic development is the introduction of so-called psychoeducational approaches with families and patients (Anderson et al., 1980; Faloon et al., 1981). All of these best treat and care for the chronically ill. I have divided these areas of knowledge into systems of care; hospital versus community care programs are essentially based on the work by Brown, Birley and Wing (1972), which demonstrated that the relapse rate for schizophrenics who were living with families exhibiting high expressed emotion (EE) but were taking medication was about the same as for those living with low-EE families and not taking medication.

Figure 7

ILLNESS COURSES OBSERVED IN 228 SWISS SCHIZOPHRENIC PATIENTS [1]

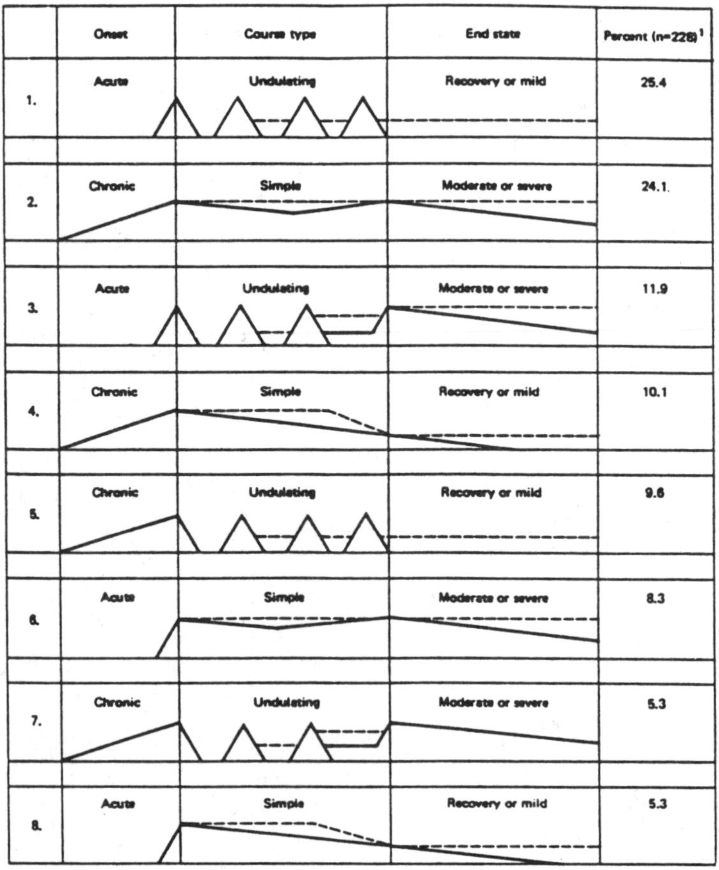

	Onset	Course type	End state	Percent (n=228)[1]
1.	Acute	Undulating	Recovery or mild	25.4
2.	Chronic	Simple	Moderate or severe	24.1
3.	Acute	Undulating	Moderate or severe	11.9
4.	Chronic	Simple	Recovery or mild	10.1
5.	Chronic	Undulating	Recovery or mild	9.6
6.	Acute	Simple	Moderate or severe	8.3
7.	Chronic	Undulating	Moderate or severe	5.3
8.	Acute	Simple	Recovery or mild	5.3

1. Source: Ciompi, (1980).

This information can be used to teach patients and families how to live with the illness and, most important, how to reduce intrafamilial stress. In addition, these approaches avoid blaming the family and instead emphasize working together to best treat and care for the chronically ill. I have divided these areas to achieve the best outcome possible. The results have been extremely encouraging, demonstrating that patients involved in such efforts have one-third to one-eighth the readmission rate of control subjects.

We also know much more now about rehabilitation of the chronically ill. For instance, we know that the severity of a person's disease state is not related to the degree of his/her disability—e.g., a person can be very sick but less disabled, or vice versa (Anthony et al., 1978). Second, we now realize that individual elements only predict themselves—e.g., previous vocational functioning predicts only future vocational functioning, not future social functioning, symptoms, etc. (Strauss and Carpenter, 1978).

Last, we know now that an individual person's level of disability depends more on his or her skills and activity than on his/her psychopathology (Anthony et al., 1978).

A final area involving treatment and care that we know much more about today than in 1978 is economics. From several comparisons of the costs of community and hospital care, several conclusions can be drawn.

1. Both forms of care for this population are costly, over $7,200 a year for community care or hospital treatment, plus traditional aftercare (Weisbrod et al., 1980). However, any comparison of community and institutional care assumes we have only one or the other, whereas we are essentially funding at least two competing systems of care. Thus, unless we abolish one or the other, we are double- funding our delivery system.

2. States save money, 65% to 80%, each time a patient is deinstitutionalized, since state hospitals are funded almost 100% from state taxes, whereas community care is financed mainly by federal and local funding—e.g., Medicaid, Medicare, and Social Security Income(SSI) (Murphy and Datel, 1976).

3. While community care saves on some costs, the savings is not great.

4. While we have greatly expanded outpatient services in the United States, their availability has not decreased the number of episodes of mental illness treated through inpatient services (Figure 8).

Figure 8
EPISODES OF CARE FOR MENTAL ILLNESS PROVIDED BY U.S. INPATIENT AND OUTPATIENT SERVICES, 1955 TO 1973[1]

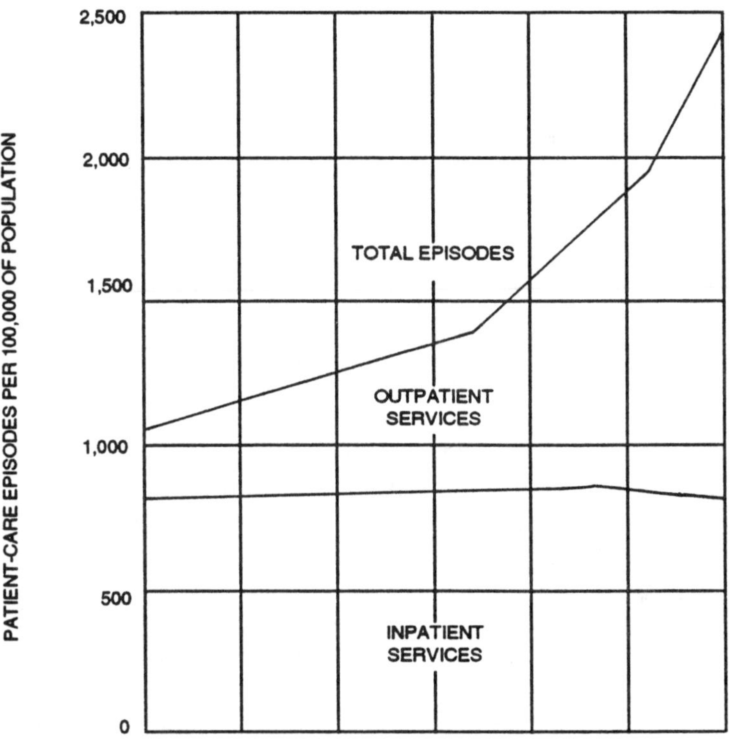

1. Source: Bassuk and Gerson, 1978, p. 52.

Principles of Successful Programs

On the basis of a variety of reviews (Bachrach, 1980; Fenton et al., 1979) it is possible to list the essential elements in successful programs serving the chronic mentally ill:

- offering lifetime access to a range of services—e.g., replacing all the services available in a hospital with the same range of services in the community under a single umbrella
- treating hospitalization as just one of the services needed by this population but ensuring that it is actually available
- treating each episode of illness or treatment as just one part of a patient's entire lifetime history of illness and need for treatment
- providing all the services available in the traditional hospital in an assertive manner— e.g., by going out and actively engaging reluctant patients
- targeting the chronic mentally ill population as a primary object of care rather than seeing it as undesirable or consisting of second-rate teaching cases
- feeling accountable for care delivered to this population and actually being held accountable
- performing internal evaluation of the program's success in meeting its goals
- making care culturally relevant—e.g., taking into account not only racial, religious factors, etc., but also relevant resources in the community
- providing a true community support system
- ensuring continuity of care through case management or resource linkage
- providing psychosocial and psychopharmacological interventions together
- utilizing skilled personnel and providing them with specialized training
- focusing on the training of patients in survival skills—e.g., the skills of every day living.

WHY CAN'T WE DO WHAT WE KNOW WORKS?

If after a decade of intense work with the chronic mentally ill we know as much as we do about the population, their optimal treatment and care, and principles of successful programs, why hasn't this knowledge been successfully translated into action? Essentially, there are seven reasons: attitudes, economic factors, governmental structure, lack of responsibility for care, people problems, legal and regulatory constraints, and research trends.

Attitudes

It is hard to think of a group of have-nots in America that has less public sympathy, less lobbying clout, and lower priority for funding than the chronic mentally ill. The negative attitudes toward the chronically ill are held by both community leaders and care givers. Community leaders want fairly simple and time- limited solutions, rather than recommendations for longer-term care. The public still believes that the mentally ill are at least partially to blame for their illnesses, unlike the mentally retarded, whose families have successfully destigmatized them over the past 25 years. The chronically ill, who have no lobbying clout, little power of taxation, and even less voting power, have insufficient voice to demand otherwise. Unfortunately, when care givers lobby, they are often seen as self- serving. Therefore, it is extremely useful when groups like the National Alliance for the Mentally Ill advocate improved services.

Care givers have somewhat different attitude problems. Most phsyicians enter medical school with a desire to cure patients, not merely care for them. Psychiatry is one of the few specialties where the most skilled practitioners take care of the fewest impaired patients. Many in the field have stated that care of the chronically ill is neither sexy nor interesting, as if we became physicians to be entertained. And there are very few rewards or thank-yous from the chronically ill.

The reasons for these negative attitudes toward the chronically ill are both neurotic and realistic. They are neurotic in that some peole are still afraid of catching mental illness from its sufferers or fear the emergence of the little bit of craziness in us all. The realistic feelings stem, however, from the fact that neither institutional nor community programs for the chronically ill have covered themselves with glory in the past 200 years, and the population is a terribly difficult one to treat and maintain interest in.

Economic Factors

The economic barriers to effecting good care and treatment of the chronic mentally ill are also substantial. First, we have no single system of care in this nation. Instead, we have mutliple systems, each competing for the same patients and resources—public (e.g., Public Health Service, VA, state hospitals, county hospitals), quasi-public (universities and voluntary non-profit institutions), and private individual hospitals and chains. Furthermore, with the establishment of each new subsystem, additional costs are generated.

Second, at each level of government (federal, state, and local) there is an inherent conflict of interest when a governmental agency chooses between operating its own facilities and contracting with community agencies. In times of scarcity, the government will direct community-designated monies back into its own facilities to save them.

Third, services are financed on a per diem basis for inpatient care and on a fee-for-service basis for outpatient care. Using these finance mechanisms rather than capitation encourages inpatient admissions rather than preventive services and maintenance in the community.

Fourth, as already stated, because of the provision of federal Medicaid, Medicare, and SSI monies, states were able to shift the economic burden for patients in state hospitals from almost 100% state taxes to largely federal funds with some local funds. The result was that patients moved out but resources did not, since they were tied to state hospital beds (Figure 9).

The total bill in 1974 for psychiatric care in this nation was approximately $37 billion (Sharfstein, 1978). About half of this went for direct services; the remainder was spent on indirect services—e.g., loss of service, loss of product. Since there are fewer than 3 million chronic mentally ill persons in this country, each person accounts for about $10,000 a year, considerably more than the $7,200 per year considered necessary for good community care Weisbrod et al.(1980).

When direct services—e.g., those paid to providers—are examined, it is apparent why the percentage of monies allocated to the chronic mentally ill is so high—i.e., 97% of the $37 billion. Over 50% goes to nursing homes and state and county hospitals, while a relatively small percentage goes to general hospitals (12%) and community mental health centers (CMHCs) (4%) (see Figure 10).

FIGURE 9
STATE AND LOCAL SHARES OF RESOURCES FOR CARE OF THE MENTALLY ILL IN NEW YORK STATE, U.S.A.

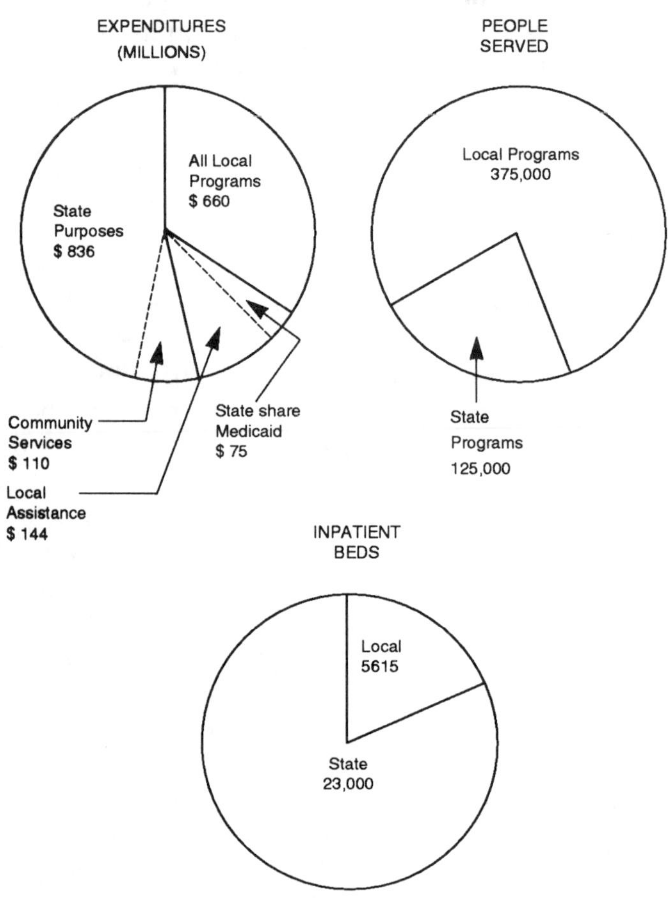

a. Source: New York State Office of Mental Health.

Figure 10
DISTRIBUTION OF 1974 U.S. EXPENDITURES FOR DIRECT CARE OF THE MENTALLY ILL BY TYPE OR LOCALE OF CARE[a]

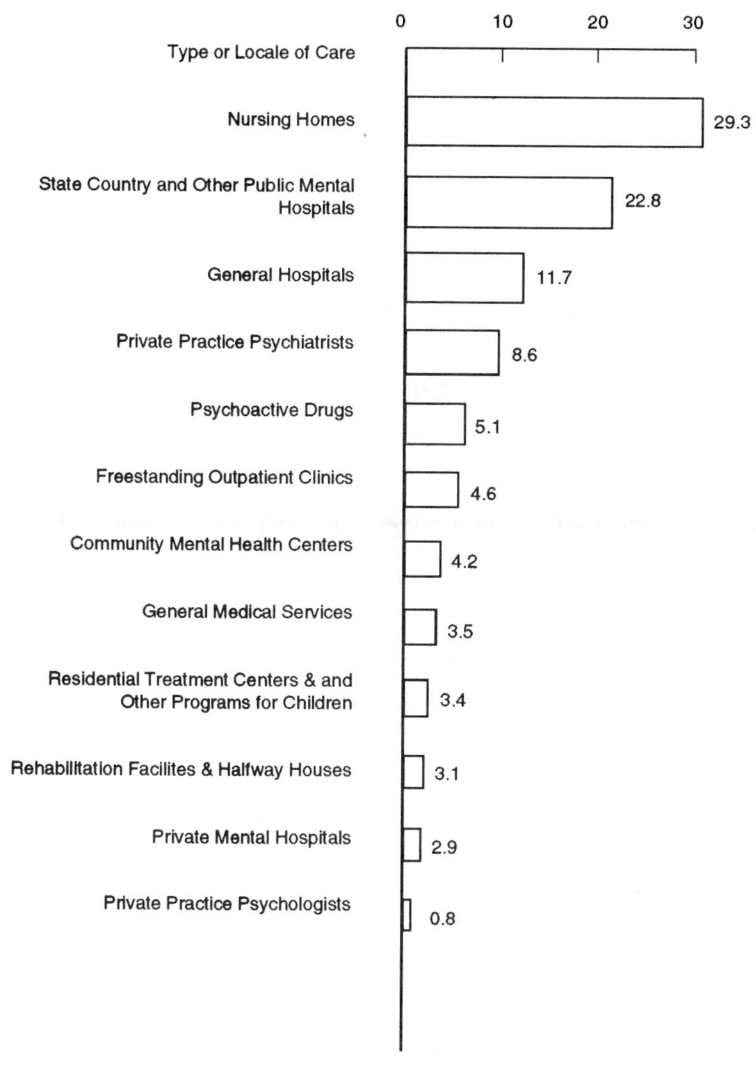

*Estimated total expendites for direct care were $145 billion

a. Source: National Institute of Mental Health, 1975.

The incentives and disincentives in the current reimbursement system are almost completely the reverse of those needed to bring about better community care for the chronically mentally ill. These systems reward

- more restrictive rather than less restrictive settings, public rather than private facilities—e.g., in New York the same phsyician seeing a patient in a hospital clinic is paid twice what he or she would receive seeing the same patient in a private office, which has much lower overhead costs
- acute rather than chronic care
- the promise of cure rather than the pursuit of care
- impatient admission rather than maintenance in the community
- direct services—e.g., contact—rather than indirect ones—e.g., coordinating with other agencies and professionals

In addition, most services needed by the chronic mentally ill are financed in a piecemeal manner rather than comprehensively, and some funding, such as nursing home funding via social service channels, is totally inaccessible to mental health officials seeking to improve these facilities. Finally, to date, no region in the country has found a mechanism to fund asylums or to adequately provide accessible low-cost housing alternatives for this population.

Governmental Structure

As already mentioned, there is no genuine system of care in this country. Instead, the structure of current government programs for mental health care resembles Figure 11. This structure invites political fights among all of the elements and, as stated before, creates inherent conflicts of interest at each level of government.

In addition, almost each need identified for the chronically ill is met by a different federal or state agency:

- Housing - Department of Housing and Urban Development

- Income - SSI
- Vocational rehabilitation - Health Resources Administration
- Social rehabilitation - Health Services Administration
- Medical and psychiatric - Medicaid and Medicare

Because of their differing legislative mandates, these agencies have differing requirements for funding and differing ideas of whom they are serving. The result is strangulating fragmentation, with multiple funding streams, multiple levels of planning, and multiple loci of implementation. All too often these funding streams reach patients separately; there is no attempt to pull them together into an accessible package that will meet patients' real needs rather than bureaucratic ideals.

Figure 11
THEORETICAL ORGANIZATION OF GOVERNMENTAL MENTAL HEALTH SERVICES IN THE UNITED STATES

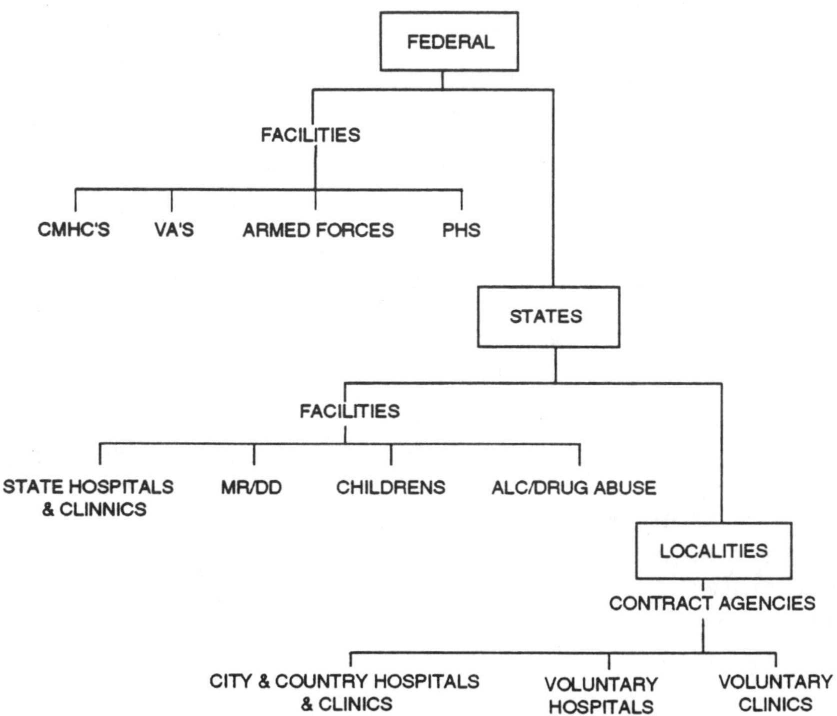

Responsibility

When we moved from a single system, the state hospital system, to multiple settings in the community, our ability to pinpoint the responsibility for care of both the entire popluation and individual patients was lost. To regain this most essential ingredient of good care, point responsibility must be established for 1) care management for each patient, 2) integrated service delivery for each group of patients, and 3) a nationwide system, involving the federal, state, and local levels, for the entire population of the chronic mentally ill. Essentially no one is in charge at present, a situation that causes endless numbers of problems.

People Problems

Barriers to more effective care and treatment of the chronically ill are also posed by several groups, including program administrators, staff members, unions, and average citizens. Leaders of programs serving the chronic mentally ill must understand the process of chronicity, be interested in persons suffering from chronic conditions, and be able to walk that fine line between expecting too much of patients, which promotes their regression, and holding up enough hope to encourage attainment of higher levels of functioning. Staff members must also recognize this balance and must be trained in modern resocialization-relearning approaches, effective rehabilitation techniqiues to use with disabled patients, techniques for teaching patients the skills of everyday living, and psychoeducational approaches with both patients and families.

Unions of employees from the governmental sector also present a sizeable obstacle to the move toward community care. In New York State, new monies for mental health helped raise the ratio of staff to patients in state psychiatric centers from 0.25 in 1955 to 1.38 in 1981. A higher ratio was promised by the most recent governor, then running for reelection, to the civil service union before any monies could be reallocated to community settings. In addition, many communities in which state hospitals are located have strenuously resisted reallocation of resources because of their dependence on these facilites for jobs, business, etc.

Legal and regulatory pressures in the past few decades, judicial findings, governmental regulations, and legal developments designed to remedy the very real abuse that existed in some facilities have often hampered quality care for the chronically ill. For instance, Soucer v. Brennan intended to remedy the peonage of state patients but instead resulted in the closing of thousands of legitimate work programs. Likewise, the multiplicity of standards promulgated by the Joint Commission on the Accreditation of Healthcare Organizations (JCAHO) and other regulatory bodies, while attempting to provide guidelines for ensuring quality of care, have often merely focused attention on what can be measured easily rather than on clinical outcome or program success. In addition, the sheer number of national, state, and local agencies (164 in New York State) that can enter any hospital, insepct it, and require it to fill out new forms, drives care toward paper compliance rather than clinical excellence. In New York, it has been calculated that 25% of all staff time and 25% of a hospital's resources go toward complying with regulatory agency standards (Hospital Association of New York State, 1979).

Research Trends

Given the current excitement in our field about the promising developments in basic research that will (soon, we hope) illuminate the etiology of the major mental illnesses, the future of effective treatment of the chronic mentally ill may hinge on basic science breakthroughs. However, while awaiting these breakthroughs, it is critical to focus attention on several unanswered questions important to the care and treatment of the chronically ill. These include:

- What causes and prevents chronicity?
- What treatment elements work for which patients in what settings?
- How many of each setting and service do we need?
- How much do they cost?
- How do we provide enough of them, especially asylum settings?

WHAT DO WE DO NOW?

I predict that, given the current political climate, economic trends, and governmental, social, mental health, and housing policies, things will get worse for the chronic mentally ill before they get better. I fear that the numbers of the homeless will continue to rise, that prison populations of the mentally ill will swell, and that scandals will become more common in facilities in both the community—e.g., nursing homes—and institutions—e.g., state hospitals.

We have already heard scattered cries for rehospitalization from, among others, the editors of the New York Times, and these will no doubt be heard again. But given the vast monies necessary—not only to rebuild the deteriorating plants in our public facilities, but to bring about effective reform of the public system—and given the fact that reinstitutionization would fly in the face of the last 25 years of scientific study and legal pressure, its actualization is unlikely. Indeed, there may be renewed calls to close state hospitals and move entirely to a community care system for the chronically ill. The Massachusetts Blue Ribbon Commission called for such a change (1981).

I believe that instead of these outcomes, we will move to a reallocation of resources and redivision of labor among the disparate parts of the mental health system. One way of conceptualizing a new breakout of functions of the traditional state facility is to divide the services into treatment and care elements, all of which should be supported by state funding but any of which can be provided in community settings.

There are several methods by which reallocation of resources and redivision of labor could be achieved. They include:

- Capitation funding as in Wisconsin (Stein and Ganser, 1983) which promotes prevention, alternatives to hospitalization, and community care.
- HMO or prepaid medical service programs, which also promote prevention, continuity of care, and indirect services.
- A voucher system that would provide each chronically mentally ill person in America one voucher for housing and another for services.

- Changes in current reimbursement mechanisms so that day hospitals, psychosocial rehabilitation programs, and other alternatives to inpatient hospitalization were more adequately reimbursed.
- A truly unified system that would incorporate all elements of our disorganized mental health programs.
- More money for the chronic mentally ill.

At this point it is impossible to predict what we as a nation will choose to do with our disjointed, negative, and inefficient mental health services. But given the huge numbers of new young chronic mentally ill persons and the rapidly increasing numbers of older persons suffering from mental illness, we are at a critical point. What we do will reveal not only our ingenuity, but our ability to act humanely in the best interests of those who cannot speak effectively for themselves.

REFERENCES

Anderson, C. M., Hogarty, G. E., Reiss, D. J.: Family treatment of acute schizophrenic patients: a psychoeducational approach. Schizophrenia Bulletin 6:490-505, 1980

Anthony, W. A., Cohen, M. R., Vitalo, R.: The measurement of rehabilitation outcome. Schizophrenia Bulletin 4:365-383, 1978

Bachrach, L. L.: Deinstitutionalization: An Analytical Review and Sociological Perspective. Rockville, Md., U.S.A., National Institute of Mental Health, 1976

Bachrach, L. L.: Overview: model programs for chronic mental patients. American Journal of Psychiatry 137:1023-1031, 1980

Bassuk, E. L.: The homelessness problem. Scientific American 251:40-45, 1984

Bassuk, E. L., Gerson, S.: Deinstitutionalization and mental health services. Scientific American 238:46-53, 1978

Bleuler, M. E.: On schizophrenic psychoses. American Journal of Psychiatry 136:1403-1409, 1979

Braun, P., Kochansky, G., Shapiro, R., et al.: Overview: deinstitutionalization of psychiatric patients, a critical review of outcome studies. American Journal of Psychiatry 138:736-749, 1981

Brown, G. W., Birley, J. L. T., Wing, J. K.: Influence of family life on the course of schizophrenic disorders: a replication. British Journal of Psychiatry 121:241-258, 1972

Carpenter, W. T., Stephens, J. P., Rey, A. C.: Early intervention vs. continuous pharmacotherapy of schizophrenia. Pharmacology Bulletin 18:21-23, 1982

Ciompi, L.: Catamnestic long-term study on the course of life and aging of schizophrenics. Schizophrenia Bulletin 6:606-618, 1980

Elpers, J. R., Crowell, A.: How many beds? an overview of resource planning. Hospital and Community Psychiatry 33:755-761, 1982

Faloon, R. H., Boyd, J. L., McGill, C. W., et al: Family management training in the community care of schizophrenia. New Directions for Mental Health Services, number 12, 1981, pp. 61-77

Fenton, F. R., Tessier, L., Struening, E. L.: A comparative trial of home and hospital psychiatric care: one-year follow-up. Archives of General Psychiatry 36:1073-1079,1979

Glick, I. D., Klar, H. M., Braff, D. L.: Guidelines for hospitalization of chronic psychiatric patients. Hospital and Community Psychiatry 35:934-936, 1984

Group for the Advancement of Psychiatry: The Chronic Mental Patient in the Community. New York, U.S.A., GAP, 1978

Gunderson, J. G., Mosher, L. R.: Psychotherapy of Schizophrenia. New York, U.S.A., Jason Aronson, 1975

Harding, C. M., Brooks, G., Ashikaga, T., et al.: Overview: the long-term course of chronic patients. Presented at the 136th annual meeting of the American Psychiatric Association, New York, U.S.A., April 30-May 6, 1983

Herz, M.: Recognizing and preventing relapse in patients with schizophrenia. Hospital and Community Psychiatry 35:344-349, 1984

Hospital Association of New York State: Cost of Regulation Study. Albany, N.Y., U.S.A., HANYS, 1979

Huber, G., Gross, G., Schuttler, R., et al.: Longitudinal studies of schizophrenic patients. Schizophrenia Bulletin 6:592-605, 1980

Kiesler, C. A.: Mental hospitals and alternative care: noninstitutionalization as potential public policy for mental patients. American Psychologist 37:349-360, 1982

Lamb, H. R.: Structure: the neglected ingredient of community treatment. Archives of General Psychiatry 37:1224-1228, 1980

Linn, M. W., Caffey, S. M., Klett, C. J., et al.: Day treatment and psychotropic drugs in the aftercare of schizophrenic patients. Archives of General Psychiatry 36:1055-1072, 1979
Massachusetts Blue Ribbon Commission on the Future of Public Inpatient Mental Health Services: Mental Health Crossroads. Boston, U.S.A., 1981

May, P. R. A.: Schizophrenia: an overview of treatment methods in Comprehensive Textbook of Psychiatry, 2nd ed., vol I. Edited by Freedman, A.M., Kaplan, H.I., Sadock, B.J. Baltimore, Md., U.S.A., Williams & Wilkins, 1975

Minkoff, K.: A map of the chronic mental patient, in The Chronic Mental Patient: Problems, Solutions, and Recommendations for a Public Policy. Edited by Talbott, J.A. Washington, D.C., U.S.A., American Psychiatric Association, 1978

Murphy, J., Datel, W.: A cost-benefit analysis of community versus institutional living. Hospital and Community Psychiatry 27:165-170, 1976

National Institute of Mental Health: Statistical Note 125. Rockville, Md., U.S.A., NIMH, Division of Biometry and Epidemiology

Pepper, B., Ryglewicz, H. (eds.): The Young Adult Chronic Patient. New Directions for Mental Health Services, number 14, 1982

Pepper, B., Ryglewicz, H. (eds.): Advances in Treating the Younger Adult Chronic Patient. New Directions for Mental Health Services, number 21, 1984

Segal, S. P., Aviram, U.: The Mentally Ill in Community-Based Sheltered Care. New York, U.S.A., John Wiley & Sons, 1978

Sharfstein, S., Turner, J. E. C., Clark, H. W.: Financing issues in providing services for the chronically mentally ill and disabled, in The Chronic Mental Patient: Problems, Solutions, and Recommendations for a Public Policy. Edited by Talbott, J.A. Washington, D.C., U.S.A., American Psychiatric Association, 1978

Stein, L. I., Ganser, L. J.: Wisconsin's system for funding mental health services, New Directions for Mental Health Services, number 18, 1983, pp.25-32

Strauss, J. S., Carpenter, W. T., Jr.: The prognosis of schizophrenia: rationale for a multidimensional concept. Schizophrenia Bulletin 4:56-67, 1978

Talbott, J. A. (ed.): The Chronic Mental Patient: Problems, Solutions, and Recommendations for a Public Policy. Washington, D.C., U.S.A., American Psychiatric Association, 1978

President's Commission on Mental Health: Report to the President. Washington, D.C., U.S.A., U.S. Government Printing Office, 1978

Talbott, J. A.: Toward a public policy on the chronically mentally ill. American Journal of Orthopsychiatry 50:43-53, 1980

Talbott, J. A. (ed.): The Chronic Mental Patient: Five Years Later. Orlando, Fla., U.S.A., Grune & Stratton, 1984

Weisbrod, B. A., Test, M. A., Stein, L. I.: Alternative to mental hospital treatment, II: economic benefit-cost analysis. Archives of General Psychiatry 37-400-405, 1980

Chapter 37

The Crisis Model's Compatibility with Meager Resources

by

Lee Ann Hoff, RN, Ph.D.
Northeastern University
College of Nursing
Boston, Massachusetts
U.S.A.

ABSTRACT

The author describes a clinically effective and cost-effective model of crisis management and illustrates its potential as a major facet of primary health care. National standards for crisis intervention exist, but widespread implementation has been delayed by the common belief that crisis intervention is a band-aid or inferior version of psychotherapy and by the lack of coordination between professionals and paraprofessionals. The four essential steps in crisis management are assessment, planning, intervention, and follow-up, which are carried out both in natural crisis management (e.g., by families) and formal crisis management (by trained crisis workers). Implementation of the crisis model depends on development and expansion of training programs, establishment of high-quality crisis services, clarification of institutional roles, and political and economic action aimed at primary prevention.

INTRODUCTION

At 11:00 p.m., police call the 24-hour telephone crisis program. A team of professional crisis workers (one, a psychiatric nurse with a master's degree; the other, a volunteer with a B.A. in psychology) is dispatched to make an outreach visit to the home of David Jones, who, the police and Mr. Jones's family believe, is acutely suicidal, uncooperative, and in need of assessment for possible involuntary hospitalization. Mr. Jones has refused to comply with police and family recommendations for treatment. The outreach team spends one and one-half hours with Mr. Jones and his family in their home. Mr. Jones is finally persuaded to go voluntarily to the emergency department of a community hospital, where he will be examined by psychiatric liaison staff for possible hospitalization. Following assessment of Mr. Jones and his family situation, he is kept overnight in the emergency department holding bed. The following morning, outpatient therapy is initiated for Mr. Jones and his family at the community mental health center with which the hospital has an interagency service contract for follow-up of such mental health emergency cases. The family is also given the telephone number of the 24-hour telephone and outreach crisis program, which the police had originally called on behalf of this family. (Adapted from Wells and Hoff, 1984)

Many family members (natural crisis managers), as well as human service professionals (formal crisis managers), will be familiar with such a crisis situation in this society. The example highlights similarities and areas of overlap between what family members and mental health professionals do in managing such a crisis—for example, listening and making judgments and decisions about what is to be done. In many respects, the work of natural and formal crisis managers is complementary in many situations (Hoff, 1984a, pp. 24-29). However, there are some differences. One of the most obvious is that the crisis outreach workers and mental health professionals in this situation are associated with formally established programs offering crisis services. These workers possess knowledge and skills regarding crisis management that go beyond what most people know about the needs of people in distress. They are skills acquired, presumably, through professional education or training.

This paper describes the crisis model, its history, major concepts and strategies related to it, and its potential as a major facet of primary health care. The focus is on American society, although the basic principles of this cost-effective model can be adapted to other cultural contexts. Also, this paper assumes that the primary consideration in applying the crisis model represents the most efficient use of meager resources because of its potential to prevent major mental illness, which is very costly in both human and financial terms.

THE CRISIS MODEL'S PLACE IN THE U.S. MENTAL HEALTH SYSTEM

Considered broadly, crisis and crisis intervention are as old as humankind. Helping people in crisis is intrinsic to the nurturing side of human character. Because of our social nature, we are able to create a culture of caring and concern for people in distress. Thus, crisis intervention can be seen as a natural human action embedded in culture.

In traditional societies, assistance and support for distressed people were available through the extended family and indigenous community leaders, such as a tribal chief or healer. In contemporary industrialized societies, however, social roles are more sharply defined and individuals are more frequently left to their own devices when troubled. Accompanying these social developments has been an expansion of the roles of professionals, including various experts trained to deal with emotional and mental upsets.

A major outgrowth of this trend is the development of crisis intervention as a distinct body of knowledge and practice. As an organized field, however, it is only a few decades old. During the 1950s, a national study of mental health in the United States found that crisis services were nonexistent for the most part. We had essentially a two-class system in which the rich could pay for services from private psychiatric resources, the poor were warehoused in large public mental hospitals, and there was little or no service between these two extremes.

To remedy this situation, the National Institute of Mental Health (NIMH) recommended that every citizen have immediate, local access to five essential mental health services:

- consultation and education
- emergency mental health service, including 24-hour crisis intervention
- out-care service
- partial hospital care
- 24-hour in-care (residential) service

Figure 1
RELATIONSHIP OF MENTAL HEALTH SERVICES CONTINUUM TO COST AND CLIENT INDEPENDENCE

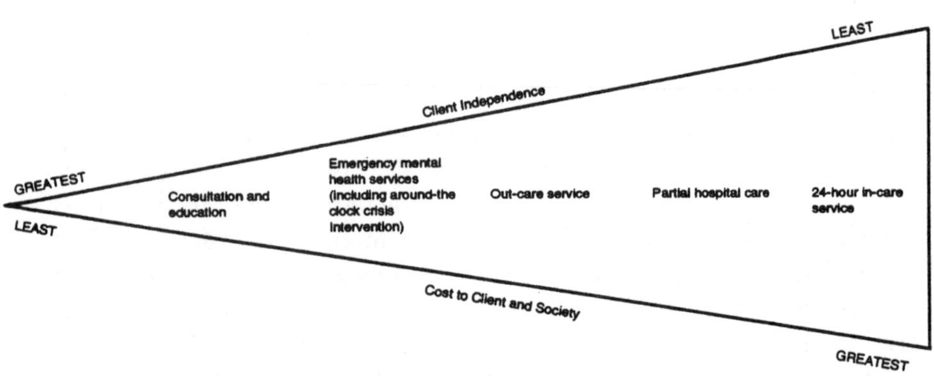

Figure 1 shows that assisting distressed people in their natural social roles (homemaker, paid worker, student) through consultation, education, and crisis services is the least costly means of service and allows the greatest client independence; institution based care is the most costly means and allows the least client independence. Primary health care, therefore, should include crisis intervention and mental health consultation and education. Crisis intervention has been hailed as the latest of three revolutionary phases that have occurred in mental and public health since the turn of the century. The first two were Freud's discovery of the unconscious and the discovery of psychotropic drugs in the 1950s.

In other words, the ideal in community mental health is that, if a person or family is experiencing an emotional crisis for any reason whatsoever, help should be available as easily and quickly as it is for someone with a broken leg, a heart attack, or other physical emergency. This ideal is illustrated in the opening case example and is akin to the current goal of the World Health Organization (WHO)— i.e., health for all by the year 2000.

To help meet this goal, in the United States we have developed national standards for crisis services and for training of health workers (Wells and Hoff, 1984). These standards state, among other things, that every health and mental health worker, including professionals with higher degrees and various paraprofessionals, should have at least 40 hours of training in crisis intervention. Sadly, however, these standards are far from being met in the United States.

Historically, paraprofessionals and lay people played a large role in responding to the need for crisis programs in the United States. The urgency of the needs for service, however, contributed to an underemphasis on the theoretical foundations of crisis work by those in the suicide prevention movement of the 1960s (Hoff, 1984a). Meanwhile, psychiatrists providing traditional services were increasingly pressured to lend their professional expertise to the growing need for crisis services, while the 1965 call for 24-hour crisis response in the federal legislation on community mental health centers went unanswered for years in all but a few communities.

One result of these historical developments has been the dichotomyzation of traditional psychiatric emergency care and crisis services provided by indigenous community sources. Various misconceptions about the crisis model have exaggerated this dichotomy. For example, popular myths about crisis intervention include the following:

- It is a useful "band-aid" until "real therapy" is available.
- It is particularly useful when poverty prevents payment for longer-term service.
- It is a shorter form of psychotherapy.

These misconceptions and the lack of coordination between professional and paraprofessional crisis workers have detrimental effects on people in crisis and have delayed the widespread implementation of primary health care crisis services that meet national standards and ideals.

MAJOR CONCEPTS IN THE CRISIS MODEL

Clarification of the major elements of the crisis model will correct some of the misconceptions and further the development of this cost-effective mode of service for troubled people. Basic to refinement of this aspect of mental health practice is recognition that crisis intervention is not merely a band-aid or an inferior version of psychotherapy, even though it uses some of the same techniques, such as listening. Rather, it is an organized approach to helping distressed people that can be mastered by lay people and professionals through a systematic educational/training program. The following definitions distinguish crisis intervention from other modes of helping distressed people (Hoff, 1984a, Chapter 1, contains further distinctions):

- Crisis: An acute emotional upset that includes a temporary inability to cope by means of one's usual problem-solving techniques.
- Crisis management: The entire process of working through a crisis to crisis resolution. It includes the efforts of the person in crisis and of people helping him/her—e.g., a family member or formal crisis worker.
- Crisis intervention: That aspect of crisis management

carried out by a crisis worker—i.e., nurse, police officer, physician, psychotherapist, counselor, or minister. It focuses on resolution of the immediate problem through the use of personal, social, environmental, and, sometimes, material resources. Crisis intervention is related to, but differs from, psychotherapy.

- Crisis counseling: The aspect of crisis management that focuses particularly on the emotional ramifications of the crisis. It is carried out by a crisis worker who also has formal preparation in counseling techniques.
- Crisis worker:. A person working on a paid or volunteer basis who has specialized knowledge and skills in crisis work, including suicide and assault prevention, who adheres to the technical and ethical standards of the field, and who spends at least part of his/her time providing crisis intervention services. Crisis workers include, but are not limited to, those who possess professional mental health degrees- -e.g., psychiatric nurse, psychiatrists, psychiatric social worker, or clinical psychologist.
- Crisis program: A generic term including emergency services of community mental health centers, suicide prevention centers, psychiatric or behavioral sections of emergency medical services, shelters for runaway teenagers, rape crisis centers, battered women's programs, and services for other victims of crime.
- Crisis model: The paradigm for the entire helping process during crisis and the theory supporting it.

Regardless of the different approaches to crisis service delivery and the different disciplines and settings involved, four essential steps characterize the crisis management process:

- Psychosocial assessment of the individual, family, or community in crisis. This always includes evaluation of the risk of suicide or assault on others.
- With the person, family, or groups in crisis, development of a plan based on assessment data.

- Implementation of the plan, drawing on personal, social, and material resources.
- Follow-up and evaluation of the crisis management process and resolution of the individual, family, or community crisis.

These steps can be followed by individuals or families in natural settings, or by trained crisis workers in telephone, office, nursing home, social agency, community hospital, or other settings. The essential steps of crisis management can also be carried out in settings specializing in crisis service, or they can be integrated with psychotherapy or other forms of human interaction. For example, in natural situations, parents who know the warning signs of suicide can implement these steps on behalf of their own child during normal parent-child interaction. In formal settings, lay volunteers, mental health professionals, nurses, police officers, clergy, or others trained in crisis theory and practice can implement the steps of crisis management as a specialized service or in concert with other kinds of needed services, e.g.,

- medical treatment of an accident victim by paramedics, nurses, and physicians
- notification of a death or rescue of a rape victim, according to policy
- comforting by a pastor or nurse of those close to a person who committed suicide
- long-term treatment of an emotionally or mentally disturbed person by technicians and other mental health workers
- social services provided to abusive parents by social workers
- support of battered women and other victims by victim advocates

Another key concept in the crisis model is the danger and opportunity that crisis presents for the individual experiencing it. The danger during crisis is that the suffering person will resolve the crisis in a very negative way, such as by suicide or an attack on others, by alcohol or other drug abuse, or through emotional or mental breakdown. The emotional pain of crisis is so severe that the person feels a great urgency to seek relief.

The opportunity during crisis is for the person to grow and develop by learning new ways of coping with the various traumas and misfortunes of life. This aspect of crisis makes crisis intervention such an appealing and rewarding way of assisting people in the mental health area. That is, if we are there when people need us and offer them no more or no less than they need, all sorts of worse trouble and pain can be avoided in most cases. In this respect, crisis intervention is truly primary health care because it can prevent the most miserable human conditions that often follow when people lack necessary assistance during crisis.

However, besides its importance in preventing long-term sociopsychological damage, crisis intervention is also a critical aspect of care for those who have already experienced emotional or mental breakdown. This is because such people are more vulnerable to further breakdowns and crises and to chronic illnesses.

The opportunity presented by crisis is related to another important facet of life crises. Crises are essentially normal experiences that people all over the world are managing in one way or another. Thus, it can be said that all people are natural crisis managers, as illustrated by the opening case example. Norris Hansell (1976), a psychiatrist who worked with Gerald Caplan (1964), sometimes called the father of crisis theory, illustrates this idea with the Bible story of Noah and the Ark. By listening to the warning signs and preparing accordingly, Noah was able to save himself and his kin from the disaster of the flood.

However, for some people, their natural crisis management skills are not enough. Because people are already vulnerable psychologically or because they lack social resources and support, they need help during crisis from people like ourselves. These people are the formal crisis managers who assisted Mr. Jones and his family when their natural resources proved insufficient. In this respect, crisis intervention is everybody's profession.

Figure 2 illustrates the complementary aspects of natural and formal crisis management with another case example, Ray and his family. It also shows how the growth and development approach, a hallmark of the crisis model differs from the traditional medical

Figure 2

NATURAL CRISIS MANAGEMENT AND TWO APPROACHES TO FORMAL CRISIS MANAGEMENT[1]

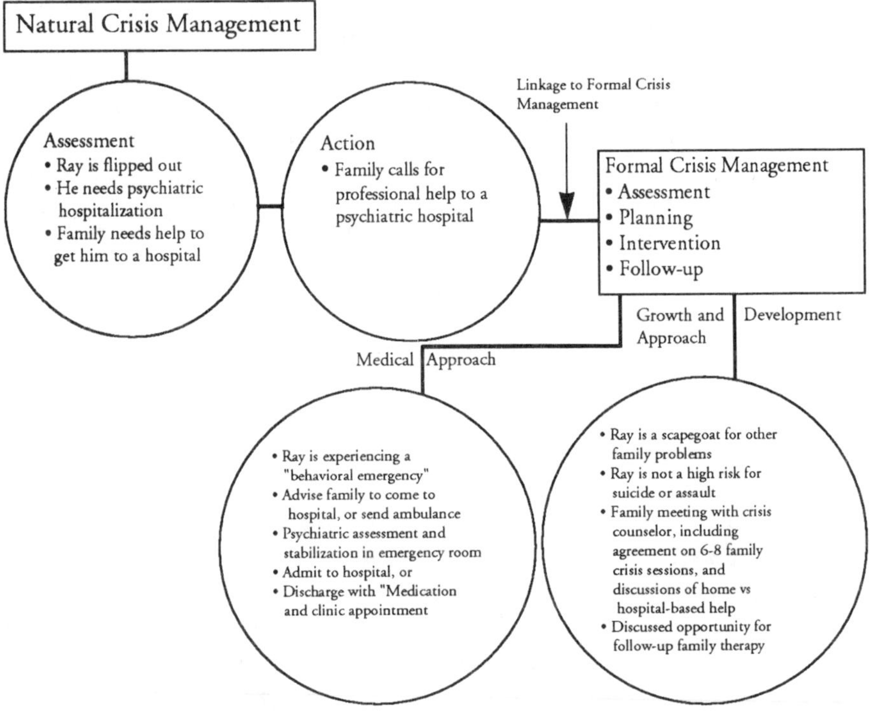

1. Source: Hoff, 1984a.

model. These core elements of the crisis model apply to a crisis worker in any discipline and to any setting in which crises occur.

During the past few decades, the popularity of this growing field of practice has been fueled by the service needs of people in crisis. It has also been strongly influenced by the need to contain costs and is thus seen as an expedient and less expensive form of treatment because of its brevity. These factors have led to an uneven development of the crisis field, and many goals are as yet unmet. Among these are:

1. development and expansion of preservice and in-service training programs for crisis practitioners in various human service disciplines, such as nursing, social work, psychology, general medical and psychiatric practice, police work, and educational, pastoral and rehabilitation counseling, and
2. establishment and refinement of programs to deliver high-quality service to people in crisis.

Accomplishment of these training and service tasks is often hindered by a chicken-and-egg dilemma confronting professional educators and program administrators in crisis work. That is, without personnel specifically prepared in crisis theory and practice, it is difficult if not impossible to establish service programs according to national standards. Conversely, the clinical training of crisis practitioners has been either nonexistent or sketchy, or supervised clinical practice settings have not been available to crisis trainees.

This dilemma is rooted primarily in the neophyte status of crisis theory and practice. Although emergency mental health/crisis service in the United States was declared an essential element of community mental health programs decades ago, comprehensive crisis services, open 7 days a week, 24 hours a day, in office and community settings, are far from routine in most American communities, as illustrated in this case example:

After an acute battering episode by her husband, Jane went by taxi to a local medical emergency facility for treatment of bruises and lacerations. While there, neither physician nor nurse inquired further about her problems when she reported that her husband had beaten her. On her own, she then went to a local community mental health center where she was given a prescription for tranquilizers and an appointment to return for counseling in one week. Jane went home feeling even more depressed than before she sought help.

Such piecemeal, ineffective approaches to people in crisis persist in spite of burgeoning public interest in the field as a response to victims of violence. During a national workshop convened by the Surgeon General of the United States in 1985, crisis intervention was highlighted as a central means of assisting victims and preventing the common secondary victimization resulting from inappropriate treatment by health and mental health professionals and the criminal justice system.

The gaps in professional training and readily available service deprives people in crisis of the assistance they are entitled to. In the long run, greater financial outlays are required for the more serious mental health problems that result from delayed responses to people in crisis. The importance of crisis intervention is thereby underscored not only in human terms but also in economic terms.

Inadequate crisis service also suggests an identity crisis in institutional roles. For example, in many American communities, basic 24- hour crisis service is provided only by police, many of whom have little or no special training. Furthermore, some police crisis work is done because mental health professionals are either untrained for or unwilling to perform this critical task. This issue is even more significant because of the life-and-death dimensions of many crisis institutions. Here the work of Morton Bard is instructive. The crisis intervention training programs for police officers developed by Bard in New York City were shown to significantly reduce the number of injuries and deaths of officers on the job. Also noteworthy, though, is that when officers made appropriate referrals of crisis cases to mental health facilities, most agencies had no crisis programs providing the immediate access to service demanded by these cases.

A related role issue in crisis work concerns the overlap between the emotional, social/political, physical, and material dimensions of particular crisis situations. For example, parents suffering the loss of an infant through sudden infant death syndrome (SIDS) need primarily emotional and social support. Unless prior psychopathology is present, peer support through a SIDS parents' group and perhaps crisis counseling for the parents often suffice. In contrast, if the crisis arises from personal injury through malice or neglect—e.g., rape or contamination of hazardous waste—some kind of social/political action is indicated in addition to the emotional support the person may need (Hoff, 1984a). Action by complementary institutions is also needed to help people who are homeless because of battering, fire or flooding, or refugee status. In these cases, material aid must be combined with emotional and social support, and political action is also needed since the origin of these crises is social (Hoff, 1984a & 1984b).

These issues underscore the multifaceted and interdisciplinary aspects of the crisis field.

Figure 3 illustrates a crisis paradigm with a sociopsychological and cultural perspective that builds on the earlier concepts proposed by Caplan (1964) and Lindemann (1944). This paradigm was developed from research with victims (Hoff, 1984b) and has been applied to a broad range of life crises (Hoff, 1984a).

Figure 3
CRISIS PARADIGM WITH A SOCIOPSYCHOLOGICAL AND CULTURAL PERSPECTIVE[1]

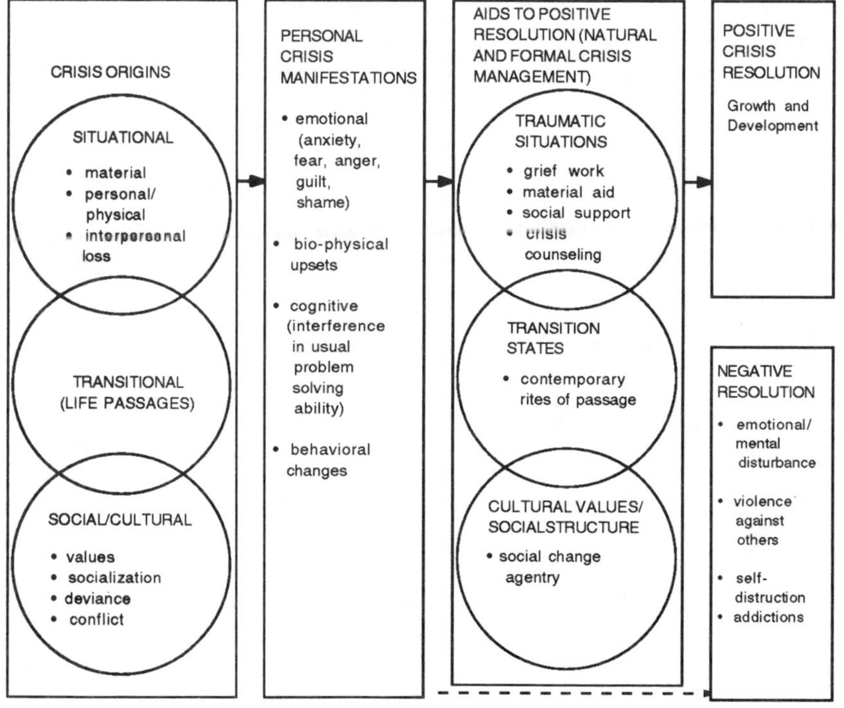

1. Source: Hoff, 1984a.

Everyone involved in the crisis field needs to acknowledge the limits of the crisis approach to human problems and the cultural meaning of the current popularity of the crisis model. While there is no substitute for the 24-hour local response to people in acute distress, the crisis model needs to be an important aspect of primary prevention, as originally proposed by Caplan (1964), as well as secondary and tertiary prevention. Particularly in American society, a disproportionate percentage of health dollars are spent on acute care while there is relative neglect of measures to prevent such acute episodes, both physical and emotional, and almost complete neglect of the political and economic aspects of primary prevention and crisis risk (McKinlay, 1979). In short, crisis management must not be regarded as a panacea for all social, emotional, and mental problems. But when it is appropriate and timely, much human pain and unnecessary financial strain can be avoided.

REFERENCES

Caplan, G.: Principles of Preventive Psychiatry. New York, U.S.A., Basic Books, 1964

Hansell, N.: The Person in Distress. New York, U.S.A., Human Sciences Press, 1976

Hoff, L. A.: People in Crisis: Understanding and helping, 2nd ed. Menlo Park, Calif., U.S.A., Addison-Wesley, 1984a

Hoff, L. A.: Violence Against Women: A Social- Cultural Network Analysis. Ph.D. dissertation, Boston University, Boston, U.S.A., 1984b

Lindemann, E.: Symptomatology and management of acute grief. American Journal of Psychiatry 101:101-148, 1944

McKinlay, J. B.: A case for refocusing upstream: the political economy of illness, in Patients, Physicians, and Illness, 3rd ed. Edited by Jacob, E.G., New York, U.S.A., Free Press, 1979

Wells, J. O. and Hoff, L. A. (eds.): Certification Standards Manual, 3rd ed. Denver, Colo., U.S.A. American Association of Suicidology, 1984

Chapter 38

Social, Ethical and Economic Issues in American Psychiatry

by

Carol C. Nadelson, MD,
Professor,
Department of Psychiatry,
Tufts University School of Medicine
and
Director of Training and Education,
Department of Psychiatry,
New England Medical Center,
Boston, Massachusetts, U.S.A.

ABSTRACT

The direct and indirect costs of mental illness and substance abuse in the United States total more than $218 billion annually, but the investment in research in these areas is only 0.5% of their cost. The clinical practice of psychiatry is directly affected by competition from physicians and nonmedical mental health practitioners. The author discusses the supply of physicians and psychiatrists and points out that the optimal psychiatrist-patient ratio cannot be determined without examining both the roles and availability of psychiatrists.

The current emphasis on competition and the private sector in U.S. health care has resulted in threats to education and research and poor access to health care for the 25 million Americans without health insurance. Another issue of concern to psychiatrists is the threat of law suits and the high cost of liability insurance. Economic factors also influence who can attend medical school and students' choices of specialty and practice setting. Despite these many pressures, however, the number and quality of students choosing psychiatry have steadily increased.

INTRODUCTION

American psychiatry is changing. As we shift from an ideologic to a scientific basis for practice, we struggle to integrate the rapidly expanding world of the neurosciences into an evolving clinical base. This explosion of knowledge, coupled with worldwide economic constraints, presents us with serious problems and challenges.

THE ECONOMICS OF U.S. PSYCHIATRY

A recent report by the U.S. Institute of Medicine estimated that in the United States the direct cost of mental and substance abuse disorders, including alcoholism, is over $50 billion annually, and the indirect costs, such as lost employment, reduced productivity, criminal activity, motor vehicle accidents, and social welfare programs, bring the cost to over $218 billion annually. In addition, schizophrenic patients occupy one-fourth of all our hospital beds. The report also noted the enormous costs, economic and social, of alcoholism and substance abuse in our young people. Since most of the funding for research, teaching, and clinical care in these areas is derived from governmental sources, there is concern about recent decisions regarding health policy and the financing of mental health services.

For example, for every patient treated for cancer in the United States, more than $300 is spent on research. For schizophrenia, the amount is about $10. The investment in alcohol, drug abuse, and mental illness research is approximately 0.5% of their cost. Most U.S.

industries, including defense, spend between 5% and 15% of their budgets on research and development. It is clear, then, that this investment for mental illness is far short of what should be expected.

Further, the recent epidemiological catchment area study conducted by the U.S. National Institute of Mental Health (NIMH) documented an almost 20% prevalence of mental and related disorders in the United States. Thus, we are dealing with pervasive difficulties that many of our government leaders, as well as our medical colleagues, have not confronted. Proposed cuts in funds allocated for research and treatment could have disastrous consequences.

In addition, our medical colleagues often compete with psychiatrists for patients because of economic pressures. They are practicing as psychotherapists and psychopharmacologists and see more than half of the psychiatric patients in the United States, while psychiatrists see about 5%. The rest are seen by a large number of nonmedical practitioners, primarily psychologists, social workers, various counselors, and nurses, many of whom have over the past two decades attained independent practitioner status and even hospital admitting privileges. This has been justified on the basis of maldistribution and undersupply of psychiatrists and the lower cost of nonpsychiatric services. It increases competition for patients and produces conflict between these practitioners. In addition, the rigorousness of credentialing among these groups varies considerably, so the quality of patient care is not assured. Public awareness and concerns about cost and the quality of medical care, however, have led to important and positive changes, particularly in the direction of more rigorous peer review.

ETHICAL AND SOCIAL ASPECTS OF HEALTH CARE TRENDS

In the 1960s, when the American medical community rejected government efforts to develop a national health service, it naively thought that the issue was put to rest. Instead, we are essentially in the process of establishing a national health service through the private sector. This has produced an overemphasis on competition to the extent that many hospitals, including academic medical centers and hospitals which treat the poor, face the threat of bankruptcy and closure and education and research may be seriously compromised. At the same time, we are also overridden with regulation, bureaucracy, and the costs of marketing and administration, which use enormous financial and human resources with little demonstrated benefit for patients.

There has been considerable discussion in the United States about whether we have an oversupply of physicians or merely a maldistribution, with lower than optimal numbers in rural and more isolated areas. The 1980 report of the Graduate Medical Education National Advisory Committee of the U.S. Department of Health and Human Services indicated that an oversupply does exist, except in a few specialties, including psychiatry and child psychiatry. Some, however, suggest that the marketplace should determine supply and that those who want to limit the numbers of practitioners merely fear competition.

While there may be some truth in this assertion, it is clearly not possible to determine the optimal psychiatrist-to-patient ratio without more clearly defining the roles and availability of psychiatrists, especially in relation to other mental health professionals and other physicians. This issue, as you know, is of worldwide concern. Our GNAC predictions were based on minimal, nonsubstitutable, and essential physician-patient contacts in the United States.

A prospective payment system based on diagnosis has been developed, although it currently excludes psychiatry. This system essentially rations health care. Although it is likely that diagnosis will fail as a basis of prospective reimbursement, a prospective reimbursement system of some type is likely to become our method of payment, and limits on access will be imposed. Yet this system has been adequately demonstrated to be ineffective, especially for psychiatry and general medicine.

Americans have not had the opportunity to examine options, to learn from others, and to build a system that considers alternatives. While we devote almost 12% of our gross national product to health care, the question of reordering priorities has not been adequately addressed by the public or the medical community. We also have not yet confronted the difficult philosophical and ethical dilemmas raised by rationing care. Nor have we made a decision about whether health care is a right or a privilege. We continue to use high-cost medical services, such as transplantation, for some while at the same time denying care to those who do not have insurance coverage for even basic care, and especially for treatment of mental illness. It is estimated that 25 million Americans are without insurance coverage. This group includes not only the poor and unemployed but also people with limited incomes, including those who are divorced or widowed and their children. Their limited access to health care, therefore, is based on income. Although it is expected that private institutions will care for those in need, there are no specific or consistent regulations or requirements, so it is possible that patients will be refused necessary care.

This situation is further complicated by the growth of for-profit or investor-owned institutions, which are responsible to their shareholders for making a profit. The question of how much free or reduced-cost care they will provide remains unanswered. Many have raised basic ethical questions regarding the role and responsibility of the private sector in U.S. health care. Indeed, we may ask whether the procompetitive medical care system represents a policy of covert social Darwinism, where only those who have access and resources have the opportunity to receive highly technical health care.

The privatization of American medicine is essentially a euphemism for major corporate control; regulation of services is increasingly in the hands of private enterprise, and the number of investor-owned or for-profit hospitals has increased dramatically in a very short time. As I have indicated, the role of the private versus public sector in providing health care for the indigent is an emerging conflict far from resolution. There is no question that the incentive provided by the private sector has stimulated progress, but many fear that the health care delivery system is governed by the accountants' bottom line rather than the quality of patient care. It seems unlikely that a national health service resembling that of any other country will evolve in the United States.

Another issue that has caused enormous concern among American psychiatrists is liability. Americans' ambivalence about their physicians is demonstrated by the belief that accidents and mistakes do not happen if physicians are competent. Americans expect a guarantee and often feel that they are owed a perfect result. On the other hand, surveys show that Americans are also in awe of their physicians and value their personal physician-patient relationship. The threat of malpractice suits has been responsible for some of the escalation in health care costs, directly or indirectly. Although some dispute it, the cost of insurance and defensive medical practices cannot be seen as trivial. This has resulted in major confrontations with lawyers and insurance companies. While psychiatrists have had fewer legal problems than their medical colleagues, change in this area is on the horizon and liability costs for psychiatrists have led the American Psychiatric Association (APA) to establish its own insurance company and program.

EDUCATION

Young people entering medicine in the United States face a world different from that a decade ago. Their educational goals are more threatened by economic, legal, and political constraints. The cost of medical education is beyond the means of most American families, and with the decrease in funds available for scholarships and even loans, it is likely that we will increasingly favor selection of students who can afford private education.

Specialty choice is also more likely to be increasingly affected by economic factors. Students graduating from medical school with enormous debts, often $100,000, tend to select fields that will provide higher salaries. Thus, psychiatry, a lower-income specialty, could be negatively affected. The impact of cost-reduction efforts, including establishment of organized care facilities, on income and choice, is not yet clear.

Many students find that the combination of debt, high liability insurance costs, and competition makes private practice unaffordable, so they have moved to organized and prepaid care settings, especially health maintenance organizations. In fact, 40% of the psychiatrists under age 35 are in salaried posts, while 20% of those 35 or older are in these positions. Since the organizations are paid in advance, they fix salaries and set up controls that may make medicine less attractive in the future.

As I indicated, the debate about whether there is an over-supply of psychiatrists in the United States or whether the problem is essentially maldistribution has not resolved. The number and quality of students choosing psychiatry, however, have steadily escalated over the past 5 years. There are now over 5,000 psychiatry residents in the United States. It does, however, continue to be difficult to interest psychiatrists in moving to rural areas. Two reasons are isolation from colleagues, and fewer opportunities for spouses and children.

The interest of young psychiatrists, including trainees, in the APA and organized psychiatry is impressive. Fifteen percent of our APA members are residents, representing almost 90% of psychiatry residents, and we have several hundred medical student members. These young members are involved in all levels of the APA, and they are clearly planning on taking a more active role in the future.

At this time, there are 216 psychiatric residence training programs in the United States, and the ratio of psychiatrists to patients is 15 per 100,000, slightly more than the estimated need. We produce an additional 500 to 600 psychiatrists each year. Thus, we are likely to have an even higher ratio in the future. Other countries estimate a much lower need. Obviously, definition of role is critical to discussion of supply.

All residency training programs in the United States are accredited by the Accreditation Council for Graduate Medical Education, a voluntary group that determines entrance requirements and training program content and maintains standards. Thus, all residents are trained in similar areas of psychiatry, although the training takes place in different institutions with different resources and philosophies.

The American Board of Psychiatry and Neurology certifies graduates of accredited programs by administering written and oral examinations. While certification is not required, it is increasingly expected in psychiatrists seeking positions and promotions.

Other efforts at assuring quality include continuing medical education. Psychiatrists participate actively in the APA annual meeting and a number of other programs, including self-assessment exams. These help members fulfill continuing education requirements and enable them to keep up with new developments in the field.

In the APA, there is developing interest in links with psychiatrists in other countries, including exchanges of fellowship and training positions. Currently, we are considering a project that will enable medical school graduates, particularly from countries that do not have the educational resources to meet their own needs, to obtain training in special areas of psychiatry in the United States. However, because of our national concern about an oversupply of physicians, licensure for foreign medical graduates is increasingly limited, especially for those who want to practice in the United States. The effort will be focused on those who will return to their own countries.

As APA President, my own personal priority was psychiatric education. One emerging concern is how to train psychiatrists to meet the needs of special populations, including the chronically mentally ill, those with alcoholism and drug abuse, and the elderly, especially with decreasing resources. A major area of controversy in the United States is whether the role of the psychiatrist should be subspecialist or generalist. The explosion of the knowledge base in psychiatry makes it difficult for residents to obtain expertise or for practitioners to be familiar with developments in all areas. There is no clear agreement as to how residents and practitioners should gain needed subspecialty experience. Most psychiatrists agree there is a danger in subspecialization and that, if we do not proceed cautiously, we may find our field incorporating the negative aspects of subspecialization, especially fragmentation of patient care, rather than fostering expertise.

Chapter 39

Payment Systems in the United States

by

Jay B. Cutler,
Director,
Office of Government Relations,
American Psychiatric Association,
Washington, D.C., U.S.A.

ABSTRACT

The author describes the need for psychiatric input into legislative and regulatory decisions on health issues and relates how the American Psychiatric Association worked to exempt psychiatry from the Medicare prospective payment system based on diagnosis-related groups (DRGs). Private plans designed to control costs include health maintenance organizations (HMOs), preferred provider organizations (PPOs), and independent provider associations (IPAs). The number of traditional insurance policies with inpatient coverage has dropped recently, and outpatient coverage is rarely comparable with medical outpatient coverage. Services are also increasingly subjected to utilization review. HMOs historically have had more limited psychiatric benefits than many commercial policies and often require the primary physician to act as gate-keeper for specialized services. Psychiatrists also face competition from nonpsychiatric physicians, who account for over half the U.S. mental health visits and are now even hiring psychologists and social workers. Nonetheless, mental illness and its treatment are receiving increasing public and legislative attention, and American psychiatry is making progress in its efforts to achieve nondiscriminatory coverage.

INTRODUCTION

This paper covers U.S. payment systems, or the new world of mental health care in the United States. This new world is inextricably bound up with a marketplace and legislative system under revolution, a revolution American-style.

To understand what is and has been happening in the Washington, D.C. world of psychiatry, patients, and politics, let me share with you the perspective of psychiatry's lobbyists in our nation's capitol using the only effective treatment modality, the therapy of reality. Let me also discuss with you how the revolution in health care in the United States has targeted medical costs, which have risen rapidly. It is changing the lives of millions of patients. Health care cost Americans an estimated $456 billion in 1985, a more than 80% increase in just the past 5 years.

Much of this change is being initiated by the federal government through major reforms in the Medicare and Medicaid programs. Many of these reforms are being duplicated by private insurance plans. In essence, they offer greater incentives to both health care providers and consumers to hold down costs. A hospital is paid on the basis of a patient's diagnosis rather than by totaling the costs of all the items on the hospital bill. And, more and more, individuals are being offered the chance to select from among several alternative health plans in an increasingly competitive and managed health care marketplace.

These changes have implications for psychiatry's role in the federal legislative and regulatory arena. We must put pressure on the Congress, since it is the key policy-making body for U.S. health care, and on the Department of Health and Human Services. We must maintain this pressure relentlessly in order to be able to shape public policy at the appropriate time. Together, individual psychiatrists throughout the United States and my staff and I maintain Congressional sensitivity to constituent grass-roots input. We are clearly perceived as psychiatry acting on behalf of psychiatric patients, with the voice of the patients themselves joining us.

THE ROLE OF THE LOBBYIST

I would like to discuss the legislative and regulatory agenda for psychiatry, its impact on U.S. payment systems, and what it means for trends in mental health care. I would also like to explain what lobbying means.

Lobbyists do the following:

- seek to educate government leaders and persuade them to become advocates for increased research funding by pointing out unprecedented major research developments. Such developments bring new methods and technology to sophisticated, objective studies of brain functioning and its link to both normal and abnormal behavior.
- seek to make leaders aware of the wide array of new and more effective treatment modalities, both somatic and psychosocial, for some of the most incapacitating forms of mental illness, including schizophrenia, major affective disorders, phobias, and panic disorder.
- focus on how appropriate treatment of mental illness has been demonstrated to be cost-effective in terms of restored productivity, reduced utilization of other health services, and lessened social dependence.
- continually try to convince members of Congress and other decision-makers that mental illness is a problem of grave concern and consequence to American society even though it is widely feared and misunderstood.

MEDICARE PAYMENT METHODS

Any discussion of trends in mental health care in the United States must address the changes in how Americans pay for medical treatment and how the new system reflects a fundamental change in the way the federal government pays for the health care of the approximately 30 million elderly and disabled Americans who are currently covered by Medicare.

What at first seemed like a minor accounting shift is proving to have the most far-reaching consequences since the federal medicare program was enacted in 1965. The key change is that, instead of reimbursing hospitals for the actual cost of treating the Medicare patient, the government now pays a set fee according to 468 diagnosis-related groups, commonly called DRGs.

However, any discussion of U.S. payment systems and trends in mental health care must include a review of the American Psychiatric Association (APA) past, present, and future activities related to the DRG prospective payment system. The Social Security Amendments of 1983 (P.L. 98-21) established the statutory framework for the Medicare hospital prospective payment system. As I mentioned, it was created to provide a prospectively determined price for each type of case, classified at discharge as one of the 468 DRGs, which the experts say were structured according to clinical coherence and similarity of resource requirements.

The APA saw this DRG legislative train pulling into the Congressional station. However, APA knew it was essential, in the interest of quality care of psychiatric patients, that psychiatric hospitals and psychiatric units of general hospitals leave that DRG train. APA's views of the adverse impact this has on patient care are now reflected in the intensity of Congressional controversy about purse tightening, which affects ways sick people are treated when they enter the nation's 5,800 hospitals. Critics focus on two main areas:

- Patients are being discharged quicker and sicker, without community support.
- Some people are denied treatment at private hospitals because they cannot afford to pay and are dumped on overburdened public hospitals.

Let me return to the APA's legislative strategy for getting off the DRG train before it left the Congressional station. At both House and Senate hearings, APA assured the Congressional station master that it was the DRGs, as constructed, that we wanted off the train and not the prospective payment scheme, which was the train's driving force.

The APA and the Congress agreed that the DRG-based prospective payment system failed to meet the treatment needs of the mentally ill. We agreed in testimony and in our lobbying that psychiatric hospitals and psychiatric units of general hospitals should only be exempt from the system until a more appropriate means of reimbursement for treatment is developed.

Thus, for any disorder included in the DRGs, Medicare now pays an amount that is published at the beginning of the year prospectively rather than cost-plus retrospectively. Psychiatric hospitals and qualifying psychiatric units in acute care hospitals are excluded, with no time limitation, from prospective payment. Nevertheless, the Secretary of the Department of Health and Human Services has been mandated to report to Congress on whether and how they can be included in the prospective payment system. According to the legislation:

> In the Annual REPORT TO CONGRESS under subparagraph (A) for 1985, the Secretary shall include the results of studies on whether and the method under which hospitals, not paid based on amounts determined under such section, can be paid for inpatient hospital services on a prospective basis as under such section.

Since implementation of DRGs for psychiatric hospitals and units could be a function of the level of Medicare funds involved, it would be helpful to know what proportion of Medicare expenditures support exempted psychiatric facilities and how it relates to the dollars for other types of health services under Medicare, especially medical and surgical procedures in acute care delivery settings. In fiscal year 1981, about 2.4% of the Medicare interim payments, or $995 million of the approximately 41 billion in total interim reimbursements, were for psychiatric services. Clearly, only a small part of the overall Medicare payments is for psychiatric services.

At the same time, psychiatrists in dialogues with legislators and the Health Care Financing Administration must continue to explain that we are not advocating returning to or maintaining a retrospective cost-plus system. Rather, we must be clear that the Tax Equity Fiscal Responsibility Act contains the rate of increase in each cost per discharge and has already placed excluded psychiatric facilities under the prospective payment system, which pays by the case. Thus, the need to develop a system of prospective payments and payments by the case is not a burning issue.

The results of the APA analysis and evaluation of psychiatric DRGs provided to the Health Care Financing Administration and key Congressional staff read, "Our study and analysis of the appropriateness of the DRG classification scheme for psychiatric patients—based upon our examination of over 1.7 million patient records—has concluded that the Congressional exemption for these facilities and units was and still is correct. DRGs are not adequate as a patient classification system for the mentally ill." The preliminary findings on this study, confirmed in other independent analyses by other health and mental health organizations, justify continuation of the exclusion until a realistic alternative is found.

Hopefully, the Health Care Financing Administration's final report will agree that, on the basis of the overwhelming research findings, DRGs as a prospective payment system are not appropriate because they do not explain variation in resource use for the psychiatric (mental and substance abuse disorders) diagnostic categories and because they allow relatively small Medicare expenditures for psychiatric services. There is a window of opportunity, and we must proceed deliberately. The political message must be clear. The window will not be open forever. The concerns about the larger health care system and about the needs of chronically disabled Medicare and Medicaid psychiatric beneficiaries can perhaps be addressed but should be addressed without undue haste.

The new medical economics, involving fierce competition between and among doctors and hospitals, dictates that all must keep one eye on healing and the other on the bottom line. It is too early to know the full impact of this focus, but questions about medical quality are just beginning to be raised. To many, the revolution is already a success. For Medicare patients, hospital time dropped from an average of 10 days in 1981 to less than 8 in 1985. Fewer people go to hospitals, since procedures such as cataract and hernia operations can be done on an outpatient basis. Most important, medical costs rose only 6.2% in 1985, compared with more than 9% every year for the last decade.

The Reagan Administration wants even more cuts in expenditures for health care. Many consumer groups and health officials worry that further cuts will erode the nation's medical standards by forcing hospitals to trim their budgets for research and new technology. Health experts, who once worried that Americans got too much health care, now fear that some will not get enough.

PRIVATE INSURANCE PLANS

Most at risk are the nearly 33 million Americans who cannot afford private health insurance but are not poor enough to qualify for Medicaid. Another 15 million do not have adequate coverage. Hospitals say they cannot afford to provide much charity care. As a result, the dumping of indigent patients from private to public hospitals has risen sharply in cities, e.g., Chicago, Dallas, and Oakland, California.

At the same time, we cannot ignore the reality that the world of medical insurance in America's private sector is changing almost every day. Suddenly, there are health maintenance organizations (HMOs), preferred provider organizations (PPOs), independent provider associations (IPAs), and a mind-numbing array of other health care options. Now you can shop among a variety of plans for the coverage that suits you best.

The first thing to understand is that, despite all the new names and initials, health insurance coverage pays for specified medical and hospital services, such as a certain number of days of hospitalization, laboratory tests and x-rays, 80% of a doctor's treatment charges, so many visits a year to a psychiatrist or to other approved mental health professionals, etc. This is the traditional Blue Cross-Blue Shield, Aetna, Prudential, or other insurance coverage, and it is still the most commonly used. Prepaid health plans provide almost all your medical care, including office visits, laboratory tests, and hospitalizations, for one fixed monthly or biweekly fee. These plans are partly old, partly new creatures, but they are the new story in U.S. health care.

An offshoot of the health maintenance organization and the

independent provider association is the preferred provider organization, which is being offered by some employers and insurance firms. There are many variants, but the employee typically receives care for a flat monthly charge if the plan's preferred hospital or preferred physicians are used. If the employee seeks treatment elsewhere, the employee pays part or all of the bill. Thus, employees have a financial incentive to stay with the preferred hospital or doctor, and the participating hospital and physicians have an incentive to provide more cost-effective treatment.

More and more employers throughout the country are offering some PPO variant. Some workers will soon not be able to choose old-style fee-for-service health insurance at all. The 6,000 United Auto Workers who work in the new General Motors Saturn plan in Tennessee will only be able to choose between an HMO and a PPO. Such changes may be just the beginning.

The number of plans in some cities may get pared down. Chicago had 25 HMOs a few years ago. Tough competition has cut the number to 10. The nation had only 50 HMOs in 1973; now it has 350, with 20 million members, and membership has been growing by 20% a year. By 1993 enrollment in these new-style plans may reach 50 million.

Insurance vis-a-vis Psychiatry

Now let me review these megatrends and the picture they paint for psychiatry. APA's nationwide analysis showed that the percentage of insurance policies with coverage of inpatient psychiatric treatment dropped between 1981 and 1984 from 58% to 48%. While the percentage of policies with outpatient coverage has actually increased, rarely is outpatient coverage for psychiatry on par with outpatient medical coverage, and we have lost ground even there. In1981, 10% of the policies had outpatient psychiatric coverage that was comparable to outpatient medical coverage, but that number is now down to 7%. The proportion of policies with no dollar maximum has also dropped. Interestingly, the coverage of alcoholism services has skyrocketed from 38% of the policies to 61%.

In addition to cutbacks within benefit packages, we see more utilization review. Many more companies and unions ask for preadmission certification for all inpatient psychiatric admissions, concurrent review, and case management. Companies that perform case management review certain cases and decide whether or not the care being given is appropriate. Such companies are growing in importance.

Alternative Health Care Plans

HMO enrollment has been increasing markedly; between 1979 and 1985, enrollment more than doubled. Most people assume that it will probably double again in 5 years. While the growth of alphabet-soup coverage affects all physicians, it affects psychiatrists more directly in that HMOs historically have had more limited benefits than many of the commercial policies or even some of the Blue Cross policies. In a study of the nation's HMOs, the typical benefit package covered 20 outpatient visits and 30 inpatient days but included various copayments and limits on use, so patients might actually be allowed less than that because of utilization review limits or incentives built into the package design. Secondly, very often the psychiatrist has to work through the primary physician who acts as a gatekeeper.

Like some of the larger hospital chains and more aggressive hospitals, PPOs have devised alternatives to inpatient care as a way of controlling costs. Along with inpatient care, provision may be made for an outpatient medical office building, partial hospitalization program, and institution's reimbursement for patients in a particular prospective community residence. So, if the payment plan is determined by diagnosis, it can control the costs for those patients. Some have predicted that prospective payment will evolve into capitation. Many of the people who are looking ahead more than 5 years are saying that in all likelihood, as prospective payment starts to eat up more and more elements within a hospital, it will evolve into capitation over a period of time.

Competition

The final megatrend facing psychiatrists, competition, could come from psychologists, social workers, and nonpsychiatric physicians. Over half the mental health visits in the country are delivered and billed by nonpsychiatric physicians. It has been forecast that they will be a more direct competitor as the oversupply of physicians increases. In many U.S. states, general practitioners are hiring their own psychologists and social workers to work in their offices and generate billings from there. As a result, insurance coverage of psychologists' services has dropped. U.S. Bureau of Labor Statistics data show an important drop in psychologists' billings as more and more companies become self-insured and do not have to comply with state laws regarding coverage of psychologists' services.

INCENTIVES AND TRENDS

No presentation on trends in mental health care in the United States should close without recognition of certain events of symbolic and legislative significance.

1. An annual Mental Illness Awareness Week was formally declared by President Reagan, and governors in 20 states have also recognized Mental Illness Awareness Week.
2. Senator Edward M. Kennedy introduced legislation that repealed the $250 limit for annual outpatient psychiatric treatment under Medicare, Part B, making outpatient psychiatric treatment equivalent to other covered outpatient medical treatment. He also introduced legislation calling for the state plan under Medicaid to include outpatient medical mental health services, including psychotherapy and drugs for the treatment of mental illness. While passage of this legislation is not expected, it is an important symbol.
3. The APA bill requiring nondiscriminatory coverage of treatment for mental illness was also introduced.
4. When APA testified before the Senate Finance Committee's Health Subcommittee on proposals to reform physician payment under Medicare, we were presented with a challenge and window of opportunity.

Senator Durenberger told APA witness John McGrath, MD, Vice Chair of the Joint Commission on Government Relations, in response to his plea for equity,

> " *Let me say to you and others, . . . now is the time to come up with some recommendations; between now and the time we start putting into effect a new system for reimbursement is the ideal time to work in mental health. . . . In competition and in consumer choice the prepaid health plans tend to discriminate against your kind of services. . . . The burden is largely on you to make recommendations to us.* "

We expect development of proposals that incrementally bring us to the goal of nondiscriminatory coverage of mental illness. As psychiatry and patients let the facts be known, politics will begin to strike a more reasonable balance between treatment for mental illness and costs.

In recent years, psychiatrists' income has improved, largely because of enhanced productivity and efficiency, diversification of treatments, work in multiple settings, expansion of group practice, and subspecialization. Although the earnings of psychiatrists are substantially lower than the earnings of physicians in the procedure oriented and surgical specialties of medicine, Astrachan and Sharfstein (1986) offered evidence that, when compared to other cognitive medical specialties, such as pediatrics and internal medicine, psychiatry is the highest paid specialty on an hourly basis. The authors were optimistic about the future of psychiatry as a medical specialty. To this, I say AMEN.

REFERENCES

Astrachan, B., Sharfstein, S.S. : The income of psychiatrists: adaptation during difficult economic times. American Journal of Psychiatry 143: 885-887, 1986

List of Participants

ABUSAH, P.Y., M.D.
Department of Psychiatry
Faculty of Medical Sciences
University of Jos
P.M.B. 2084
Jos, NIGERIA

ACUDA, S. Wilson, M.D.
Chairman
Department of Psychiatry
Faculty of Medicine
University of Nairobi
Kenyatta National Hospital
P.O. Box. 30588
Nairobi, KENYA

ANNABI, Salim, M.D.
Hospital Razi
La Manouba
TUNISIA

ASSEN, G.P., M.D.
Hooischelf 8
6581 SM MALDEN
NETHERLANDS

ASUNI, Tolani, Professor
Department of Psychiatry
College of Medicine
University of Lagos, P.M.B. 12003
Lagos, NIGERIA

BANTA, Lawrence E., M.D.
Department of Psychiatry
Creighton University
819 Dorcas
Omaha, Nebraska 68108
U.S.A.

BEIGEL, Allan, M.D.
30 Camino Espanol
Tucson, Arizona 85716
U.S.A.

BELL, Carl C., M.D.
Community Mental Health Council
1001 East 87th Street
Chicago, Illinois 60619
U.S.A.

BINITIE, Ayo, Professor
Department of Mental Health
College of Medical Sciences
University of Benin Teaching
Hospital, P.M.B. 1111
Benin City, NIGERIA

BOROFFKA, A., M.D.
Segebergerstrasse 17
2300 Kiel 14
FEDERAL REPUBLIC OF
GERMANY

BOSSA, Steven, Professor
Department of Psychiatry
Makerere University
P.O. Box 7072
Kampala, UGANDA

BRYAN, Kathleen, Director
Office of Meetings Management
American Psychiatric Association
1400 K Street, NW
Washington, DC 20005
U.S.A.

BUGAISA, G.M., S.R.N.
P.O. Box 65252
Da} es Salaam, TANZANIA

CLAVER, B., M.D.

CUTLER, Jay, Director
Office of Government Relations
American Psychiatric Association
1400 K Street, NW
Washington, DC 20005
U.S.A.

DA COSTA, G.A., M.D.
Staff Psychiatrist
Child and Family Studies Center
Clarke Institute of Psychiatry
250 College Street
Toronto M5T lR8, CANADA

DAVIS, Joseph, M.D.
1305 Franklin Street
Suite 401
Oakland, California 94612
U.S.A.

DAVIS, King E., Ph.D.
Galt Professor of Public Mental Health
Medical College of Virginia
P.O. Box 1797
Richmond, Virginia 23214
U.S.A.

DHADPHALE, Manohar, M.D.
Department of Psychiatry
Faculty of Medicine
University of Nairobi
Kenyatta National Hospital
P.O. Box 30588
Nairobi, KENYA

DIXIE-BELL, Dora, M.D.
5514 South Cornell
Chicago, Illinois 60637
U.S.A.

DUDLEY, Richard G., Jr., M.D.
416 West 144th Street
New York, New York 10031
U.S.A.

EARLS, Felton, M.D.
Blanche F. Ittleson Professor of Psychiatry
Washington University School of Medicine , 4940 Audubon Avenue
St. Louis, Missouri 63110
U.S.A.

EBIE, J.C., Professor
Department of Mental Health
College of Medical Sciences
University of Benin Teaching
Hospital, P.M.B. 1111
Benin City, NIGERIA
FEKSI, A.T., M.D.
Nairobi, KENYA

FIELDS, Richard A., M.D.
Superintendent's Office
Georgia Regional Hospital
Box 370407
3073 Panthersville Road
Decatur, Georgia 20037
U.S.A.

FRANKLIN, John, M.D.
16 Lake Street - 5G
White Plains,
New York 10603
U.S.A.

FREEMAN, Linda M., M.D.
Department of Psychiatry
Rush-Presbyterian-St. Luke's
Medical Center
912 South Wood Street.
Chicago, Illinois 60612
U.S.A.

GATERE, Samuel, M.D.
Nairobi, KENYA

GERMAN, Allen G., Professor
Department of Psychiatry
University of Western Australia
Nedlands, Western Australia 6009
AUSTRALIA

GOTTLIEB, Fred, M.D.
3170 Antelo Road
Los Angeles, California 90077
U.S.A.

GRIFFITH, Ezra E.H., M.D.
Department of Psychiatry,
Yale University School of Medicine
34 Park Street
New Haven, Connecticut 06519
U.S.A.

GUINNESS E.A., M.D.
Consultant Psychiatrist
Matsapa Mental Hospital
P.O. Box 424
Manzini, SWAZILAND

HAJI, A., M.D.
Nairobi, KENYA

HAMMERSLEY, Donald H., M.D.
Deputy Medical Director,
Office of Psychiatric Services
American Psychiatric Association
1400 K Street, NW
Washington, DC 20005 U.S.A.

HARRIS, Hiwatha, M.D.
1127 Wilshire Boulevard
Suite 1404
Los Angeles, California 90017
U.S.A.

HARRIS, Thelissa A., M.D.
200 Retreat Avenue
Hartford, Connecticut 06106
U.S.A.

HAULI, I.G., M.D.
Department of Psychiatry
Muhimbili Medical Centre
P.O. Box 65293
Dar es Salaam, TANZANIA

HAWKINS, David R., M.D.
Department of Psychiatry
Michael Reese Hospital
29th and Ellis Avenue
Chicago, Illinois 60616
U.S.A.

HAWORTH, A., Professor
Chairman Hills Hospital
P.O. Box 30043
Lusaka, ZAMBIA

HOFF, Lee Ann, RN, Ph.D.
Associate Professor
Northeastern University
College of Nursing
360 Huntington Avenue
Boston, Massachusetts 02115
U.S.A.

JACOBS, Rosevelt, Ph.D.
Assistant Professor of Psychiatry and Human Behavior
Charles R. Drew Post Graduate Medical School
1621 East 120th Street
Los Angeles, California 90059
U.S.A.

JOHNSON, Attah, M.D.
Department of Psychiatry
Faculty of Medical Sciences
University of Jos, P.M.B. 2084
Jos, NIGERIA

JOHNSON, Bertha, M.D.
P.M.B. 2008
Yaba, NIGERIA

JOHNSON, Joyce M., D.O.
St. Elizabeth's Hospital
200 Barton Hall
2700 Martin Luther King Avenue,SE
Washington, DC 20032
U.S.A.

JONES, Billy E., M.D., Director
Department of Psychiatry
Lincoln Hospital
234 East 149th Street
Bronx, New York 10451
U.S.A.

KILONZO, G.P., M.D.
Department of Psychiatry
Muhimbili Medical Centre
P.O. Box 65293
Dar es Salaam, TANZANIA

KING, Richard D., M.D.
752 Clipper Street
San Francisco, California 94132
U.S.A.

LAWSON, William, Ph.D., M.D.
Psychiatry Service
VA Medical Service
5901 East 7th Street
Long Beach, California 90822
U.S.A.

LOZA, Nasser, M.D.
Institute of Psychiatry
de Crespigny Park London
SE5 8AZ UNITED KINGDOM

LUKWAGO, Miriam G., Ph.D.
Nairobi, KENYA

MAHY, George, M.D.
Queen Elizabeth Hospital
St. Michael, BARBADOS

MAJID, A., M.D.
Department of Psychological
Medicine, St. Luke's Hospital
Middlesborough
Cleveland T54 3AF
UNITED KINGDOM

MAKANJUOLA, J.D.A., M.D.
Director of Research and Training
Neuropsychiatric Hospital
Aro, Abeokuta
NIGERIA

MANLEY, Myrl, M.D.
Lecturer in Psychiatry
Godfrey Huggins School of
Medicine
P.O. Box A 178
Avondale, Harare
ZIMBABWE

MARKS-BROWN, Shirley F., M.D.
2600 S Loop W, Suite 220
Houston, Texas 77054
U.S.A.

MATETE, F.G., M.D.
Nairobi, KENYA

MBUGUA, C., M.D.
Nairobi, KENYA

MENGECH, Haroun H.K. arap,
M.D.
Nairobi, KENYA

MENNINGER, Roy, M.D.,
President
The Menninger Foundation
P.O. Box 829
Topeka, Kansas 66601
U.S.A.

MERCER, Ellen, Director
Office of International Affairs
American Psychiatric Association
1400 K Street, NW
Washington, DC 20005
U.S.A.

MULINDI, Sobbie, Ph.D.
Nairobi, KENYA

MULUKA, Evan P., M.D.
Nairobi, KENYA

MUSTAFA, Gulam, M.D.
Nairobi, KENYA

MUYA, Willy J., M.D.
Nairobi, KENYA

NADELSON, Carol C., M.D.
Department of Psychiatry
Tufts New England Medical Center
171 Harrison Avenue
Boston, Massachusetts 02111
U.S.A.

NADELSON, Theodore, M.D.
Psychiatrist-in-Chief
Boston Medical Center
150 South Huntington Avenue
Boston, Massachusetts 01230
U.S.A.

NDETEL, David M., M.D.
Nairobi, KENYA

NJENGA, F.G., M.D.
Nairobi, KENYA

NYAKIAMO, Peter, E.C.H.., M.P.
Minister of Health
Ministry of Health
P.O. Box 30016
Nairobi, KENYA

ODEJIDE, A.O., Professor
Department of Psychiatry
University of Ibadan
University College Hospital
Ibadan, NIGERIA

ODIASE, G.I., M.D.
Department of Mental Health
College of Medical Sciences
University of Benin Teaching Hospital
Benin City, NIGERIA

OGBOLU, Irene N., S.R.N.
49 Park Avenue G.R.A.
P.O. Box 1309
Enugu, NIGERIA

OKASHA, Ahmed, Professor
3 Sahwarby Street, Kas-el-Nil
Cairo, EGYPT

OKOKO, A.E.J., M.D.
Department of Physiology
Faculty of Medical Sciences
P.M.B. 2084
Jos, NIGERIA
OKONJI, M., M.D.
Nairobi, KENYA

OKPAKU, Samuel O., M.D., Ph.D
Institute for Public Policy Studies
Vanderbilt University
1218 18th Avenue South
Nashville, Tennessee 37212
U.S.A.

PARDES, Herbert, M.D.
Professor and Chairman
Department of Psychiatry
College of Physicians and Surgeons
Columbia University
722 West 168th Street
New York, New York 10032
U.S.A.

PARKS, Gilbert R., M.D.
P.O. Box 1321
Topeka, Kansas 66601
U.S.A.

PASNAU, Robert O., M.D.
UCLA Neurospsychiatric Institute
760 Westwood Plaza
Los Angeles, Carlifornia 90024
U.S.A.

PELTZER, Karl, Ph.D.
Department of Psychology
University of Malawi
P.O. Box 280
Zomba, MALAWI

PIERCE, Chester M., M.D.
Professor of Education and Psychiatry
Harvard Graduate School of Education
Nichols House, Appian Way
Cambridge, Massachusetts 02138
U.S.A.

PINDERHUGHES, Charles, M.D.
VA Hospital
200 Springs Road
Bedford, Massachusetts 01730
U.S.A.

PLATMAN, Stanley R., M.D.
3915 North Charles Street
Baltimore, Maryland 21218
U.S.A.

RAJAH, S.G., M.D.
Consultant Psychiatrist
Ministry of Health
Brown Sequard Hospital
Beau Bassin, MAURITIUS

RATAEMANE, S., M.D.
Department of Psychiatry
Johannesburg Hospital
Johannesburg 2000
SOUTH AFRICA

RUGEIYAMU, KRoeber F., M.D.
P.O. Box 65252
Dar es Salaam, TANZANIA

RWEGELLERA, George, M.D.
Department of Psychiatry
Makerere University Medical School
P.O. Box 7072
Kampala, UGANDA

SMITH, Quentin T., M.D.
2750 Ridge Valley Road, NW
Atlanta, Georgia 30327
U.S.A.

SPURLOCK, Jeanne, M.D.
Deputy Medical Director
Office of Minority/National Affairs
American Psychiatric Association
1400 K Street, NW
Washington, DC 20005
U.S.A.

STATON, Robert Dennis, M.D.
Chief, Psychiatry Service
VA Medical Center
Fargo, North Dakota 58102
U.S.A.

SULIMAN, H., M.D.
Chief Consultant in NeuroPsychiatry
Mental Health
P.O. Box 183A
Khartoum, SUDAN

SUMBA, R. Onyango, M.D.
Nairobi, KENYA

TALBOTT, John A., M.D.
200 Goodwood Gardens
Baltimore, Maryland 2120
U.S.A.

TARDY, Walter J., M.D.
Green Oaks Hospital
7808 Clodus Fields Drive
Dallas, Texas 75251
U.S.A.

WEISE, Maurice, M.D.
5987 Peacock Ridge Road
Rancho Palos Verdes
Carlifornia 90274
U.S.A.

WOODBURY, Arline, M.D.
U.S.A.

WORKINEH, Fikre, Professor
Addis Ababa University
Faculty of Medicine
Department of Psychiatry
P.O. Box 1176
Addis Ababa, ETHIOPIA

WRIGHT, Harry H., M.D.
Assistant Professor
USC School of Medicine
P.O. Box 202
Columbia, South Carolina 29202
U.S.A.

YAMBO, M., Ph.D.
Nairobi, KENYA

YIPTONG, Charles C., M.D.
1 Francis Street
North Bay, Ontario
CANADA

Index

D

E

F

G

H

I

J

K

L

M

N